Pulsed Field Ablation

Editors

FENGWEI ZOU
LUIGI DI BIASE

CARDIAC ELECTROPHYSIOLOGY CLINICS

www.cardiacEP.theclinics.com

Consulting Editors
LUIGI DI BIASE
EMILY P. ZEITLER

June 2025 • Volume 17 • Number 2

ELSEVIER

1600 John F. Kennedy Boulevard • Suite 1800 • Philadelphia, Pennsylvania, 19103-2899

http://www.theclinics.com

CARDIAC ELECTROPHYSIOLOGY CLINICS Volume 17, Number 2
June 2025 ISSN 1877-9182, ISBN-13: 978-0-443-34705-4

Editor: Joanna Gascoine
Developmental Editor: Sukirti Singh

Publication information: *Cardiac Electrophysiology Clinics* (ISSN 1877-9182) is published quarterly by Elsevier Inc., 1600 John F. Kennedy Boulevard, Suite 1600, Philadelphia, PA 1910, United States. Periodicals postage paid at New York, NY and additional mailing offices. USA POSTMASTER: Send address changes to *Cardiac Electrophysiology Clinics*, Elsevier Customer Service Department, 3251 Riverport Lane, Maryland Heights, MO 63043, USA Months of issue are March, June, September, and December. Subscription prices are $267.00 per year for US individuals, $291.00 per year for Canadian individuals, $355.00 per year for international individuals, and $100.00 per year for US, Canadian and international students/residents. For institutional access pricing please contact Customer Service via the contact information below. To receive student/resident rate, orders must be accompanied by name of affilliated institution, date of term, and the signature of program/residency coordinator on institution letterhead. Orders will be billed at individual rate until proof of status is received. Foreign air speed delivery is included in all Clinics subscription prices. All prices are subject to change without notice. Orders, claims, and journal inquiries: Please visit our Support Hub page https://service.elsevier.com for assistance.

Reprints. For copies of 100 or more of articles in this publication, please contact the Commercial Reprints Department, Elsevier Inc., 360 Park Avenue South, New York, NY 10010-1710. Tel.: 212-633-3874; Fax: 212-633-3820; E-mail: reprints@elsevier.com.

Cardiac Electrophysiology Clinics is covered in *MEDLINE/PubMed (Index Medicus)*.

Printed in the United States of America.

Contributors

CONSULTING EDITORS

LUIGI DI BIASE, MD, PhD, FACC, FESC, FHRS
Section Head of Electrophysiology, Director of Arrhythmia Services, Professor of Medicine (Cardiology), Montefiore-Einstein Center for Heart and Vascular Care, Montefiore Medical Center, Albert Einstein College of Medicine, Bronx, New York, USA

EMILY P. ZEITLER, MD, MHS, FHRS
Cardiac Electrophysiology, Assistant Professor of Medicine, Geisel School of Medicine, Hanover, New Hampshire, USA; Assistant Professor of Health Care Policy, The Dartmouth Institute, Dartmouth-Hitchcock Medical Center, Lebanon, New Hampshire, USA

EDITORS

FENGWEI ZOU, MD
Fellow, Department of Medicine/Cardiology, Montefiore-Einstein Center for Heart and Vascular Care, Montefiore Medical Center, Bronx, New York, USA

LUIGI DI BIASE, MD, PhD, FACC, FESC, FHRS
Section Head of Electrophysiology, Director of Arrhythmia Services, Professor of Medicine (Cardiology), Montefiore-Einstein Center for Heart and Vascular Care, Montefiore Medical Center, Albert Einstein College of Medicine, Bronx, New York, USA

AUTHORS

AMIN AL-AHMAD, MD
Electrophysiologist, Department of Clinical Cardiac Electrophysiology, Texas Cardiac Arrhythmia Institute, St David's Medical Center, Austin, Texas, USA

RESHMA AMIN, MD
Doctor, Department of Electrophysiology, AZ Sint-Jan Hospital, Bruges, Belgium

T. JARED BUNCH, MD
Associate Chief of Cardiology, Division of Cardiovascular Medicine, Department of Internal Medicine, University of Utah Health, Salt Lake City, Utah, USA

J. DAVID BURKHARDT, MD
Electrophysiologist, Department of Clinical Cardiac Electrophysiology, Texas Cardiac

Arrhythmia Institute, St David's Medical Center, Austin, Texas, USA

MARÍA CESPÓN-FERNÁNDEZ, MD, PhD
Electrophysiologist, Department of Cardiology, Heart Rhythm Management Centre, European Reference Networks Guard-Heart, Universitair Ziekenhuis Brussel Heart Rhythm Research Brussels, Postgraduate Program in Cardiac Electrophysiology and Pacing, Vrije Universiteit Brussel, Brussels, Jette, Belgium

GAETANO CHIRICOLO, MD
Interventional Cardiologist, Division of Cardiology, Department of Biomedicine and Prevention, Policlinico Tor Vergata, Roma, Italy

KYOUNG-RYUL JULIAN CHUN, MD
Cardiologist, Department of Cardiology, Cardioangiologisches Centrum Bethanien, Frankfurt/Main, Germany; Clinic for

Rhythmologie, University Hospital Lübeck, Schleswig-Holstein, Lübeck, Germany

THOMAS F. DEERING, MBA, MD
Cardiologist, Department of Electrophysiology, Piedmont Heart of Buckhead Electrophysiology, Piedmont Heart Institute, Atlanta, Georgia, USA

LUIGI DI BIASE, MD, PhD, FACC, FESC, FHRS
Section Head of Electrophysiology, Director of Arrhythmia Services, Professor of Medicine (Cardiology), Montefiore-Einstein Center for Heart and Vascular Care, Montefiore Medical Center, Albert Einstein College of Medicine, Bronx, New York, USA

MATTIAS DUYTSCHAEVER, MD, PhD
Professor, Department of Electrophysiology, AZ Sint-Jan Hospital, Bruges, Belgium

MORITOSHI FUNASAKO, MD, PhD
Physician, Department of Cardiology, Charles University, Na Homolce Hospital, Prague, Czech Republic

CAROLA GIANNI, MD
Clinical Research Fellow, Department of Clinical Cardiac Electrophysiology, Texas Cardiac Arrhythmia Institute, St David's Medical Center, Austin, Texas, USA

RAJESH KABRA, MD
Cardiac Electrophysiologist, Department of Clinical Electrophysiology, Kansas City Heart Rhythm Institute, Overland Park, Kansas, USA

AASHISH KATAPADI, MD
Department of Clinical Electrophysiology, Kansas City Heart Rhythm Institute, Overland Park, Kansas, USA

JOSEF KAUTZNER, MD, PhD
Director, Department of Cardiology, Institute for Clinical and Experimental Medicine (IKEM), Prague, Czech Republic

JACOB S. KORUTH, MD
Associate Professor, Director, Department of Cardiology, Experimental Lab Helmsley Electrophysiology, Helmsley Electrophysiology Center, Mount Sinai Fuster Heart Hospital, Icahn School of Medicine at Mount Sinai, New York, New York, USA

VINCENZO MIRCO LA FAZIA, MD
Clinical Research Fellow, Department of Clinical Cardiac Electrophysiology, Texas Cardiac Arrhythmia Institute, St David's Medical Center, Austin, Texas, USA

DHANUNJAYA LAKKIREDDY, MBA, MD
Executive Medical Director, Department of Clinical Electrophysiology, Kansas City Heart Rhythm Institute, Overland Park, Kansas, USA

KERRI LEVERENCE, BA
Principal Field Clinical Specialist, Abbott, Plymouth, Minnesota, USA

MONICA LO, MD, FHRS, FACC
Physician, Department of Electrophysiology, Arkansas Heart Hospital, Little Rock, Arkansas, USA

JACOPO MARAZZATO, MD, PhD
Cardiologist, Department of Cardiology, Montefiore Medical Center, Bronx, New York, USA; Electrophysiology and Cardiac Pacing Unit, Humanitas Mater Domini, Varese, Italy

MOHAMAD MDAIHLY, MD
Postdoctoral Research Fellow, Cardiac Electrophysiology and Pacing Section, Department of Cardiovascular Medicine, Cleveland Clinic, Cleveland, Ohio, USA

ANDREAS METZNER, MD
Head of Electrophysiology, Department of Cardiology, University Heart and Vascular Center, Hamburg, Germany

AMBER MILLER, PhD
Associate Director of Clinical Research, Abbott, Plymouth, Minnesota, USA

SANGHAMITRA MOHANTY, MD
Director of Translational Research, Department of Clinical Cardiac Electrophysiology, Texas Cardiac Arrhythmia Institute, St David's Medical Center, Austin, Texas, USA

ANDREA NATALE, MD
Full Professor, Division of Cardiology, Department of Biomedicine and Prevention, Policlinico Tor Vergata, Roma, Italy; Executive Medical Director, Texas Cardiac Arrhythmia Institute, St David's Medical Center, Austin, Texas, USA

PETR NEUZIL, MD, PhD
Professor, Head, Department of Cardiology,
Charles University, Na Homolce Hospital,
Prague, Czech Republic

MORITZ NIES, MD
Electrophysiology Fellow, Electrophysiology
Resident, Department of Cardiology, University
Medical Center Hamburg-Eppendorf,
University Heart and Vascular Center,
Hamburg, Germany; Postdoctoral Research
Fellow, Department of Cardiology,
Experimental Lab Helmsley Electrophysiology,
Helmsley Electrophysiology Center, Mount
Sinai Fuster Heart Hospital, Icahn School of
Medicine at Mount Sinai, New York, New York,
USA

CHARBEL NOUJAIM, MD
Internal Medicine Resident, Cardiac
Electrophysiology and Pacing Section,
Department of Cardiovascular Medicine,
Cleveland Clinic, Cleveland, Ohio, USA

CONNOR P. OATES, MD
Cardiac Electrophysiology Fellow, Department
of Cardiology, Helmsley Electrophysiology
Center, Icahn School of Medicine at Mount
Sinai, New York, New York, USA

KISHAN PADALIA, MD
Fellow of Clinical Cardiac Electrophysiology,
Division of Cardiology, Department of
Medicine, University of Colorado, Anschutz
Medical Campus, Aurora, Colorado, USA

PETR PEICHL, MD, PhD
Cardiac Electrophysiology Specialist,
Department of Cardiology, Institute for Clinical
and Experimental Medicine (IKEM), Prague,
Czech Republic

JAN PETRU, MD
Head of EP Lab, Department of Cardiology,
Charles University, Na Homolce Hospital,
Prague, Czech Republic

ANDREAS RILLIG, MD
Deputy Head of Electrophysiology,
Department of Cardiology, University Heart
and Vascular Center, Hamburg, Germany

PASQUALE SANTANGELI, MD, PhD
Cardiac Electrophysiologist,
Cardiac Electrophysiology and Pacing
Section, Department of Cardiovascular
Medicine, Cleveland Clinic, Cleveland, Ohio,
USA

ANDREA SARKOZY, MD, PhD, FEHRA
Director, Department of Cardiology,
Ventricular Arhythmia and Sudden Cardiac
Death Unit Heart, Rhythm Management
Centre, European Reference Networks Guard-
Heart, Universitair Ziekenhuis Brussel Heart
Rhythm Research Brussels, Postgraduate
Program in Cardiac Electrophysiology and
Pacing, Vrije Universiteit Brussel, Brussels,
Jette, Belgium

D. SCHAACK, MD
Cardiologist, Department of Cardiology,
Cardioangiologisches Centrum Bethanien,
Frankfurt/Main, Germany

BORIS SCHMIDT, MD, FHRS
Professor of Medicine, Department of
Cardiology, Cardioangiologisches Centrum
Bethanien, Frankfurt/Main, Germany;
Department of Cardiology, University Hospital
Frankfurt, Frankfurt, Germany

ALEXANDRA STEYER, MD
Doctor, Department of Cardiology,
Cardioangiologisches Centrum Bethanien,
Frankfurt/Main, Germany

GIUSEPPE STIFANO, MD
Electrophysiologist, Division of Cardiology,
Department of Biomedicine and Prevention,
Policlinico Tor Vergata, Roma, Italy

CHADI TABAJA, MD
Internal Medicine Resident, Cardiac
Electrophysiology and Pacing Section,
Department of Cardiovascular Medicine,
Cleveland Clinic, Cleveland, Ohio, USA

MOHIT K. TURAGAM, MD, FACC, FHRS
Associate Professor, Department of
Cardiology, Helmsley
Electrophysiology Center, Icahn School of
Medicine at Mount Sinai, New York, New York,
USA

WENDY S. TZOU, MD
Professor, Division of Cardiology,
Electrophysiology Section, Department of

Medicine, Director, Cardiac Electrophysiology, University of Colorado School of Medicine, Aurora, Colorado, USA

OUSSAMA M. WAZNI, MD, MBA
Section Head, Cardiac Electrophysiology and Pacing Section, Department of Cardiovascular Medicine, Cleveland Clinic, Cleveland, Ohio, USA

XIAODONG ZHANG, MD, PhD
Assistant Professor, Department of Cardiology, Montefiore Medical Center, Bronx, New York, USA

FENGWEI ZOU, MD
Fellow, Department of Medicine/Cardiology, Montefiore-Einstein Center for Heart and Vascular Care, Montefiore Medical Center, Bronx, New York, USA

Contents

High-voltage electric fields can lead to increased permeability of cell membranes—a phenomenon called electropermeabilization. The mechanisms contributing to this effect are electroporation, membrane lipid peroxidation, oxidative stress, and structural changes in membrane proteins. If extensive cell damage occurs, cell death ensues (irreversible electroporation). Calcium levels and adenosine triphosphate supply are crucial in deciding whether cells undergo apoptosis or necrosis. Myocytes are particularly susceptible for electropermeabilization. This facilitates tissue-specific ablation and offers safety advantages over thermal ablation. Each ablation system has its unique waveform that influences ablation efficacy, effects on nonmyocardial tissue, and intraprocedural behavior of the ablation catheter.

Pulsed field ablation (PFA) has emerged as a promising, nonthermal technique for arrhythmia ablation, leveraging high-voltage electrical fields to induce electroporation and create precise ablation lesions. Unlike traditional thermal methods such as radiofrequency ablation (RFA) and cryoablation, PFA selectively targets myocardial cells while sparing surrounding tissues, reducing the risk of collateral damage. This review focuses on the key characteristics of PFA lesion formation, drawing comparisons with RFA and cryoablation based on histopathology, imaging, and electroanatomical mapping.

Over the last 2 decades, thermal-based catheter ablation has remained the mainstay treatment of cardiac arrhythmias. Although rare, thermal ablation can extend beyond the myocardium resulting in serious adverse events namely pulmonary vein stenosis, esophagus and phrenic nerve injury. In contrast, pulsed field ablation (PFA) has emerged as a promising technique that creates nonthermal lesions in cardiac tissue through the mechanism of irreversible electroporation (IRE). IRE involves the application of short-duration high-voltage pulsed electrical fields leading to cell death through membrane destabilization in a tissue-specific manner. This article discusses the mechanisms of electroporation while highlighting the tissue selectivity of PFA.

Vincenzo Mirco La Fazia, Carola Gianni, Giuseppe Stifano, Sanghamitra Mohanty, Gaetano Chiricolo, J. David Burkhardt, Amin Al-Ahmad, and Andrea Natale

Pulsed field ablation (PFA) is an innovative technology for the ablation of atrial fibrillation (AF), characterized by its ability to create tissue-selective lesions while minimizing collateral damage to surrounding structures. Isolation of the pulmonary veins (PVs) remains the cornerstone of AF ablation; however, recent evidence underscores the significance of extra-PV triggers, such as those from the posterior wall of the left atrium, the superior vena cava, the coronary sinus, and the left atrial appendage. While preliminary data suggest that PFA may enhance safety outcomes compared to traditional thermal techniques, further studies needed to validate its efficacy in non-PV areas.

Kishan Padalia and Wendy S. Tzou

Pulsed field ablation, in commercially available formulations, is as effective as thermal ablation in controlling atrial fibrillation. In contrast to thermal ablation, pulsed field ablation has preferential tissue selectivity and reduces risk of injury to adjacent non-myocardial structures (eg, esophagus, phrenic nerve), and its mechanism of myocyte injury reduces risk of pulmonary vein stenosis. Pulsed field ablation may reduce overall procedure time, although often at the cost of increased fluoroscopy use, compared to thermal ablation. Pulsed field ablation incurs risks of coronary vasospasm and acute kidney injury from hemolysis, which must be considered and proactively managed.

Alexandra Steyer, Kyoung-Ryul Julian Chun, D. Schaack, and Boris Schmidt

The viability of pulsed field ablation (PFA) for the treatment of atrial fibrillation has been demonstrated in several trials. The good safety profile paired with procedural streamlining has contributed to the overall efficiency of this energy source. In terms of lesion durabilitiy and reduced arrhythmia burden, PFA appears largely comparable to established thermal ablation. There is however, a need for larger, systematic remapping trials with longer follow-up duration. Furthermore, the release of optimized catheters and wave-forms requires further attention in terms of general performance in future.

Jacopo Marazzato, Fengwei Zou, Xiaodong Zhang, and Luigi Di Biase

Pulsed electrical field energy is a highly customizable, minimally thermal energy source associated with a myriad of potential ablation recipes that would hypothetically limit the importance of catheter-tissue contact on lesion formation. However, recent preclinical studies conducted on ventricular swine models suggest that contact force is pivotal in achieving adequate lesion formation even during pulsed field ablation. Despite the accruing preclinical evidence, clinical data on ablation targets beyond pulmonary veins are lacking and vast, and prospective human studies are required to better explore the clinical outcome of patients undergoing contact-force-guided pulsed field ablation for cardiac arrhythmias.

Josef Kautzner and Petr Peichl

Pulsed field ablation (PFA) is a novel nonthermal energy source for catheter ablation, which is potentially useful also for ablation of ventricular arrhythmias since it mitigates the risk of collateral damage to adjacent tissues and may better penetrate through the scar tissue. Solid-tip PFA within the great cardiac vein appears to be advantageous for arrhythmias originating from the left ventricular summit. The use of a large-footprint catheter that toggles between radiofrequency current and PFA may provide an additional advantage since it allows the development of larger lesions to modify myocardial substrate. More experience is expected in the next few years.

Current Safety Profile of Pulse Field Ablation: Not Everything that Shines Is Gold   213

Aashish Katapadi, T. Jared Bunch, Rajesh Kabra, Thomas F. Deering, and Dhanunjaya Lakkireddy

Pulse field ablation is a novel, non-thermal alternative for catheter ablation of atrial fibrillation. Preclinical and early clinical studies have demonstrated a favorable safety profile with significant reductions in esophageal and pulmonary vein injury compared to radiofrequency ablation. However, there are still procedural and energy-related complications inherent to electroporation, tissue selectivity, and energy-dosing. Minimizing the frequency of application and extent of energy, as well as careful selection of the energy source, may mitigate these adverse events. There remains controversy and a lack of long-term outcomes, highlighting the need for further evaluation.

Pulsed Field Ablation Using a Lattice-Tip Catheter for Treatment of Ventricular Tachycardias   227

Moritz Nies, Andreas Metzner, and Andreas Rillig

The inability to create durable, high-quality lesions in the ventricles has limited ventricular tachycardia (VT) ablation outcomes. With pulsed field ablation (PFA), a new modality offers the potential to overcome limitations of conventional, thermal ablation. The lattice-tip catheter's design makes it a promising and versatile tool for ventricular ablation. Preclinical studies have shown that PFA using this system can penetrate scar and fat, create deep lesions, and address difficult ablation targets. Clinical data are scarce but suggest acute feasibility and safety. More research is necessary to evaluate whether this novel ablation system could take VT ablation to the next level.

Catheters and Tools with Pulsed Field Ablation—Pulmonary Vein Isolation with Focal Lattice-Tip Affera Sphere 9   239

María Cespón-Fernández and Andrea Sarkozy

The Affera system features a versatile and large footprint catheter with a lattice-tip design that is capable of delivering both pulsed field and radiofrequency energy. It provides precise mapping and ablation capabilities, demonstrating high acute success rates and durable lesion formation, with excellent safety profile in both radiofrequency and pulsed field ablation modes. Preclinical and clinical studies have shown high lesion durability, reduced procedural time, and promising outcomes in pulmonary vein isolation with minimal complications.

Safety, Effectiveness, and Clinical Workflow with a Balloon-Based Pulsed Field Ablation System: A Single-Center Experience   251

Monica Lo, Amber Miller, and Kerri Leverence

A balloon-based pulsed field ablation (PFA) system with tissue proximity and mapping integration is currently undergoing clinical study. The initial 47 cases performed by a single operator identified important procedural workflow and system features that allow for the efficient adoption of this new catheter ablation technology resulting in an average procedure time including a 20 minute waiting period of

CARDIAC ELECTROPHYSIOLOGY CLINICS

Foreword
The Future Is Upon Us

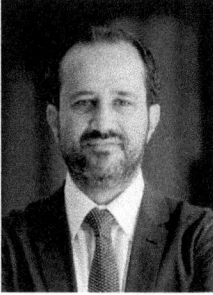

Luigi Di Biase, MD, PhD, FACC, FESC, FHRS   Emily P. Zeitler, MD, MHS, FHRS   Fengwei Zou, MD

Consulting Editors

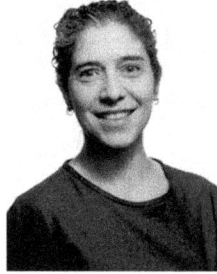

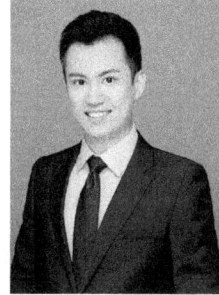

Since atrial fibrillation (AF) was first recognized, clinicians, including electrophysiologists (EPs), have attempted to tame this beast. We have come a long way from controlling ventricular rate with nodal blocking agents and mastering atrial antiarrhythmic medications to effectively utilizing direct current cardioversion and routinely performing intracardiac catheter ablations to reduce arrhythmia substrate.

While techniques for AF catheter ablation are refined, including exploration of treatment of nonpulmonary vein triggers, we embrace a technological advance that has the potential to change the landscape of AF management: pulsed field ablation (PFA). Using ultrashort high-energy bursts delivered in microseconds to nanoseconds, PFA creates ablation lesions through electroporation.

Contrary to conventional thermal energy–based ablation approaches, electroporation allows for faster procedures, and it appears to be more forgiving in terms of technical characteristics like lesion duration. Its ability to create durable lesions by controlling operator-dependent variables may help resolve some of the critiques of older trials with variable outcomes in effectiveness of targeting nonpulmonary vein triggers. An improved understanding of appropriate ablation targets will improve ablation success. Moreover, PFA's streamlined approach offers an excellent training platform for EP fellows, increasing opportunities for hands-on experience and elevating

the overall standard of care in AF ablation, especially as ablation becomes a first-line therapy for AF rhythm management.

Ultimately, the improved efficiency offered by PFA expands our ability to reach more patients as the population eligible for this treatment continues to grow. The future is upon us.

Luigi Di Biase, MD, PhD, FACC, FESC, FHRS
Albert Einstein College of Medicine
at Montefiore Health System
New York, NY 10467, USA

Emily P. Zeitler, MD, MHS, FHRS
Dartmouth Health Lebanon
The Dartmouth Institute
Lebanon, NH, USA

The Geisel School of Medicine at Dartmouth
Hanover, NH, USA

Fengwei Zou, MD
Albert Einstein College of Medicine at Montefiore
Health System
New York, NY
10467, USA

E-mail addresses:
dibbia@gmail.com (L. Di Biase)
emily.p.zeitler@hitchcock.org (E.P. Zeitler)
fzou@montefiore.org (F. Zou)

Card Electrophysiol Clin 17 (2025) xiii
https://doi.org/10.1016/j.ccep.2025.03.002
1877-9182/25/© 2025 Published by Elsevier Inc.

Preface
Pulsed Field Ablation

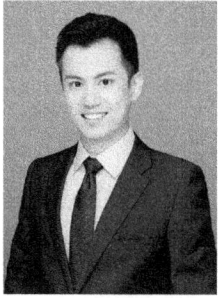

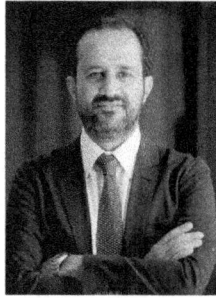

Fengwei Zou, MD   Luigi Di Biase, MD, PhD, FACC, FESC, FHRS

Editors

Pulsed field ablation (PFA) is one of the most anticipated advances in electrophysiology for the past two decades, and the field has witnessed an explosion of evidence already accumulated not long since its inception. Some of the biggest merits of PFA are its customizability of power, pulse duration, number of pulses delivered, catheter shape, and more. However, at the early stage of technological development, high degrees of variability can be detrimental, as this hinders unbiased understanding of safety and efficacy of PFA. Currently, there are four FDA-approved PFA systems in the United States, each with its own configuration and pulsed field parameters: Pulse-Select and Affera from Medtronic, Farapulse from Boston Scientific, and Varipulse from Johnson & Johnson.

In this issue of *Cardiac Electrophysiology Clinics*, we bring to you a comprehensive collection of articles touching upon every aspect of PFA from key investigators that shaped the current landscape of evidence. For starters, we investigate the basic science behind electroporation, its biophysics, and its impact on lesion characteristics and tissue selectively. This foundational understanding of PFA enables scientific hypothesis generation and testing. We then move on to the early application of PFA in both atrial and ventricular arrhythmias with an emphasis on safety, efficacy, and the need for contact force. From these initial preclinical animal studies and pivotal human trials, we can better grasp how this new technology is different from traditional thermal ablations and its potential pitfalls. The next section focuses on the initial experience of each individual FDA-approved PFA system as well as ones in development, providing direct comparison between each system. We hope this issue can provide you with a thorough insight into PFA and its promising future.

Dr. Zou would like to dedicate this issue to his parents and his family. Dr. Di Biase would like to dedicate this issue to his lovely wife, his beautiful son, his parents, and his family.

Fengwei Zou, MD
Department of Medicine/Cardiology
Montefiore-Einstein Center
for Heart and Vascular Care
Montefiore Medical Center
Bronx, NY, USA

Luigi Di Biase, MD, PhD, FACC, FESC, FHRS
Montefiore-Einstein Center for Heart and
Vascular Care
Montefiore Medical Center
Bronx, NY, USA

E-mail addresses:
fzou@montefiore.org (F. Zou)
dibbia@gmail.com (L. Di Biase)

Card Electrophysiol Clin 17 (2025) xv
https://doi.org/10.1016/j.ccep.2025.03.001
1877-9182/25/© 2025 Published by Elsevier Inc.

Biophysics of Electroporation and Pulsed Field Ablation

Moritz Nies, MD[a,b], Jacob S. Koruth, MD[a],*

KEYWORDS

• Electroporation • Catheter ablation • Arrhythmia • Myocardium • Electropermeabilization

KEY POINTS

- High-voltage electric fields lead to increased cell membrane permeability via electroporation as well as membrane lipid peroxidation, and structural changes to membrane proteins (electropermeabilization).
- Osmotic stress, adenosine triphosphate-depletion, and oxidative stress damage the affected cells. If a certain threshold of damage is exceeded, cell damage becomes irreversible, and cell death ensues.
- Due to their relative susceptibility with endocardial delivery, cardiomyocytes are ideal targets for electropermeabilization. The primary mechanisms for cell death in vivo however remain debated.
- The extent of cell death is largely determined by tissue penetration of the lethal electric field which depends on the voltage delivered, stable contact, pulse and catheter design. These variables have to be carefully designed to avoid for thermal damage, muscle/nerve capture, and loss of tissue specificity.
- Current pulsed field generators allow for mostly fixed output and only pulse repetition can provide for limited additional lesion depth.

ELECTROPORATION/ELECTROPERMEABILIZATION

When eukaryotic cells are exposed to short, high-voltage electric impulses, their cellular membranes' permeability increases.[1,2] Technically, the term electroporation in its narrow definition describes the formation of pores in cellular membranes—but this is only one of several mechanisms involved in cell death after exposure to electric fields.[1,3] Thus, the term electropermeabilization is more accurate as it encompasses all the mechanisms that contribute to increased membrane permeability.

High-voltage electric fields charge the plasma membrane (PM) which can be thought to function as a capacitor.[4] This induces a transmembrane voltage (TMV) gradient that is proportional to the external electric field and is considered the main driver for electropermeabilization in eukaryotic cells.[1,5] It is important to note that several mechanisms contribute to the increase in membrane permeabilization.

Pore Formation in Cell Membranes

Molecular dynamic models have shown that when a sufficiently high TMV is achieved, water molecules reorient their dipoles to align with the local

a Department of Cardiology, Experimental Lab Helmsley Electrophysiology, Helmsley Electrophysiology Center, Icahn School of Medicine at Mount Sinai, New York, NY, USA; b Department of Cardiology, University Heart and Vascular Center, University Medical Center Hamburg-Eppendorf, Martinistraße 52, 20246 Hamburg, Germany
* Corresponding author. Experimental Lab Helmsley Electrophysiology, Helmsley Electrophysiology Center, Mount Sinai Fuster Heart Hospital, Department of Cardiology, Icahn School of Medicine at Mount Sinai, One Gustave L. Levy Place, Box 1030, New York, NY 10029.
E-mail address: jacob.koruth@mountsinai.org

Card Electrophysiol Clin 17 (2025) 125–135
https://doi.org/10.1016/j.ccep.2025.02.001
1877-9182/25/© 2025 Elsevier Inc. All rights are reserved, including those for text and data mining, AI training, and similar technologies.

Abbreviations

ATP   adenosine triphosphate
PFA   pulsed field ablation
PM   plasma membrane
ROS   reactive oxygen species
TMV   transmembrane voltage

electric field. This results in small "water fingers" protruding into the hydrophobic core of the bilayer lipid membrane. When these water fingers span through the entire bilayer membrane, they initially form a small hydrophopic pores capable of conducting ions ("water column," **Fig. 1**A, B).[6–8] Lipid molecules adjacent to the hydrophobic pores then realign, pointing their polar headgroups toward the hydrophobic pores. The resulting hydrophilic pores (**Fig. 1**C-E) are more stable, larger (up to ~100 nm in diameter), and can be considered the final stage of cell membrane electroporation.[9]

Effects on Membrane Lipids

It has been shown that strong electric fields lead to the generation of reactive oxygen species (ROS) and induce peroxidation of unsaturated lipids within the cellular membrane (**Fig. 2**).[10,11] This has been associated with increased membrane permeability, increased membrane resealing time, and cell damage.[10–12] The generation of ROS does not seem to be a direct effect of the electric field, but the exact mechanisms have not been described conclusively thus far and it remains unclear to what extent lipid peroxidation contributes to electropermeabilization.[12,13] However, studies have shown that larger amounts of peroxidized lipids within a bilayer lipid membrane result in a much higher membrane permeability and predisposes the membrane to pore formation.[14–16]

Effects on Membrane Proteins

As membrane permeability remains increased even after aqueous pores in the lipid bilayer have resealed, additional factors seem to be involved that are independent of bilayer pore formation.[17–19] High-amplitude electric fields can alter the conductivity of transmembrane ion transporters, which has been reported for Na^+/K^+-ATPase and other proteins in studies using mostly submicrosecond electric pulses (**Fig. 3**).[18,20–22] It is hypothesized that these structural protein changes are the result of thermal denaturation which is brought about by electric current passing through the proteins, driven by the high TMV.[23] This increased permeability of structurally altered membrane proteins might be an additional contributing factor in electropermeabilization.[24]

Mechanisms of Cell Damage via Electropermeabilization

Several mechanisms are involved in causing cell damage via electropermeabilization (**Fig. 4**): (i) Calcium influx from the extracellular space triggers intracellular signal cascades and causes osmotic imbalance as well as cell swelling.[3] (ii) Adenosine triphosphate (ATP)-depletion occurs via direct leakage through pores, increased ATP-consumption by active repair mechanisms, and inhibited mitochondrial ATP-production.[25–27] (iii) The generation of ROS is triggered by pulsed electric fields, leading to oxidative stress.[28,29] (iv) Nanosecond-scale pulses have been hypothesized to affect intracellular membranes as well, specifically to damage mitochondria.[30,31] (v) Direct damage to DNA and to intracellular proteins has been described/suggested by molecular dynamics models but the exact mechanisms remain unclear.[32–34]

As many of these processes occur simultaneously and are interdependent, it is challenging to ascertain or predict which is the main driver for cell damage observed in vivo.

Reversible versus Irreversible Electropermeabilization

Electropermeabilization occurs only when a certain threshold of TMV is surpassed.[35,36] All 3 mechanisms outlined earlier (electroporation, lipid peroxidation, protein denaturation) are potentially reversible as pores can reseal, and altered membrane lipids and proteins are eventually replaced. Repairing physiologic membrane function is crucial to preserve cell viability after electropermeabilization. Several different repair mechanisms are employed.

Very small pores (few nanometers) in the lipid bilayer may reseal spontaneously after the TMV ceases.[3] For larger membrane defects, active repair mechanisms are necessary: Small defects less than 100 nm are repaired via exocytosis of lysosomes that reduce membrane tension and promote pore resealing. Excreted lysosomal contents then trigger endocytosis and degradation of altered membrane sections.[37,38] Medium-sized pores up to few micrometers are resealed via protein (mostly annexin) clogging and consecutive shedding of the membrane segment.[38] Membrane defects larger than few micrometers are patched by cytoplasmic vesicles that fuse and then merge with the damaged membrane to seal the hole.[38] A detailed description of the repair mechanisms is beyond the scope of this article, but it should be noted that the active repair mechanisms are activated by intracellular calcium and require ATP.

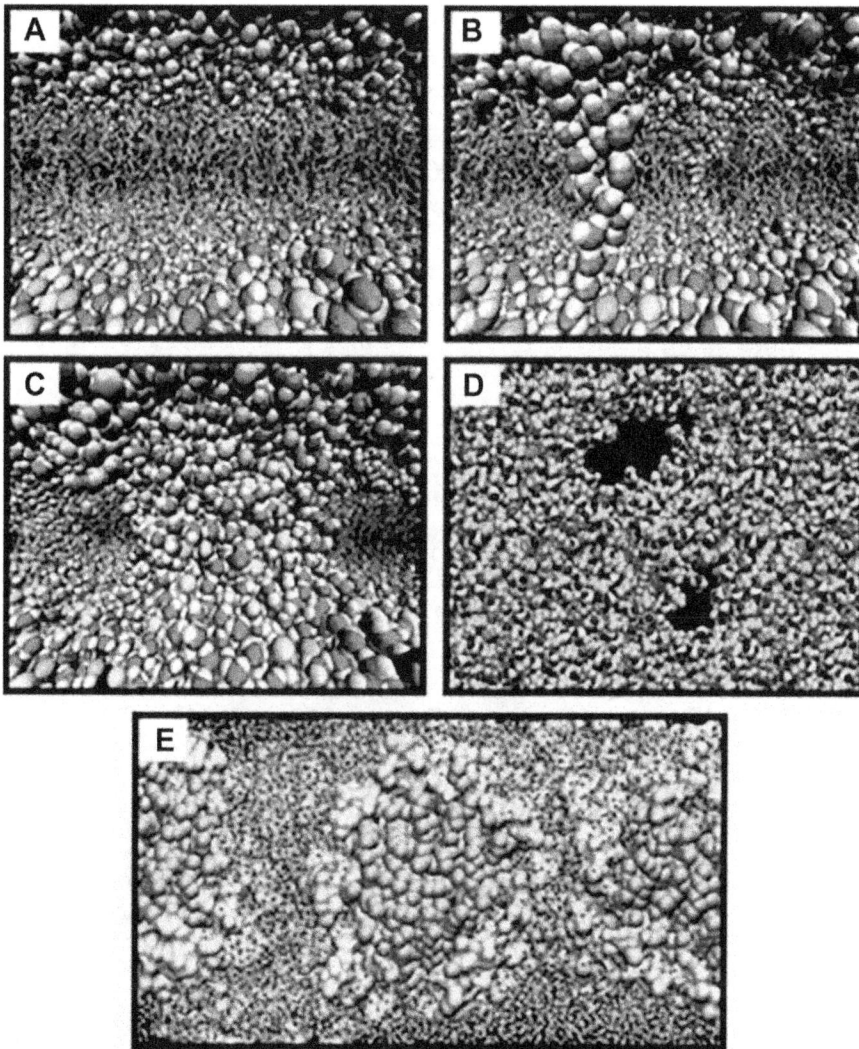

Fig. 1. Molecular dynamics model showing configurations for a dimyristoyl-phosphatidylcholine bilayer. (*A*) Bilayer membrane at baseline. (*B*) Water columns form during the first stage after exposure of the bilayer membrane to a transverse electric field. (*C*) Subsequently, the simulation shows larger water pores that are stabilized by lipid headgroups. (*D*) Superior view on the water pores in the bilayer; (*E*) Side view. A to C, water molecules; O, red globes; H, white globes; lipid phosphate, yellow globes; nitrogen, green globes; acyl chains, cyan (stick representation). (*Data from* Tarek M. Membrane electroporation: a molecular dynamics simulation. Biophys J. 2005;88(6):4045–4053. doi:https://doi.org/10.1529/biophysj.104.050617; with permission.)

As mentioned before, the extent of membrane damage and the dimension of pores brought about via electroporation largely depend on the field intensity/TMV.

If cell damage after electropermeabilization becomes too extensive, repair mechanisms are insufficient to preserve cell viability, and cell death ensues (irreversible electroporation).[3] The thresholds for the occurrence of electropermeabilization and for irreversible cell damage mostly depend on field intensity, but there are a number of other contributing factors such as cell type, cell size, membrane geometry, and duration of exposure.[1,39–41] For eukaryotic cells in cell suspension, electropermeabilization was detectable at a TMV of hundreds of millivolts, and irreversible cell damage typically occurs when the TMV is futher increased 3- to 5-fold.[1]

Cell Death After Electropermeabilization

Several types of cell death have been observed after exposure to electric fields. Which form of cell death an affected cell will undergo is dependent on a number of factors such as TMV, pulse waveform, cell type, treatment conditions, and more.[3]

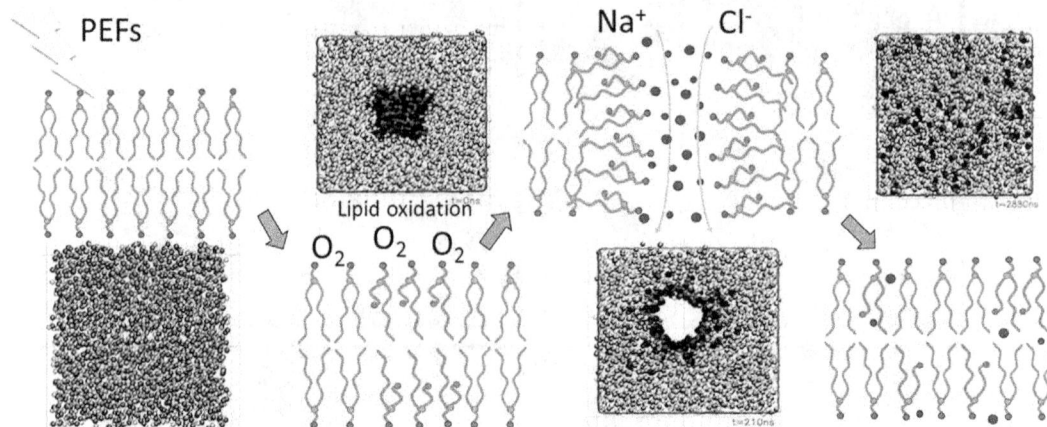

Fig. 2. Lipid oxidation and its effects on the permeability of membranes. Pulsed electric fields lead to lipid oxidation which propagates membranous pore formation. PEF, pulsed electric fields. (*Data from* Wiczew D, Szulc N, Tarek M. Molecular dynamics simulations of the effects of lipid oxidation on the permeability of cell membranes. Bioelectrochemistry. 2021;141:107869. doi:https://doi.org/10.1016/j.bioelechem.2021.107869; with permission.)

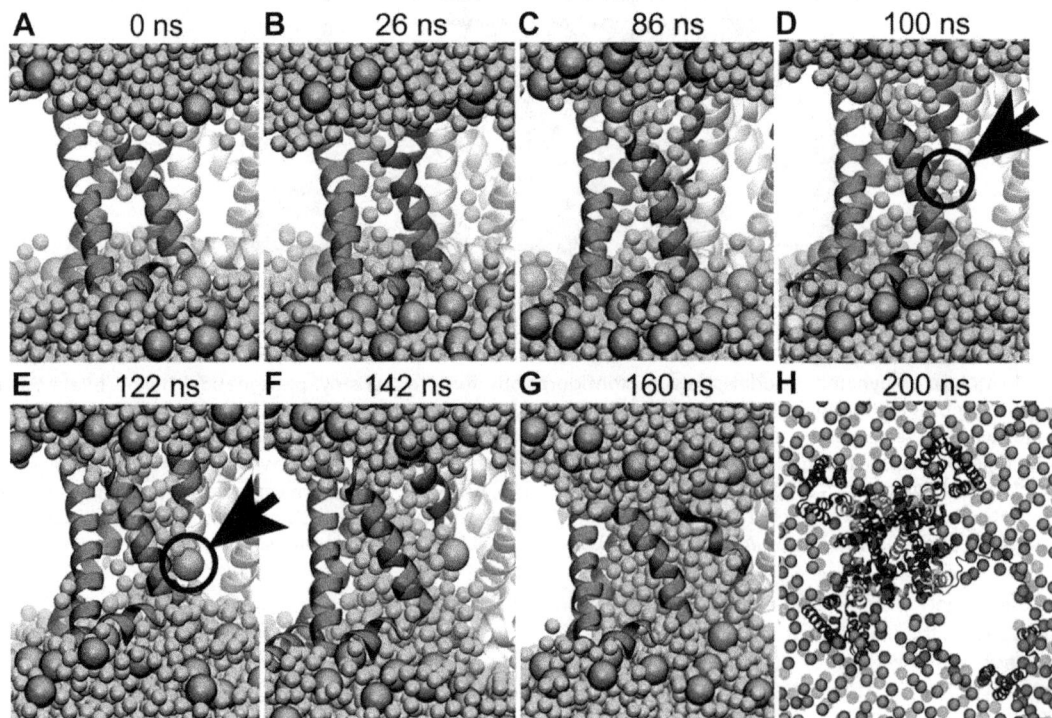

Fig. 3. Complex pore formation within a transmembrane protein (ion channel) after exposure to an electric field. (*A*) Hydrated membrane protein at baseline. (*B*) and (*C*) After application of the electric field, water molecules (blue globes) enter the protein channel. (*D*) A chloride ion (green globe; black circle and arrow) passes through the transmembrane protein ~90 ns after application. (*E*) and (*F*) More water and ions enter the protein, and a complex pore within the protein channel forms. The black circle and arrow in (*E*) mark the first lipid headgroup (large golden globe) moving into the pore. (*G*) The complex pore expands, and the membrane protein starts unfolding from the channel. (*H*) Unfolded protein channel, seen from extracellular. Sodium ions, yellow globes. (*From* Rems L, Kasimova MA, Testa I, Delemotte L. Pulsed electric fields can create pores in the voltage sensors of voltage-gated ion channels. Biophysical journal. 2020;119(1):190-205. https://doi.org/10.1016/j.bpj.2020.05.030.)

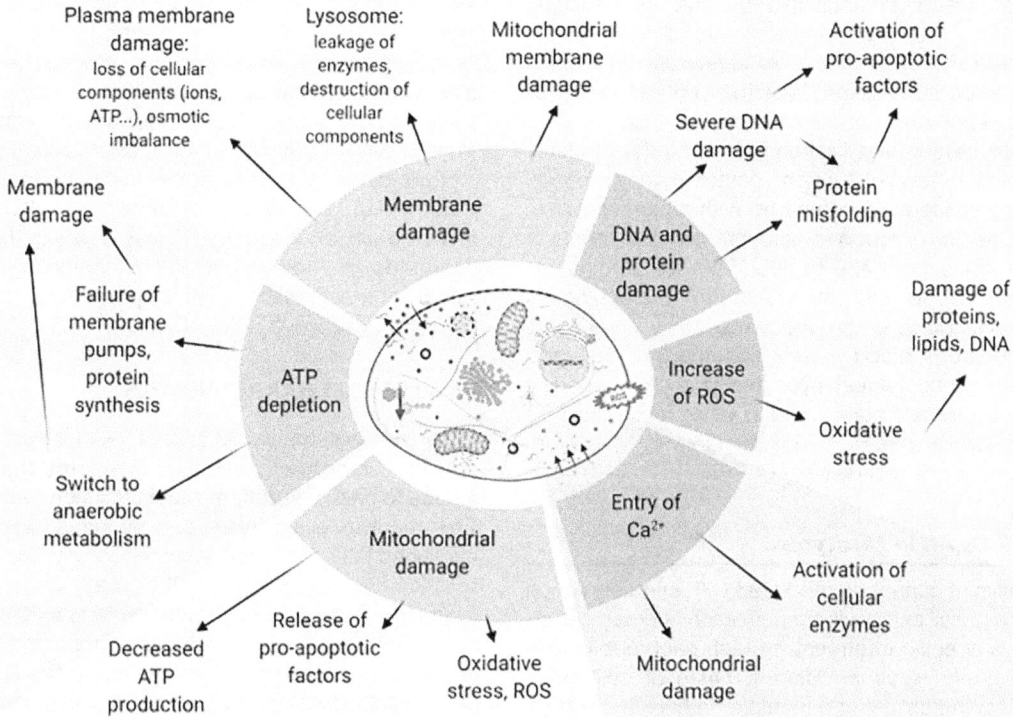

Fig. 4. Different mechanisms of cell injury after electropermeabilization. (*Data from* Batista Napotnik T, Polajzer T, Miklavcic D. Cell death due to electroporation - A review. Bioelectrochemistry. 2021;141:107871. https://doi.org/10.1016/j.bioelechem.2021.107871; with permission.)

Apoptosis

This programmed, regulated cell death has been considered the predominant mechanism after electropermeabilization.[3,42,43] Especially nanosecond electropermeabilization has been described to affect cell organelles and preferentially induce apoptosis.[30,44] Apoptotic cells typically show cell shrinkage, apoptotic fragmentation, and DNA condensation.[3] Apoptosis is an energy-dependent process, so cells are less likely to enter apoptosis if extensive ATP-depletion occurs.[45,46]

Necrosis

Necrotic cells undergo a rapid, uncontrolled cell death, and show a typical morphologic pattern: Osmotic imbalance leads to cell swelling that includes intracellular organelles like the endoplasmic reticulum and mitochondria. This is accompanied by random degeneration of DNA. Finally, the PM ruptures, and cellular contents are released into the extracellular space.[3,47]

Among the aforementioned mechanisms for cell damage, ATP-depletion seems to be crucial in deciding which type of cell death takes place.[46,48,49] More extensive electropermeabilization that typically occurs in areas with high electric field intensity leads to severe ATP-depletion, limiting the membrane repair mechanisms' abilities to restore cell integrity.[50] When necrosis occurs, the uncontrolled spilling of intracellular molecules into the extracellular space typically triggers a marked inflammatory response.[3,48]

Other Types of Cell Death

Recently, other forms of cell death have been described and might occur after electropermeabilization.[51] Necroptosis is triggered by death receptor activation and initiates a process that morphologically mimics necrosis.[3,52] Pyroptosis is triggered by caspase activation and ends in pore formation and cell membrane rupture as well.[53] Lastly, ferroptosis is a form of programmed cell death triggered by oxidative stress and iron-dependent lipid peroxidation.[54,55] As most studies about electropermeabilization have been performed before these new forms were described, their contribution remains unclear.

Targeting Cardiomyocytes (Pulsed Field Ablation)

The utilization of short, high-voltage electric field to induce electropermeabilization for catheter ablation of cardiac arrhythmias is currently referred to as pulsed field ablation (PFA). This novel ablation modality has been integrated into clinical practice rapidly due to its favorable safety and efficiency. Several considerations have to be noted for electro-permeabilization of cardiomyocytes:

Electropermeabilization is an attractive modality for the ablation of cardiomyocytes as they are relatively susceptible compared with other cell types. Studies have reported field intensity thresholds in the range from 400 to 600 V/cm for cardiomyocytes, depending on waveform characteristics such as pulse length and number.[56,57] Thresholds for neurons, blood vessels/endothelium, red blood cells, or esophageal myocytes have been reported to be approximately 2-fold to 4-fold higher than for cardiomyocytes.[57–60] This is particularly relevant with endocardial delivery of PFA.

Cell Death in Myocytes

In vivo, it cannot be predicted with certainty which type of cell death will occur in each affected cell after a specific treatment. In fact, each application will likely result in different types of cell death within the tissue, and multiple pathways might be triggered simultaneously.[54]

Apoptosis has generally been considered the main mechanism of cell death after electropermeabilization.[3] However, recent data question the validity of this observation for catheter ablation as they describe predominant cardiomyocyte necrosis after PFA.[61,62] Currently available catheter ablation systems deliver PFA from a single catheter tip.[63] Therefore, the generated electric field intensity will be highest in the lesion center, decreasing with more distance to the catheter tip. Myocytes located close to the ablation electrodes are exposed to stronger electric fields and subsequent TMV values, leading to more extensive cell damage. In these central areas, necrosis is the main mechanism of cell death.[64] Toward the lesion's periphery, a certain area will experience irreversible but less extensive cell damage, and apoptosis might be observed. In fact, apoptosis-like features have been documented in histologic and ultrastructural microscopy assessments of PFA lesions,[64,65] but the observed contribution of apoptosis-like cell death to the lesion has been inconsistent. Some studies reported large areas with apoptosis-like cell death,[64] while others described that most ablated cardiomyocytes showed necrosis-like features even in the lesion's periphery.[65]

As the electric field intensity diminishes further toward the edge of the lesion, there will most likely be cardiomyocytes that undergo reversible electroporation after PFA. This area will appear ablated acutely but regain physiologic function over time. As mentioned earlier, the exact threshold for reversible and irreversible electroporation depends on several waveform characteristics—details which remain proprietary for all currently available systems. It is, therefore, currently impossible to predict the chronic PFA lesion size in vivo intraprocedurally, and to define lesion endpoints. Determining the extent of reversibly affected myocardium after each PFA-lesion would be a huge step to improve our understanding of PFA lesion characteristics, define procedural endpoints, and improve lesion durability.

WAVEFORM CHARACTERISTICS

Many details in the application of PFA for catheter ablation comprise a specific waveform that is unique to each currently available ablation system. The most relevant waveform features will be explained later. However, exact waveform characteristics are proprietary for all clinically approved systems. This still limits our understanding of lesion formation and precludes transferring the knowledge gained using one system to the application of another.

Pulse Amplitude

As explained before, the TMV is the main driver for electropermeabilization. Its amplitude is proportional to the voltage output during PFA. Based on the disclosed information, currently available systems deliver pulses with an amplitude between 0.5 and 2 kV.[63] However, new systems featuring higher pulse amplitudes are under investigation. Increasing the voltage output boosts electropermeabilization effects and ablation efficacy, but comes with the risk of more pronounced thermal effects and of losing tissue specificity.[66] When considering tissue heating, the pulse amplitude should be put into context with the pulse duration as heating is determined by the total energy transferred to tissue during the pulse.

Pulse Duration/Pulse Width

The pulse duration or pulse width is the time during which the electric field is applied for each singular pulse (**Fig. 5**). Long pulse durations increase the pulse's electropermeabilization efficacy, causing larger lesions or facilitating irreversible electroporation with lower pulse amplitudes.[40] However, long application times also induce more Joule heating and local impedance changes.[66] Long pulse durations also increase muscle and nerve capture which is a limitation for their clinical use.[67] It is crucial to find a combination of pulse

Monophasic waveform

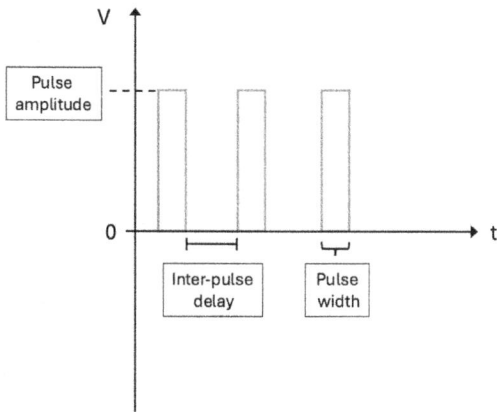

Biphasic waveform

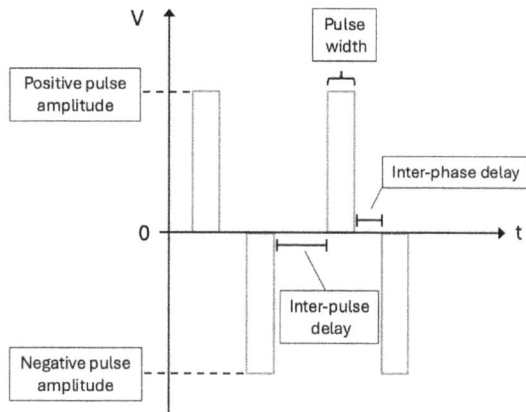

Fig. 5. Monophasic and biphasic waveforms. Shown are examples of a monophasic (*left*) and biphasic waveform (*right*). In both examples, rectangular pulses are used in which the field is applied and stopped rapidly. In monophasic PFA, repetitive pulses with the same polarity are delivered. In biphasic PFA, the electric field polarity is alternated within each respective pulse.

width and pulse amplitude that allows for effective electropermeabilization without significant tissue heating and minimal muscle/nerve capture.[66] Microsecond-scale pulses with amplitudes in the low kilovolt range have been used in clinical cancer therapy and are applied in commercially available PFA systems as well.[63,68]

Microsecond pulses are longer than the PM's charging time.[1] Therefore, the membrane acts as a capacitor, and the TMV predominantly affects the PM. With modern pulse generators, submicrosecond pulses (eg, nanosecond pulses) can be created with a sufficient amplitude for irreversible electroporation. These pulses are shorter than the PM's charging time and can, therefore, affect intracellular organelles as well.[3,30] A novel ablation system using this different mechanism for electroporation is currently under investigation for PFA.[69]

Monophasic/Biphasic Pulsed Field Ablation

In monophasic pulses, the electric field is applied unidirectionally for each pulse and returns to 0 V between pulses. Monophasic waveforms pose fewer technical requirements for the pulse generator and ablation system and have been used in vitro for decades. However, strong muscle capture limits their clinical use in clinical applications.[70,71] Conversely, in biphasic pulses, the electric field's charge and directionality is alternated with each respective pulse (see **Fig. 5**). Biphasic waveforms can overcome impedance variations in heterogeneous tissue and attenuate muscle capture as compared with monophasic pulses.[70–72] Biphasic pulses are standard for most modern PFA systems for atrial ablation.[63]

Monopolar/Bipolar Pulsed Field Ablation

Analogous to radiofrequency ablation, the distinction between monopolar and bipolar PFA refers to the position of the reference/grounding electrode in the circuit. Monopolar PFA is applied between the catheter tip and a grounding patch on the body surface.[73] The result is a large electric field that dissipates with increasing distance from the catheter tip. This large field can cause more muscle and nerve capture as compared with bipolar PFA.[73] However, monopolar PFA can be delivered from the whole catheter tip, and the large distance to the grounding electrode attenuates the risk for arching. Therefore, PFA can be delivered more reliably even if the catheter tip is deformed (eg, when pressed against tissue).

In bipolar PFA, both poles are integrated into the catheter tip. This can be achieved via 2 large ablation electrodes or with multielectrode catheters in which 2 ablation electrodes are paired, respectively. The resulting electric field is more condensed around the catheter tip and, therefore, muscle and nerve capture are attenuated.[73,74] However, if the paired electrodes are situated too closely together when PFA is applied, arching can occur. Ablation systems will abort the application when arching is detected, which can hinder ablation when the catheter tip is deformed (eg, in anatomically challenging areas).

Pulse Repetition

To achieve clinically significant irreversible electroporation with a single pulse would require voltages and pulse durations associated with unacceptable thermal effects or deviation from the biphasic design.[66] Striking examples are the first DC-ablations in the 1980s, in which a single shock was delivered via a 2-mm catheter using a standard DC-defibrillator (typically 1000–3000 V, 5–15 ms duration, 200–360 J).[73,75,76] This strong pulse sometimes led to blood vaporization, gas expansion, and significant barotrauma.[73] Applying pulses repetitively has an additive effect, so PFA can be amplified using repetitive, short pulses.[5,77] Pulse repetition also allows for effective ablation while limiting detrimental effects (heating, muscle capture).[66] Each clinical PFA application typically consists of multiple pulse bursts, each containing many pulses (see **Fig. 5**).

SUMMARY

During myocardial PFA, myocyte ablation is achieved via electroporation and other mechanisms of membrane damage. The design of the waveform has to ensure effective ablation while retaining advantages like nonthermal ablation and relative myocardial specificity. The introduction of PFA into clinical atrial fibrillation ablation has increasingly been viewed as a significant advance in terms of procedural safety and efficiency. Further research and technological innovation are necessary to allow us to optimize PFA waveforms and catheter designs to achieve the right balance of safety, efficacy, and efficiency.

CLINICS CARE POINTS

- The cellular response to high-voltage electric fields is complex and not fully elucidated thus far. Electroporation is one of the several mechanisms that lead to increased membrane permeability and ultimately cell death after exposure to strong electric fields.

- The waveform design largely determines each ablation system's characteristics in terms of lesion formation, thermal effects, muscle/nerve capture, and tissue specificity.

- Cardiomyocytes are ideal targets for pulsed field ablation as they have a significantly higher susceptibility for irreversible electroporation as compared with surrounding non-myocardial tissue like nerves or blood vessels. This is the basis for PFA's superior safety profile.

DISCLOSURE

Dr M. Nies has received a scholarship from the German Research Foundation (Deutsche Forschungsgemeinschaft). Dr J.S. Koruth has served as a consultant for, received grant support and equity from Affera-Medtronic, Field Medical, and Pulse Biosciences and serves as a consultant with grant support from CardioFocus, Abbott, Boston Scientific, Biosense Webster, CathVision, Kardium, and Medtronic.

REFERENCES

1. Kotnik T, Rems L, Tarek M, et al. Membrane Electroporation and electropermeabilization: Mechanisms and models. Annu Rev Biophys 2019;48:63–91.
2. Neumann E, Rosenheck K. Permeability changes induced by electric impulses in vesicular membranes. J Membr Biol 1972;10(3):279–90.
3. Batista Napotnik T, Polajzer T, Miklavcic D. Cell death due to electroporation - a review. Bioelectrochemistry 2021;141:107871.
4. Hibino M, Shigemori M, Itoh H, et al. Membrane conductance of an electroporated cell analyzed by submicrosecond imaging of transmembrane potential. Biophys J 1991;59(1):209–20.
5. Kotnik T, Miklavčič D, Slivnik T. Time course of transmembrane voltage induced by time-varying electric fields—a method for theoretical analysis and its application. Bioelectrochem Bioenerg 1998;45(1):3–16.
6. Delemotte L, Tarek M. Molecular dynamics simulations of lipid membrane electroporation. J Membr Biol 2012;245(9):531–43.
7. Ho MC, Casciola M, Levine ZA, et al. Molecular dynamics simulations of ion conductance in field-stabilized nanoscale lipid electropores. J Phys Chem B 2013;117(39):11633–40.
8. Tokman M, Lee JH, Levine ZA, et al. Electric field-driven water dipoles: nanoscale architecture of electroporation. PLoS One 2013;8(4):e61111.
9. Tieleman DP. The molecular basis of electroporation. BMC Biochem 2004;5:10.
10. Benov LC, Antonov PA, Ribarov SR. Oxidative damage of the membrane lipids after electroporation. Gen Physiol Biophys 1994;13(2):85–97.
11. Maccarrone M, Bladergroen MR, Rosato N, et al. Role of lipid peroxidation in electroporation-induced cell permeability. Biochem Biophys Res Commun 1995;209(2):417–25.
12. Gabriel B, Teissie J. Generation of reactive-oxygen species induced by electropermeabilization of Chinese hamster ovary cells and their consequence on cell viability. Eur J Biochem 1994;223(1):25–33.
13. Pakhomova ON, Khorokhorina VA, Bowman AM, et al. Oxidative effects of nanosecond pulsed electric field exposure in cells and cell-free media. Arch Biochem Biophys 2012;527(1):55–64.
14. Rems L, Viano M, Kasimova MA, et al. The contribution of lipid peroxidation to membrane permeability

in electropermeabilization: a molecular dynamics study. Bioelectrochemistry 2019;125:46–57.

15. Vernier PT, Levine ZA, Wu YH, et al. Electroporating fields target oxidatively damaged areas in the cell membrane. PLoS One 2009;4(11):e7966.

16. Wiczew D, Szulc N, Tarek M. Molecular dynamics simulations of the effects of lipid oxidation on the permeability of cell membranes. Bioelectrochemistry 2021;141:107869.

17. Tsong TY. On electroporation of cell membranes and some related phenomena. J Electroanal Chem Interfacial Electrochem 1990;299(3):271–95.

18. Nesin V, Bowman AM, Xiao S, et al. Cell permeabilization and inhibition of voltage-gated Ca(2+) and Na(+) channel currents by nanosecond pulsed electric field. Bioelectromagnetics 2012;33(5):394–404.

19. Rems L, Kasimova MA, Testa I, et al. Pulsed electric fields can create pores in the voltage sensors of voltage-gated ion channels. Biophys J 2020;119(1):190–205.

20. Teissie J, Tsong TY. Evidence of voltage-induced channel opening in Na/K ATPase of human erythrocyte membrane. J Membr Biol 1980;55(2):133–40.

21. Chen W, Han Y, Chen Y, et al. Electric field-induced functional Reductions in the K^+ channels mainly Resulted from supramembrane potential-mediated electroconformational changes. Biophys J 1998;75(1):196–206.

22. Chen W, Zhongsheng Z, Lee RC. Supramembrane potential-induced electroconformational changes in sodium channel proteins: a potential mechanism involved in electric injury. Burns 2006;32(1):52–9.

23. Tsong TY. Electroporation of cell membranes. Biophys J 1991;60(2):297–306.

24. Silkuniene G, Mangalanathan UM, Rossi A, et al. Identification of proteins Involved in cell membrane Permeabilization by nanosecond electric pulses (nsEP). Int J Mol Sci 2023;24(11):9191.

25. Rols MP, Teissie J. Electropermeabilization of mammalian cells. Quantitative analysis of the phenomenon. Biophys J 1990;58(5):1089–98.

26. Gibot L, Montigny A, Baaziz H, et al. Calcium Delivery by electroporation induces in vitro cell Death through mitochondrial Dysfunction without DNA damages. Cancers 2020;12(2):425.

27. Brookes PS, Yoon Y, Robotham JL, et al. Calcium, ATP, and ROS: a mitochondrial love-hate triangle. Am J Physiol Cell Physiol 2004;287(4):C817–33.

28. Rajagopalan NR, Munawar T, Sheehan MC, et al. Electrolysis products, reactive oxygen species and ATP loss contribute to cell death following irreversible electroporation with microsecond-long pulsed electric fields. Bioelectrochemistry 2024;155:108579.

29. Asadipour K, Hani MB, Potter L, et al. Nanosecond pulsed electric fields (nsPEFs) modulate electron Transport in the plasma Membrane and the mitochondria. Bioelectrochemistry 2024;155:108568.

30. Beebe SJ, Sain NM, Ren W. Induction of cell death Mechanisms and Apoptosis by nanosecond pulsed electric fields (nsPEFs). Cells 2013;2(1):136–62.

31. Batista Napotnik T, Wu YH, Gundersen MA, et al. Nanosecond electric pulses cause mitochondrial membrane permeabilization in Jurkat cells. Bioelectromagnetics 2012;33(3):257–64.

32. Beebe SJ, Fox PM, Rec LJ, et al. Nanosecond pulsed electric field (nsPEF) effects on cells and tissues: apoptosis induction and tumor growth inhibition. IEEE Trans Plasma Sci 2002;30(1):286–92.

33. Marracino P, Apollonio F, Liberti M, et al. Effect of high exogenous electric Pulses on protein conformation: Myoglobin as a case study. J Phys Chem B 2013;117(8):2273–9.

34. Hekstra DR, White KI, Socolich MA, et al. Electric-field-stimulated protein mechanics. Nature 2016;540(7633):400–5.

35. Towhidi L, Kotnik T, Pucihar G, et al. Variability of the minimal transmembrane voltage resulting in detectable membrane electroporation. Electromagn Biol Med 2008;27(4):372–85.

36. Teissie J, Rols MP. An experimental evaluation of the critical potential difference inducing cell membrane electropermeabilization. Biophys J 1993;65(1):409–13.

37. Andrews NW, Corrotte M. Plasma membrane repair. Curr Biol 2018;28(8):R392–7.

38. Jimenez AJ, Perez F. Plasma membrane repair: the adaptable cell life-insurance. Curr Opin Cell Biol 2017;47:99–107.

39. Ĉemazĉ̂r M, Jarm T, Miklavĉiĉ D, et al. Effect of electric-field intensity on electropermeabilization and electrosensitmty of various tumor-cell lines in vitro. Electro- and Magnetobiology 1998;17(2):263–72.

40. Rols M-P, Teissié J. Electropermeabilization of mammalian Cells to macromolecules: Control by pulse duration. Biophys J 1998;75(3):1415–23.

41. Vernier PT, Aimin L, Marcu L, et al. Ultrashort pulsed electric fields induce membrane phospholipid translocation and caspase activation: differential sensitivities of Jurkat T lymphoblasts and rat glioma C6 cells. IEEE Trans Dielectr Electr Insul 2003;10(5):795–809.

42. Hofmann F, Ohnimus H, Scheller C, et al. Electric field pulses can induce apoptosis. J Membr Biol 1999;169:103–9.

43. Zhou W, Xiong Z, Liu Y, et al. Low voltage irreversible electroporation induced apoptosis in HeLa cells. J Cancer Res Therapeut 2012;8(1):80–5.

44. Beebe SJ, Fox PM, Rec LJ, et al. Nanosecond, high-intensity pulsed electric fields induce apoptosis in human cells. FASEB J 2003;17(11):1–23.

45. Elmore S. Apoptosis: a review of programmed cell death. Toxicol Pathol 2007;35(4):495–516.

46. Proskuryakov SY, Konoplyannikov AG, Gabai VL. Necrosis: a specific form of programmed cell death? Exp Cell Res 2003;283(1):1–16.

47. Nirmala JG, Lopus M. Cell death mechanisms in eukaryotes. Cell Biol Toxicol 2020;36(2):145–64.

48. Festjens N, Berghe TV, Vandenabeele P. Necrosis, a well-orchestrated form of cell demise: signalling cascades, important mediators and concomitant immune response. Biochim Biophys Acta Bioenerg 2006;1757(9–10):1371–87.

49. Qian T, Herman B, Lemasters JJ. The mitochondrial permeability transition mediates both necrotic and apoptotic death of hepatocytes exposed to Br-A23187. Toxicol Appl Pharmacol 1999;154(2):117–25.

50. Leist M, Single B, Castoldi AF, et al. Intracellular adenosine triphosphate (ATP) concentration: a switch in the decision between apoptosis and necrosis. J Exp Med 1997;185(8):1481–6.

51. Galluzzi L, Vitale I, Aaronson SA, et al. Molecular mechanisms of cell death: recommendations of the Nomenclature Committee on Cell Death 2018. Cell Death Differ 2018;25(3):486–541.

52. Frank D, Vince JE. Pyroptosis versus necroptosis: similarities, differences, and crosstalk. Cell Death Differ 2019;26(1):99–114.

53. Man SM, Karki R, Kanneganti TD. Molecular mechanisms and functions of pyroptosis, inflammatory caspases and inflammasomes in infectious diseases. Immunol Rev 2017;277(1):61–75.

54. Liu D, Li Y, Zhao Q. Effects of inflammatory cell death Caused by catheter Ablation on atrial fibrillation. J Inflamm Res 2023;16:3491–508.

55. Dixon SJ, Lemberg KM, Lamprecht MR, et al. Ferroptosis: an iron-dependent form of nonapoptotic cell death. Cell 2012;149(5):1060–72.

56. Baena-Montes JM, O'Halloran T, Clarke C, et al. Electroporation Parameters for human cardiomyocyte ablation in vitro. J Cardiovasc Dev Dis 2022;9(8):240.

57. Hunter DW, Kostecki G, Fish JM, et al. In vitro cell Selectivity of Reversible and irreversible: Electroporation in cardiac tissue. Circ Arrhythm Electrophysiol 2021;14(4):e008817.

58. Casciola M, Keck D, Feaster TK, et al. Human cardiomyocytes are more susceptible to irreversible electroporation by pulsed electric field than human esophageal cells. Phys Rep 2022;10(20):e15493.

59. Moshkovits Y, Grynberg D, Heller E, et al. Differential effect of high-frequency electroporation on myocardium vs. non-myocardial tissues. Europace 2023;25(2):748–55.

60. Kinosita K Jr, Tsong TY. Formation and resealing of pores of controlled sizes in human erythrocyte membrane. Nature 1977;268(5619):438–41.

61. Im SI, Higuchi S, Lee A, et al. Pulsed field Ablation of left ventricular Myocardium in a swine infarct model. JACC Clin Electrophysiol 2022;8(6):722–31.

62. Nakagawa H, Farshchi-Heydari S, Maffre J, et al. Evaluation of ablation Parameters to predict irreversible lesion size during pulsed field ablation. Circulation: Arrhythmia and Electrophysiology 2024;17(8):e012814.

63. Kawamura I, Koruth J. Novel ablation Catheters for atrial fibrillation. Rev Cardiovasc Med 2024;25(5):187.

64. Nakagawa H, Castellvi Q, Neal R, et al. Effects of contact Force on lesion size during pulsed field catheter ablation: histochemical Characterization of ventricular lesion boundaries. Circulation: Arrhythmia and Electrophysiology 2024;17(1):e012026.

65. Kawamura I, Wang BJ, Nies M, et al. Ultrastructural insights from myocardial ablation lesions from microsecond pulsed field vs radiofrequency energy. Heart Rhythm 2024;21(4):389–96.

66. Davalos RV, Rubinsky B, Mir LM. Theoretical analysis of the thermal effects during in vivo tissue electroporation. Bioelectrochemistry 2003;61(1):99–107.

67. Cvetkoska A, Maček-Lebar A, Trdina P, et al. Muscle contractions and pain sensation accompanying high-frequency electroporation pulses. Sci Rep 2022;12(1):8019.

68. Geboers B, Scheffer HJ, Graybill PM, et al. High-voltage electrical Pulses in oncology: irreversible electroporation, electrochemotherapy, gene electrotransfer, electrofusion, and electroimmunotherapy. Radiology 2020;295(2):254–72.

69. Nies M, Watanabe K, Kawamura I, et al. Ablating myocardium using nanosecond pulsed electric fields: preclinical Assessment of feasibility, safety, and durability. Circ Arrhythm Electrophysiol 2024;17(7):e012854.

70. Arena CB, Sano MB, Rossmeisl JH Jr, et al. High-frequency irreversible electroporation (H-FIRE) for non-thermal ablation without muscle contraction. Biomed Eng Online 2011;10:102.

71. Arena CB, Sano MB, Rylander MN, et al. Theoretical considerations of tissue electroporation with high-frequency bipolar pulses. IEEE Trans Biomed Eng 2011;58(5):1474–82.

72. Fusco R, Di Bernardo E, D'Alessio V, et al. Reduction of muscle contraction and pain in electroporation-based treatments: An overview. World J Clin Oncol 2021;12(5):367–81.

73. Bradley CJ, Haines DE. Pulsed field ablation for pulmonary vein isolation in the treatment of atrial fibrillation. J Cardiovasc Electrophysiol 2020;31(8):2136–47.

74. Stewart MT, Haines DE, Verma A, et al. Intracardiac pulsed field ablation: Proof of feasibility in a

chronic porcine model. Heart Rhythm 2019;16(5): 754–64.

75. Gallagher JJ, Svenson RH, Kasell JH, et al. Catheter technique for closed-chest ablation of the atrioventricular conduction system. N Engl J Med 1982; 306(4):194–200.

76. Scheinman MM, Morady F, Hess DS, et al. Catheter-induced ablation of the atrioventricular junction to control refractory supraventricular arrhythmias. JAMA 1982;248(7):851–5.

77. Tarek M. Membrane electroporation: a molecular dynamics simulation. Biophys J 2005;88(6):4045–53.

Lesion Characteristics of Pulsed Field Ablation

Charbel Noujaim, MD, MSc, Chadi Tabaja, MD, Oussama M. Wazni, MD, Pasquale Santangeli, MD, PhD*

KEYWORDS

- Pulsed field ablation • Electroporation • Atrial fibrillation • Nonthermal ablation • Lesion formation
- Histopathology • Pulmonary vein isolation

KEY POINTS

- Pulsed field ablation (PFA) is a nonthermal technique that uses high-voltage electrical fields to induce electroporation, selectively targeting myocardial cells while sparing surrounding tissues.
- PFA lesions are well-demarcated with preserved extracellular matrix, leading to less chronic fibrosis and edema compared with traditional thermal ablation methods like radiofrequency and cryoablation.
- Imaging studies show that PFA-induced lesions exhibit unique characteristics, making traditional late gadolinium enhancement-MRI less accurate for assessing lesion formation compared with thermal methods.
- Electroanatomical mapping studies demonstrate high rates of durable pulmonary vein isolation with PFA, achieving success rates up to 96% to 97% in some trials.
- Optimization of ablation parameters, such as contact force and pulse settings, is crucial for consistent lesion formation and maximizing the efficacy of PFA procedures.

INTRODUCTION

In recent years, pulsed field ablation (PFA) has emerged as a novel, nonthermal approach that utilizes high-voltage electrical fields to create ablation lesions through electroporation.[1] This technique selectively targets myocardial cells while sparing surrounding tissues, offering a potentially safer and more precise alternative to conventional thermal ablation methods.[2,3] Despite its promise, the histopathological, imaging, and electroanatomical characteristics of PFA-induced lesions and their clinical implications remain areas of active investigation.

The purpose of this review is to examine the characteristics of lesion formation with PFA, focusing specifically on histopathological features, imaging findings, and electroanatomical mapping outcomes. By comparing PFA-induced lesions to those created by radiofrequency ablation (RFA) and cryoablation, we aim to provide a comprehensive understanding of how PFA differs from traditional methods and to highlight its potential advantages in the field of catheter ablation.

BASICS OF ENERGY DELIVERY

To comprehend the impact of different ablation modalities on the myocardium, it is essential to first understand their underlying energy delivery mechanisms. RFA works by generating alternating current which is delivered from the catheter tip to the surrounding myocardial tissue. This process induces ionic agitation and frictional heating, ultimately leading to coagulative necrosis.[4] Several factors influence the size and depth of ablation lesions, including contact force, duration of energy application, and electrode size. To prevent overheating

Cardiac Electrophysiology and Pacing Section, Department of Cardiovascular Medicine, Cleveland Clinic, Cleveland, OH, USA
* Corresponding author. 9500 Euclid Avenue, Cleveland, OH 44195.
E-mail address: santanp3@ccf.org

Card Electrophysiol Clin 17 (2025) 137–145
https://doi.org/10.1016/j.ccep.2025.02.002
1877-9182/25/© 2025 Elsevier Inc. All rights reserved, including those for text and data mining, AI training, and similar technologies.

Abbreviations	
CF	contact force
IRE	irreversible electroporation
LGE	late gadolinium enhancement
PFA	pulsed field ablation
PV	pulmonary vein
PW	posterior wall
RFA	radiofrequency ablation
TZ	transition zone

and charring, irrigated-tip catheters are commonly used.[5–9]

Cryoablation, in contrast, delivers energy by cooling cardiac tissue to subzero temperatures. The catheter tip is cooled using a refrigerant gas, typically nitrous oxide or argon, which absorbs heat from the surrounding tissue. This process induces cellular death through the formation of ice crystals, which disrupts cellular membranes and intracellular structures. Additionally, cryoablation causes vascular stasis and ischemia, contributing further to tissue injury.[10]

PFA, unlike traditional methods, is a nonthermal ablation modality. It operates on the fundamental principle of inducing tissue damage through the application of high-voltage electrical fields in close proximity to the myocardium. The primary mechanism of injury is known as electroporation, which involves the increased permeability of plasma membranes when subjected to an electrical field. This process results in the formation of pores within the lipid bilayer, caused by the variation in potential across the cell membrane, leading to enhanced membrane permeability.[11,12] The goal of PFA is to induce irreversible pore formation and cell death through various mechanisms, including the downstream inactivation of membrane proteins and the initiation of apoptosis.[13–16] This technology is characterized by negligible heating, owing to the short pulse duration and the efficient dissipation of any generated heat through conduction and convection cooling effects.[17] This results in the theoretic selective targeting of cell membranes while sparing the extracellular matrix, which underpins the marketed tissue specificity of PFA.[18–20] However, after the membrane reseals and regains selective permeability, the cells return to normal function. This is a direct result of reversible electroporation, as demonstrated through theoretic models, such as the Hodgkin–Huxley-type model, and in vitro studies on single cells and cell monolayers mimicking cardiac tissue. In the context of PFA using a focal catheter, the resulting lesion typically has a central zone of irreversible damage surrounded by a rim of reversibly electroporated cells.

This means that the final PFA lesion develops over time. Consequently, despite the high acute procedural success, such as immediate pulmonary vein (PV) isolation observed in clinical studies, PFA may not necessarily lead to superior long-term outcomes.[3,21,22]

EVALUATION OF ABLATION LESION FORMATION

The gold standard for evaluating ablation lesion formation remains direct visualization through histopathology. While some postmortem studies have examined lesion formation using gross pathology and histologic examination, this method is most commonly employed in animal models where ablation is performed, and tissue is assessed ex vivo. Although histopathology is highly precise, it cannot be used to evaluate lesions postprocedurally in live human patients.

In the research setting, alternate validated modalities are available, with late gadolinium enhancement-MRI (LGE-MRI) being the most widely used. LGE-MRI relies on the delayed washin and washout mechanics of gadolinium, where delayed washin occurs in fibrotic or scarred ablated tissue, and subsequent delayed washout is detected on MRI, accurately highlighting ablation lesions.[23–25] T2-weighted imaging is another valuable tool for assessing acute tissue injury immediately postablation.[26] Electroanatomical mapping (or remapping) is a fundamental tool for assessing acute procedural success in terms of electrical isolation. However, while it provides a general indication of lesion formation, it may not accurately reflect the full impact of ablation on the myocardium.[27–30]

Other imaging modalities that have been employed to assess lesion delivery and scar formation include contrast-enhanced computed tomography, contrast-enhanced ultrasound, intracardiac echocardiography, optical coherence tomography, and intracardiac myocardial elastography, but are much less used in practice and in research.

CONVENTIONAL ENERGY DELIVERY METHODS AND LESION FORMATION

To gain a better understanding of PFA lesion formation, it is essential to first review the process as it occurs with the most widely used ablation tools, RFA and cryoablation. These established methods provide a well-documented reference point for comparison. Deneke and colleagues evaluated the histopathology of radiofrequency-induced ablation lesions in a series of 7 patients who died 2 to 22 days after undergoing permanent atrial fibrillation ablation. Barkagan and colleagues investigated RFA in a swine model with chronic infarction, focusing on heterogenous ventricular scar tissue as well as healthy ventricular myocardium. Gross examination generally revealed well-delineated lesions, characterized by whitish areas with hemorrhagic borders, with depths reaching up to 5.5 mm in the atrium and 9.3 mm in the ventricle. Histologically, the lesions exhibited a core of coagulative necrosis surrounded by an outer rim of contraction necrosis. Connective tissue appeared more resistant to thermal injury compared with cardiomyocytes. Additionally, lesion formation in damaged or scarred myocardium lacked a distinct architecture, making it challenging to predict.[31,32] Cryoablation-induced lesions are generally believed to have a smaller surface area but achieve similar depths compared with those created by RFA. Histologically, these lesions tend to preserve ultrastructural integrity better than RFA-induced lesions, as fibroblasts and collagen fibers are more resistant to the effects of hypothermia.[10] On LGE-MRI, acute edema is generally more prominent with RFA compared with other ablation modalities.[33] RFA and cryoablation lesions typically appear as the areas of hyperenhancement on LGE-MRI, with subtle differences observed during the early phases of scar formation. While this provides a general overview of ablation lesions produced by the 2 most widely used energy delivery methods, it is important to note that scar formation is influenced by a multitude of factors, which will not be the focus of this review.[33–35]

LESION CHARACTERISTICS OF PULSED FIELD ABLATION
Histopathological Features of Pulsed Field Ablation Lesion Formation

Multiple studies have been conducted to investigate the histologic characteristics of PFA-induced ablation lesions. In the early stages of PFA development, Lavee and colleagues performed beating-heart surgical epicardial ablations of the right and left atrial appendages in a swine model. They used direct current pulses applied between 2 4-cm long parallel electrodes connected to an irreversible electroporation (IRE) generator. The study reported clearly demarcated ablation lesions with complete transmural destruction of atrial tissue at the electrode application sites, with a mean lesion depth of 0.9 cm.[36] Similarly, most studies examining the gross pathology of PFA lesions have observed a clear demarcation between the ablation lesions and the surrounding normal tissue.[37–40] Wittkampf and colleagues conducted ablation procedures in an in vivo porcine model, targeting

the left ventricular epicardium with devices mimicking a 20-mm diameter 7F circular ablation catheter. Histologic analysis revealed that all lesions exhibited complete replacement of cardiomyocytes with granulation tissue composed of fibroblasts, loose collagen fibers, and capillaries.[39] Grimaldi and colleagues utilized a multichannel IRE generator system and a multielectrode circular IRE catheter with 10 ablation electrodes (Biosense Webster, CA, USA) to create lesions in the right and left atria of 10 swine models, divided into subchronic (7-day) and chronic (30-day) cohorts. Their study once again demonstrated well-demarcated lesions on gross pathology. Histologically, all ablated cardiac sites showed discrete zones of myocardial fiber and smooth muscle cell loss, while preserving overall tissue architecture. This resulted in fibrocellular replacement, neovascularization, and neocollagen deposition, thereby confirming the findings of Wittkampf and colleagues and supporting the previous literature.[39,41,42] The subchronic group showed evidence of mineralization, often associated with inflammation, which was not observed in the chronic group. In both groups, arterioles and autonomic nerves were generally preserved. In the chronic group, inflammation and mineralization had largely resolved, and there was evidence of endocardial healing, which was absent at 7 days. Most studies concur that IRE lesions are histologically characterized by the elimination of cardiomyocytes while preserving the structural extracellular matrix, with residual fibrosis and fibroblasts present.[22,43,44]

Comparative Histopathology of Pulsed Field Ablation and Radiofrequency Ablation Lesion Formation

Hong and colleagues conducted the first comparison between RFA and PFA lesions in a sheep model, where they created epicardial lesions using bipolar clamp or linear surface probe devices at multiple cardiac locations, as well as RFA lesions. Pulses were delivered in 3 or 5 trains at a frequency between 1 and 5 Hz, with each train consisting of 10 to 40 pulses. IRE lesions were characterized by edema or hemorrhage in the interstitial spaces, contraction band formation, or myofiber breakup, with cell swelling of cardiomyocytes and a loss of native myofiber birefringence under polarized light. In contrast, RF lesions exhibited contraction bands restricted to the outer rim of the lesion and coagulation necrosis in the core. Additionally, RFA lesions consistently showed more severe blood vessel damage compared with IRE lesions.[45] Stewart and colleagues conducted ablations in 6 pigs using a circular PV ablation catheter, with the energy source randomized to deliver either PFA or RFA to 3 atrial endocardial sites. Histologic evaluation at 2 weeks revealed that PFA resulted in more uniform fibrotic remodeling compared with RFA. Unlike RFA, PFA lesions rarely contained isolated viable myocytes and did not induce epicardial fat inflammation, which was observed with RFA. Additionally, intralesional arteries remained unaffected by PFA; medial hyperplasia and thrombosis, commonly seen with RFA, were absent. Moreover, PFA lesions showed no evidence of myocardial sparing around large intralesional arteries.[22,40]

Imaging Features of Pulsed Field Ablation Lesion Formation

While LGE-MRI remains an invaluable tool for assessing lesion and scar formation in both the ventricles and atria when thermal energy is used, its accuracy in evaluating lesions created by PFA is controversial. As discussed in the histopathology section, acute PFA lesions are typically characterized by interstitial edema and contraction band formation, while preserving tissue structural integrity. This preservation may result in less extensive scar tissue formation through replacement fibrosis, and PFA could also induce varying degrees of reactive fibrosis.[46]

LGE-MRI relies on the accumulation of contrast agents in the extracellular space, which does not penetrate intact cellular membranes. Typically,

LGE highlights areas of fibrosis and scarring by exploiting the expanded extracellular space and reduced capillary density, leading to prolonged contrast washout and hyperintensity on MRI sequences. This method effectively differentiates between healthy and scarred myocardium, a principle validated for ablation-induced fibrosis with thermal energy delivery.[23,47,48]

However, as gadolinium—the primary contrast agent—accumulates in the extracellular space and does not cross intact cell membranes, the mechanics of PFA suggest there may be less available extracellular space for gadolinium to accumulate due to the preservation of the extracellular matrix. This difference poses a challenge in accurately evaluating lesion formation on LGE-MRI when PFA is used, as compared with RFA.[46]

Sohns and colleagues conducted atrial fibrillation (AF) ablation in 10 patients using a 31-mm pentaspline PFA catheter. They performed 8 PFA applications—4 in a flower configuration and 4 in a basket configuration—along with 8 additional applications in the flower configuration for concomitant posterior wall (PW) isolation. LGE-MRI was conducted 3 months postprocedure, revealing a mean total LA scar burden of $8.1 \pm 2.1\%$ and a mean scar width of 12.8 ± 2.1 mm. In the posterior LA, $22.6 \pm 2.2\%$ of the anatomic segment developed chronic scar tissue, primarily concentrated at the PW[49] (**Fig. 1**). Nakatani and colleagues compared the effects of PFA and thermal ablation (radiofrequency and

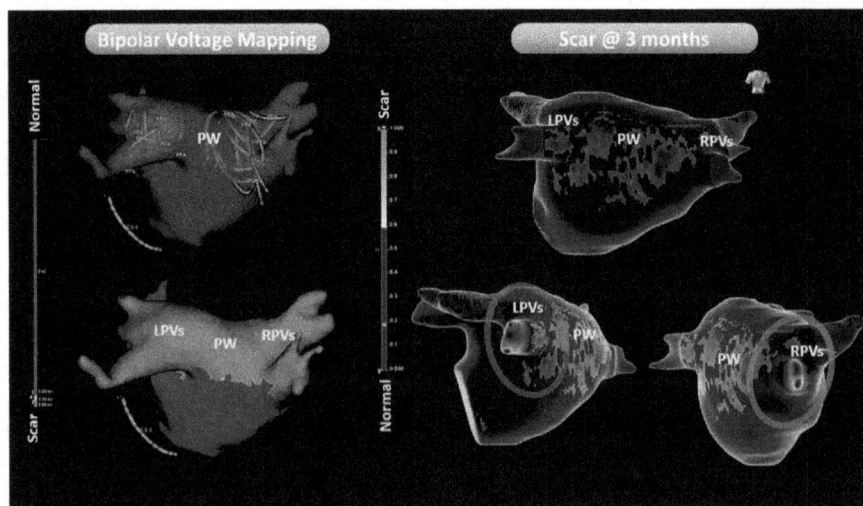

Fig. 1. Visualization of PFA treatment sites and lesion development assessed by electroanatomical mapping and LGE cardiovascular magnetic resonance imaging (CMR) at 3 months postablation. *Left panel*: Displays the PFA catheter positioned at the ostium of each PV and along the PW, illustrating the ablation sites targeted during the procedure. *Right panel*: Shows the resulting left atrial scar formation as detected by LGE CMR imaging, indicating areas of successful ablation and tissue remodeling. (*Data from* Fink T, Sciacca V, Neven K, Didenko M, Sommer P, Sohns C. Pulsed field ablation for atrial fibrillation – lessons from magnetic resonance imaging. Pacing Clin Electrophysiol. 2023;46(12):1586–1594. doi:https://doi.org/10.1111/pace.14864. © 2024, John Wiley and Sons.)

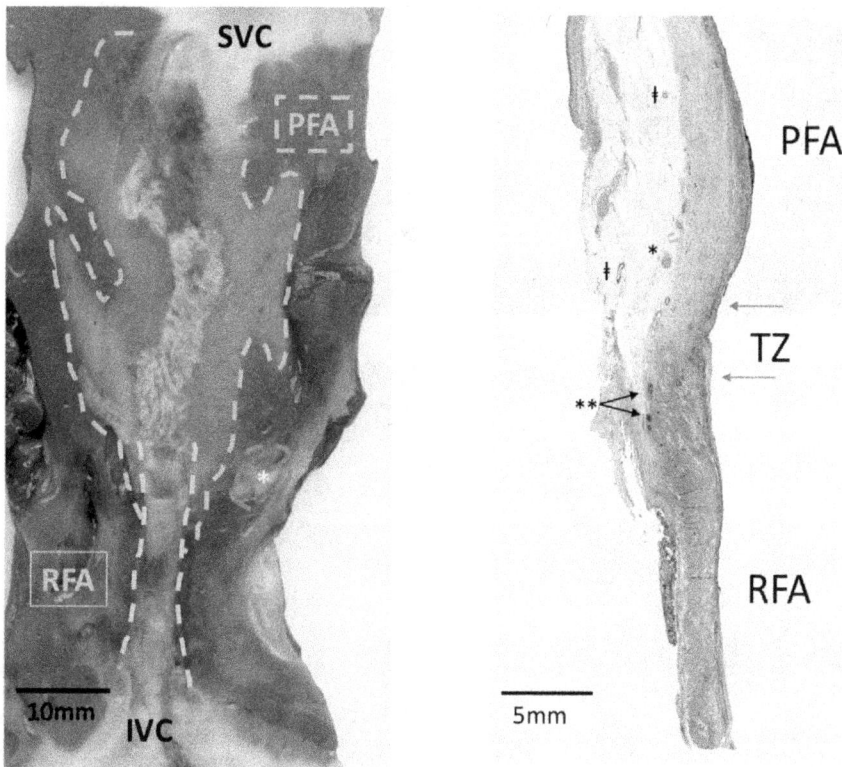

Fig. 2. Histologic examination of the right atrium following ablation procedures. *Left image*: Gross pathology of the intercaval line is displayed. Areas treated with PFA are outlined with green-dotted lines, while regions subjected to RFA are marked with orange-dotted lines. The transition zone (TZ) marker lesions are encircled in red. *Right image*: A histopathological section stained using Masson's trichrome technique. The upper section reveals collagen deposition and fibrosis characteristic of PFA-induced injury. Blood vessels (†) and nerves (*asterisk*) remain largely unaffected. In the central portion of the histology, the TZ exhibits evidence of 2 injury types: predominant PFA injury with hemorrhagic and thermal effects (indicated by *blue arrows*) and damaged nerves (*double asterisk*). The lower section shows contraction bands and cell necrosis, which are consistent with thermal injury caused by RFA. The magnification used is ×20. Abbreviations: IVC, inferior vena cava; SVC, superior vena cava. (*Data from* Younis A, Santangeli P, Garrott K, et al. Impact of contact force on pulsed field ablation outcomes using focal point catheter. Circulation: Arrhythmia Electrophysiol. 2024;17(6):e012723. https://doi.org/10.1161/CIRCEP.123.012723. © 2024, Wolters Kluwer Health, Inc.)

cryoablation) in 41 patients with paroxysmal atrial fibrillation undergoing PV isolation. Cardiac magnetic resonance imaging (LGE, T2-weighted, cine) was performed preablation, acutely (<3 hours), and 3 months postablation. The findings revealed that PFA resulted in a 60% larger acute late gadolinium enhancement (LGE) volume compared with thermal ablation, but with 20% less edema and more homogeneous tissue changes, without signs of microvascular damage or intramural hemorrhage. In the chronic stage, most acute LGE from PFA disappeared, whereas it persisted after thermal ablation. Additionally, measures of left atrial function declined acutely after both ablation types but recovered only with PFA at the chronic stage. The study concluded that PFA induces large acute LGE without long-term tissue damage, suggesting a reparative process with less chronic fibrosis,

potentially preserving tissue compliance and left atrial function.[50]

Electroanatomical Assessment of Pulmonary Vein Isolation Durability with Pulsed Field Ablation

One of the key objectives of PFA is to achieve durable PV isolation. While remapping studies may not fully capture lesion formation, they remain an important tool for evaluating outcomes in humans, as they are one of the few modalities available for this purpose. The majority of remapping studies have demonstrated impressive pulmonary vein isolation (PVI) durability with commercially available PFA systems. For instance, Reddy and colleagues employed a 9-mm lattice tip catheter in 178 patients with paroxysmal or persistent AF,

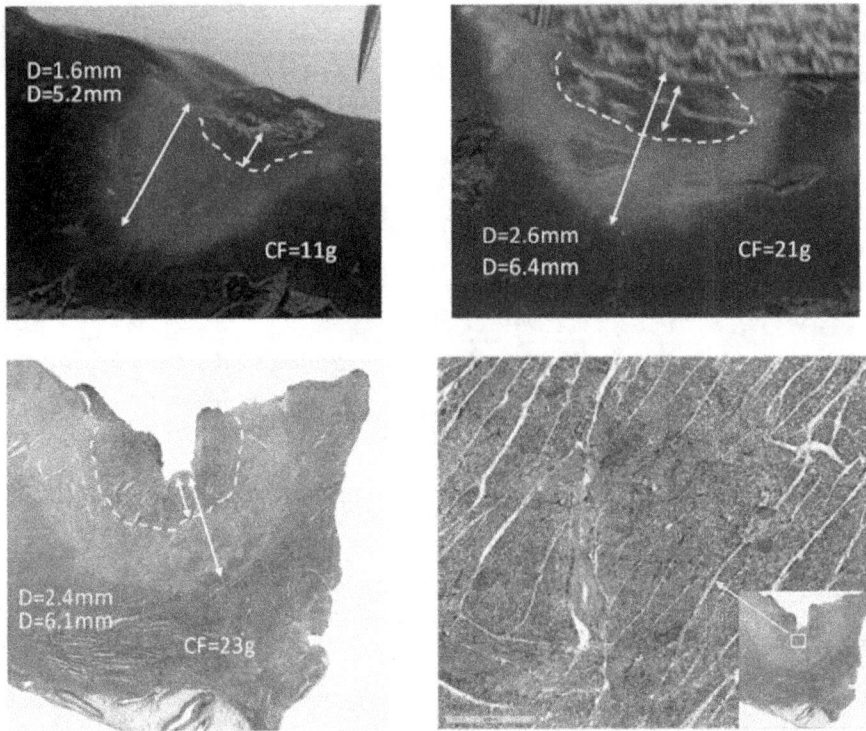

Fig. 3. This figure presents pathology images of PFA lesions generated using different CFs, alongside their corresponding histologic analyses. *Top panels*: Gross pathology images of 2 distinct PFA lesions created with varying CFs. These images reveal 2 types of tissue injuries: shallow and deeper lesions. The deeper injury is highlighted by a white line indicating its maximum depth. A superficial, brown-colored area is outlined with dotted yellow lines, representing the shallower lesion. *Bottom panels*: Histologic sections stained with Masson's trichrome dye. The larger area exhibits collagen deposition and fibrosis typical of PFA-induced injury. In contrast, the smaller area enclosed by dotted yellow lines shows superficial coagulative necrosis, indicative of a minor thermal effect. The images on the left are magnified at ×20, while those on the right are at ×60 magnification. (*Data from* Younis A, Santangeli P, Garrott K, et al. Impact of contact force on pulsed field ablation outcomes using focal point catheter. Circulation: Arrhythmia Electrophysiol. 2024;17(6):e012723. https://doi.org/10.1161/CIRCEP.123.012723. © 2024, Wolters Kluwer Health, Inc.)

testing various waveforms: PULSE1 (3-s to 5.5-s lesions; saline at 4–30 mL/min), PULSE2 (4-s lesions; saline at 15 mL/min), and PULSE3 (4-s lesions; saline at 15 mL/min). Remapping at 3 months postablation showed that, with the optimal waveform, PVI durability reached 97%.[51] In the 1-year outcome study of the (a safety and feasibility study of the IOWA approach endocardial ablation system to treat atrial fibrillation [IMPULSE]), (a safety and feasibility study of the FARAPULSE endocardial ablation system to treat paroxysmal atrial fibrillation [PEFCAT]), and (expanded safety and feasability study of the FARAPULSE endocardial multi ablation system to treat paroxysmal atrial fibrillation [PEFCAT II]) trials, Reddy and colleagues used a basket or flower PFA catheter for AF ablation in 1212 patients, with remapping performed 2 to 3 months postprocedure. Their findings demonstrated a PVI durability of 96% when the optimized biphasic energy

PFA waveform was employed.[52] Similarly, the (pulsed field ablation in patients with persistent atrial fibrillation [PersAFOne]) study utilized a biphasic bipolar PFA multispline catheter for PV and left atrial PW ablation in 25 patients. Remapping performed 2 to 3 months postprocedure demonstrated durable isolation in 96% of PVs and 100% of the left atrial PW treated with the pentaspline catheter.[53] Other studies, such as the (European real-world outcomes with pulsed field ablation in patients with symptomatic atrial fibrillation [EUPORIA]) registry and the (pulsed field or conventional thermal ablation for paroxysmal atrial fibrillation [ADVENT]) trial, reported lower rates of PV isolation on remapping, with 72% and 65%, respectively.[3,54] However, it is important to note that remapping in these studies was not protocol-mandated and was conducted only in patients with AF recurrence requiring a repeat ablation procedure.

ABLATION PARAMETERS INFLUENCING LESION FORMATION

Lesion creation in PFA is influenced by a multitude of ablation parameters, including amplitude, pulse width, number of pulses, polarity, and pulse cycle, all of which constitute the waveform. Additionally, catheter characteristics such as shape and the distance between the cardiac tissue and the catheter also play a crucial role in lesion formation. It is important to note that most pulse parameters are preselected by manufacturers and may vary between different PFA systems. These parameters are carefully chosen to balance the effectiveness of the ablation while minimizing the risk of unwanted and potentially dangerous effects, such as electrical breakdown, bubble formation, thermal damage, arcing, barotrauma, and emboli.[21]

From the variables that are within operator control, contact force and burst pulses seem to significantly impact lesion formation. Nakagawa and colleagues used a 7.5 F catheter with a 3.5-mm ablation electrode and a contact force (CF) sensor was connected to a PFA system and tested in 11 closed-chest swine. Biphasic PFA current was applied at 219 sites in the left and right ventricles using 12, 18, and 24 burst pulses and various CF levels: low (4–15 g), moderate (16–30 g), high (32–65 g), and no electrode contact. The swine were euthanized 2 hours postablation, and lesion sizes were assessed using triphenyl tetrazolium chloride staining. They reported that lesion depth increased significantly with increasing CF and PFA burst pulses, and that impedance decrease, and electrode temperatures were poor predictors of lesion size. There were also no detectable lesions when there was no contact between the catheter and the myocardium.[55] In a related study, Di Biase and colleagues utilized a CF-sensing OMNYPULSE catheter to deliver predefined PFA applications ($\times 3$, $\times 6$, $\times 9$, and $\times 12$) at varying CF levels—low (5–25 g), high (26–50 g), and very high (51–80 g)—to the ventricular myocardium of 11 swine. Lesion depth was assessed at necropsy following the procedure. Their findings indicate that, rather than CF or PFA dose alone, it is the combination of both, quantified through a pulsed field index, that significantly influences lesion depth, following an asymptotically increasing relationship.[56] Similarly, Younis and colleagues conducted an in vivo study involving 8 swine to evaluate atrial and ventricular lesion formation using an investigational dual-energy CF focal catheter with local impedance. The study comprised 2 experiments: In the first experiment, a point-by-point approach was used to create an intercaval line in the atria, with half of the lesions created using RF and PFA. PF ablation produced significantly wider lesions compared with RF, with both modalities achieving complete transmural ablation, as confirmed by histology (**Fig. 2**).

In the second experiment, PFA was used to create discrete ventricular lesions at varying CF levels (low: 5–15 g, medium: 20–30 g, high: 35–45 g). The results demonstrated that lesion depth increased significantly with higher CF levels, with a mean depth of 6.4 mm observed at moderate CF[57] (**Fig. 3**).

SUMMARY

In conclusion, PFA represents a promising non-thermal approach to cardiac ablation, characterized by its unique ability to selectively target myocardial cells while preserving the structural integrity of the extracellular matrix. The review of available studies highlights the distinct histologic and imaging characteristics of PFA-induced lesions, including their well-demarcated borders, uniform fibrotic remodeling, and reduced likelihood of collateral damage compared with traditional thermal ablation methods. While PFA demonstrates high rates of durable PV isolation, particularly with optimized waveforms, variability in lesion formation and durability has been observed across different studies. As PFA technology continues to evolve, further research is necessary to refine lesion creation parameters and to better understand the long-term outcomes associated with this novel ablation modality. Ultimately, PFA has the potential to significantly advance the safety and efficacy of ablation procedures, offering a valuable demarcation from conventional thermal techniques.

CLINICS CARE POINTS

- Pulsed field ablation (PFA) offers a safer alternative to thermal ablation by minimizing collateral damage to surrounding tissues, which is particularly beneficial in areas near critical structures.

- Clinicians should be aware that traditional imaging modalities like late gadolinium enhancement-MRI may not accurately reflect PFA lesion formation due to preserved extracellular matrix.

- Optimization of ablation parameters is essential; factors like contact force and pulse number significantly influence lesion depth and efficacy in PFA.

- Familiarity with the unique characteristics of PFA-induced lesions will aid clinicians in interpreting postprocedural assessments and improving patient outcomes.

DISCLOSURE

The authors have nothing to disclose.

REFERENCES

1. Tabaja C, Younis A, Hussein AA, et al. Catheter-based electroporation. JACC (J Am Coll Cardiol): Clinical Electrophysiology 2023;9(9):2008–23.
2. Reddy VY, Neuzil P, Koruth JS, et al. Pulsed field ablation for pulmonary vein isolation in atrial fibrillation. J Am Coll Cardiol 2019;74(3):315–26.
3. Reddy VY, Gerstenfeld EP, Natale A, et al. Pulsed field or conventional thermal ablation for paroxysmal atrial fibrillation. N Engl J Med 2023;389(18):1660–71.
4. Hussein AA, Saliba WI, Barakat A, et al. Radiofrequency ablation of persistent atrial fibrillation. Circulation: Arrhythmia and Electrophysiology 2016;9(1):e003669.
5. Nakagawa H, Yamanashi WS, Pitha JV, et al. Comparison of in vivo tissue temperature profile and lesion geometry for radiofrequency ablation with a saline-irrigated electrode versus temperature control in a canine thigh muscle preparation. Circulation 1995;91(8):2264–73.
6. Avitall B, Mughal K, Hare J, et al. The effects of electrode-tissue contact on radiofrequency lesion generation. Pacing Clin Electrophysiol 1997;20(12):2899–910.
7. Wittkampf FHM, Nakagawa H. RF catheter ablation: lessons on lesions. Pacing Clin Electrophysiol 2006;29(11):1285–97.
8. Nakagawa H, Jackman WM. The role of contact force in atrial fibrillation ablation. J Atr Fibrillation 2014;7(1):1027.
9. Calkins H, Hindricks G, Cappato R, et al. 2017 HRS/EHRA/ECAS/APHRS/SOLAECE expert consensus statement on catheter and surgical ablation of atrial fibrillation. Heart Rhythm 2017;14(10):e275–444.
10. Andrade JG, Khairy P, Dubuc M. Catheter cryoablation. Circulation: Arrhythmia and Electrophysiology 2013;6(1):218–27.
11. Weaver JC. Electroporation of cells and tissues. IEEE Trans Plasma Sci 2000;28(1):24–33.
12. Krassowska W, Filev PD. Modeling electroporation in a single cell. Biophys J 2007;92(2):404–17.
13. Frandsen SK, Gissel H, Hojman P, et al. Direct therapeutic applications of calcium electroporation to effectively induce tumor necrosis. Cancer Res 2012;72(6):1336–41.
14. Nesin V, Bowman AM, Xiao S, et al. Cell permeabilization and inhibition of voltage-gated Ca(2+) and Na(+) channel currents by nanosecond pulsed electric field. Bioelectromagnetics 2012;33(5):394–404.
15. Chen W. Electroconformational denaturation of membrane proteins. Ann N Y Acad Sci 2005;1066:92–105.
16. Matsuki N, Ishikawa T, Imai Y, et al. Low voltage pulses can induce apoptosis. Cancer Lett 2008;269(1):93–100.
17. Davalos RV, Mir IL, Rubinsky B. Tissue ablation with irreversible electroporation. Ann Biomed Eng 2005;33(2):223–31.
18. Koruth J, Kuroki K, Iwasawa J, et al. Preclinical evaluation of pulsed field ablation: electrophysiological and histological assessment of thoracic vein isolation. Circ Arrhythm Electrophysiol 2019;12(12):e007781.
19. Cochet H, Nakatani Y, Sridi-Cheniti S, et al. Pulsed field ablation selectively spares the oesophagus during pulmonary vein isolation for atrial fibrillation. Europace 2021;23(9):1391–9.
20. Golberg A, Yarmush ML. Nonthermal irreversible electroporation: fundamentals, applications, and challenges. IEEE Trans Biomed Eng 2013;60(3):707–14.
21. Chun K-RJ, Miklavčič D, Vlachos K, et al. State-of-the-art pulsed field ablation for cardiac arrhythmias: ongoing evolution and future perspective. EP Europace 2024;26(6). https://doi.org/10.1093/europace/euae134.
22. Bradley CJ, Haines DE. Pulsed field ablation for pulmonary vein isolation in the treatment of atrial fibrillation. J Cardiovasc Electrophysiol 2020;31(8):2136–47.
23. Marrouche NF, Wilber D, Hindricks G, et al. Association of atrial tissue fibrosis identified by delayed enhancement MRI and atrial fibrillation catheter ablation: the DECAAF study. JAMA 2014;311(5):498–506.
24. Akoum N, Fernandez G, Wilson B, et al. Association of atrial fibrosis quantified using LGE-MRI with atrial appendage thrombus and spontaneous contrast on transesophageal echocardiography in patients with atrial fibrillation. J Cardiovasc Electrophysiol 2013;24(10):1104–9.
25. Fukumoto K, Habibi M, Gucuk Ipek E, et al. Comparison of preexisting and ablation-induced late gadolinium enhancement on left atrial magnetic resonance imaging. Heart Rhythm 2015;12(4):668–72.
26. Hopman LHGA, van Pouderoijen N, Mulder MJ, et al. Atrial ablation lesion evaluation by cardiac magnetic resonance: review of imaging strategies and histological correlations. JACC (J Am Coll Cardiol) 2023;9(12):2665–79.
27. Rolf S, Hindricks G, Sommer P, et al. Electroanatomical mapping of atrial fibrillation: review of the current techniques and advances. J Atr Fibrillation 2014;7(4):1140.
28. Narayan SM, John RM. Advanced electroanatomic mapping: current and emerging approaches. Curr Treat Options Cardiovasc Med 2024;26(4):69–91.
29. Parmar BR, Jarrett TR, Burgon NS, et al. Comparison of left atrial area marked ablated in electroanatomical maps with scar in MRI. J Cardiovasc Electrophysiol 2014;25(5):457–63.
30. Harrison JL, Jensen HK, Peel SA, et al. Cardiac magnetic resonance and electroanatomical mapping of acute and chronic atrial ablation injury: a

histological validation study. Eur Heart J 2014; 35(22):1486–95.

31. Barkagan M, Leshem E, Shapira-Daniels A, et al. Histopathological characterization of radiofrequency ablation in ventricular scar tissue. JACC Clin Electrophysiol 2019;5(8):920–31.

32. Deneke T, Khargi K, Müller KM, et al. Histopathology of intraoperatively induced linear radiofrequency ablation lesions in patients with chronic atrial fibrillation. Eur Heart J 2005;26(17):1797–803.

33. Yamashita K, Kholmovski E, Ghafoori E, et al. Characterization of edema after cryo and radiofrequency ablations based on serial magnetic resonance imaging. J Cardiovasc Electrophysiol 2019;30(2):255–62.

34. Khurram IM, Catanzaro JN, Zimmerman S, et al. MRI evaluation of radiofrequency, cryothermal, and laser left atrial lesion formation in patients with atrial fibrillation. Pacing Clin Electrophysiol 2015;38(11):1317–24.

35. Kurose J, Kiuchi K, Fukuzawa K, et al. Lesion characteristics between cryoballoon ablation and radiofrequency ablation with a contact force-sensing catheter: late-gadolinium enhancement magnetic resonance imaging assessment. J Cardiovasc Electrophysiol 2020;31(10):2572–81.

36. Lavee J, Onik G, Mikus P, et al. A novel nonthermal energy source for surgical epicardial atrial ablation: irreversible electroporation. Heart Surg Forum 2007; 10(2):E162–7.

37. Deodhar A, Dickfeld T, Single GW, et al. Irreversible electroporation near the heart: ventricular arrhythmias can be prevented with ECG synchronization. AJR Am J Roentgenol 2011;196(3):W330–5.

38. Neven K, van Driel V, van Wessel H, et al. Myocardial lesion size after epicardial electroporation catheter ablation after subxiphoid puncture. Circulation 2014; 7(4):728–33.

39. Wittkampf FH, van Driel VJ, van Wessel H, et al. Myocardial lesion depth with circular electroporation ablation. Circ Arrhythm Electrophysiol 2012;5(3):581–6.

40. Stewart MT, Haines DE, Verma A, et al. Intracardiac pulsed field ablation: proof of feasibility in a chronic porcine model. Heart Rhythm 2019;16(5):754–64.

41. Sugrue A, Vaidya V, Witt C, et al. Irreversible electroporation for catheter-based cardiac ablation: a systematic review of the preclinical experience. J Interv Card Electrophysiol 2019;55(3):251–65.

42. Grimaldi M, Di Monaco A, Gomez T, et al. Time course of irreversible electroporation lesion development through short- and long-term follow-up in pulsed-field ablation–treated hearts. Circulation 2022;15(7): e010661.

43. Wittkampf FH, van Driel VJ, van Wessel H, et al. Feasibility of electroporation for the creation of pulmonary vein ostial lesions. J Cardiovasc Electrophysiol 2011;22(3):302–9.

44. Witt CM, Sugrue A, Padmanabhan D, et al. Intrapulmonary vein ablation without stenosis: a novel balloon-based direct current electroporation approach. J Am Heart Assoc 2018;7(14). https://doi.org/10.1161/jaha.118.009575.

45. Hong J, Stewart MT, Cheek DS, et al. Cardiac ablation via electroporation. Annu Int Conf IEEE Eng Med Biol Soc 2009;2009:3381–4.

46. Fink T, Sciacca V, Neven K, et al. Pulsed field ablation for atrial fibrillation – lessons from magnetic resonance imaging. Pacing Clin Electrophysiol 2023; 46(12):1586–94.

47. Oakes RS, Badger TJ, Kholmovski EG, et al. Detection and quantification of left atrial structural remodeling with delayed-enhancement magnetic resonance imaging in patients with atrial fibrillation. Circulation 2009;119(13):1758–67.

48. Akoum N, Wilber D, Hindricks G, et al. MRI assessment of ablation-induced scarring in atrial fibrillation: analysis from the DECAAF study. J Cardiovasc Electrophysiol 2015;26(5):473–80.

49. Sohns C, Fink T, Braun M, et al. Lesion formation following pulsed field ablation for pulmonary vein and posterior wall isolation. Pacing Clin Electrophysiol 2023;46(7):714–6.

50. Nakatani Y, Sridi-Cheniti S, Cheniti G, et al. Pulsed field ablation prevents chronic atrial fibrotic changes and restrictive mechanics after catheter ablation for atrial fibrillation. Europace 2021;23(11):1767–76.

51. Reddy VY, Peichl P, Anter E, et al. A focal ablation catheter toggling between radiofrequency and pulsed field energy to treat atrial fibrillation. JACC (J Am Coll Cardiol) 2023;9(8, Part 3):1786–801.

52. Reddy VY, Dukkipati SR, Neuzil P, et al. Pulsed field ablation of paroxysmal atrial fibrillation: 1-year outcomes of IMPULSE, PEFCAT, and PEFCAT II. JACC (J Am Coll Cardiol) 2021;7(5):614–27.

53. Reddy VY, Anic A, Koruth J, et al. Pulsed field ablation in patients with persistent atrial fibrillation. J Am Coll Cardiol 2020;76(9):1068–80.

54. Schmidt B, Bordignon S, Neven K, et al. EUropean real-world outcomes with Pulsed field ablatiOn in patients with symptomatic atRIAl fibrillation: lessons from the multi-centre EU-PORIA registry. EP Europace 2023; 25(7). https://doi.org/10.1093/europace/euad185.

55. Nakagawa H, Farshchi-Heydari S, Maffre J, et al. Evaluation of ablation parameters to predict irreversible lesion size during pulsed field ablation. Circ Arrhythm Electrophysiol 2024;17(8):e012814.

56. Di Biase L, Marazzato J, Govari A, et al. Pulsed field ablation index–guided ablation for lesion formation: impact of contact force and number of applications in the ventricular model. Circulation 2024;17(4):e012717.

57. Younis A, Santangeli P, Garrott K, et al. Impact of contact force on pulsed field ablation outcomes using focal point catheter. Circulation 2024;17(6):e012723.

Tissue Selectivity of Pulsed Field Ablation

Chadi Tabaja, MD[1], Mohamad Mdaihly, MD[1], Charbel Noujaim, MD,
Oussama M. Wazni, MD, MBA, Pasquale Santangeli, MD, PhD*

KEYWORDS

- Pulsed field ablation • Electroporation • Atrial fibrillation • Arrhythmia

KEY POINTS

- Pusled field ablation utilizes pulsed electric fields that induce tissue-specific lesions without increasing the risk of thermal collateral damage.
- PFA minimizes thermal effects, producing efficient myocardial ablation without the significant temperature rise observed in traditional methods.
- Recent evidence from clinical trials demonstrate that PFA is noninferior to traditional radiofrequency and cryoballoon ablation in terms of safety and atrial fibrillation recurrence.

INTRODUCTION

Catheter ablation using thermal energy such as radiofrequency (RF) and cryothermy is currently the mainstay treatment of cardiac arrhythmias.[1] Despite advances in thermal techniques, safety remains a major concern as thermal ablation can extend beyond the myocardium, which can result in rare, but potentially serious complications including phrenic nerve injury resulting in diaphragmatic paralysis, pulmonary veins (PVs) stenosis, and atrio-esophageal fistula.[2,3] In contrast, pulsed field ablation (PFA) is a novel ablation strategy that uses irreversible electroporation (IRE) that selectively ablates cardiomyocytes while avoiding damage to the surrounding tissue.[4,5] IRE involves the application of short-duration high-voltage pulsed electrical fields (PEF) resulting in cell death through membrane destabilization in a tissue-specific manner. This effect occurs only when the electroporation threshold of the targeted cell is reached, such as those in the esophagus and phrenic nerve, are more resistant to these changes. This tissue specificity underscores the potential role of PFA in minimizing collateral damage.

In the last decade, several preclinical studies demonstrated that PFA causes selective cell death, targeting key arrhythmogenic lesions, while preserving its surrounding environment.[6-8] On the other hand, recent clinical trials data demonstrated favorable safety and efficacy profiles, positioning PFA as a competitive alternative to traditional ablation techniques.[9,10]

Since the regulatory approval of the first pentaspline catheter in 2021, PFA has seen rapid clinical adoption, with over 20,000 procedures performed globally. Notably, the 2023 ADVENT randomized trial provided robust evidence that PFA is noninferior to RF and cryoballoon (CB) ablation in terms of procedural safety, efficiency, and freedom from atrial fibrillation (AF) recurrence.[10,11] This pivotal trial was instrumental in securing Food and Drug Administration approval for PFA in 2024, paving the way for its widespread clinical use in the United States.

Cardiac Electrophysiology and Pacing Section, Department of Cardiovascular Medicine, Cleveland Clinic, Cleveland, OH, USA
[1] Chadi Tabaja and Mohamad Mdaihly are co-first authors.
* Corresponding author. Cleveland Clinic, 9500 Euclid Avenue, Cleveland, OH 44195.
E-mail address: santanp3@ccf.org

Card Electrophysiol Clin 17 (2025) 147–154
https://doi.org/10.1016/j.ccep.2025.02.003

Abbreviations	
AF	atrial fibrillation
CB	cryoballoon
CMR	cardiac magnetic resonance
GP	ganglionated plexi
ICANS	intrinsic cardiac autonomic nervous system
IRE	irreversible electroporation
LEF	lethal electric field
OR	odds ratio
PEF	pulsed electric fields
PFA	pulsed field ablation
PVs	pulmonary veins
RF	radiofrequency
TMV	transmembrane voltage

This review aims to discuss the mechanisms of electroporation while highlighting the tissue selectivity of PFA.

MECHANISM OF ELECTROPORATION

Electroporation is the process of increasing cell membrane permeability through the application of high voltages or currents between electrodes over a short period of time (microseconds or nanoseconds).[4,12,13] As charges are redistributed across the cell membrane, a transmembrane voltage (TMV) is induced. Nanopores are formed within the lipid bilayer when the voltage exceeds 100 mv.[4,13,14] The membranous defects caused by nanopores allow water and impermeable ions to penetrate into the cell leading to programmed cell death and apoptosis[12,13] (**Fig. 1**). Tokman and colleagues proposed that water molecules form energetically favorable column-like structures, with their dipoles reorienting with the field at the water-lipid or water-vacuum interface.[15] Other proposed mechanisms include damage to the embedded membrane proteins, lipid peroxidation, disruption of intracellular calcium mechanisms, and the depletion of ATP. These overlapping pathways intersect to result in cellular death predominantly through apoptosis.[12,16,17]

Electroporation can induce either reversible or irreversible damage. Short, reversible pulses generate sublethal electric fields that temporarily increase cell membrane permeability without causing cell death, a process known as reversible electroporation, which has been utilized for gene transfer and drug delivery for decades.[17]

PFA uses irreversible electroporation to induce tissue destruction by generating an electric field around the catheter electrodes, with lesions forming when the field exceeds a threshold influenced by factors such as tissue type and pulse parameters like voltage, duration, and repetition.[13] As tissues have specific electroporation thresholds, PFA causes preferential ablation to the cardiomyocytes, given their lower tissue threshold compared to surrounding key structures such as the pulmonary veins and the esophagus, sparing the surrounding from critical damage.[18] Pierucci and colleagues explained the principle of selective electroporation, which is based on the cell size and type, as crucial for targeting myocardial cells without causing collateral damage.[19]

TISSUE SPECIFICITY

The lethal electric field (LEF) threshold at which TMV induces cell membrane breakdown and subsequent cell death, ranges between 500 and 1000 V/cm (**Fig. 2**).[20] In a study on porcine and human hearts, the LEF for the proprietary biphasic Medtronic waveform was 535 V/cm in porcine hearts and 416 V/cm in human hearts, which is lower than most other tissues reported in the literature except for skeletal muscle.[20] While the LEF threshold is a tissue property, the overall effect of electroporation depends on various waveform parameters, including pulse amplitude (voltage), polarity (monophasic or biphasic), number of pulses, pulse width, and cycle period, as well as catheter geometry and the distance of cells or tissues from the electrode.[13,14] Studies have shown that increasing the voltage and pulse duration increases the magnitude of the delivered electric field and subsequently the electroporation effect.[21,22]

PFA is often considered nonthermal as most heat is dissipated through conduction and convection cooling.[23] However, some degree of heating at the catheter tip is inevitable. Heat generation follows Joule heating, where tissue temperature rises when currents pass through a resistive load. Younis and colleagues demonstrated histologic evidence of superficial coagulative necrosis with PFA, indicating a minimal but present risk of thermal effects.[24] Verma and colleagues found that PEF ablation of muscle tissue caused only a minimal temperature increase (max 2.8°C), insufficient for stromal protein coagulation, whereas RF ablation led to a significant rise (max 39.8°C).[25]

Although severe complications from thermal ablation are rare, PV stenosis, phrenic nerve injury, and atrio-esophageal fistula remain significant safety concerns.[4,26] Preclinical studies have demonstrated the safety of PFA in avoiding collateral thermal tissue damage to the PVs, esophagus, coronary arteries, and phrenic nerves.[6,27–29] Recent studies have also shown lower rates of phrenic nerve injury[30,31] and esophageal injuries[32,33] when compared to RF or CB ablation.

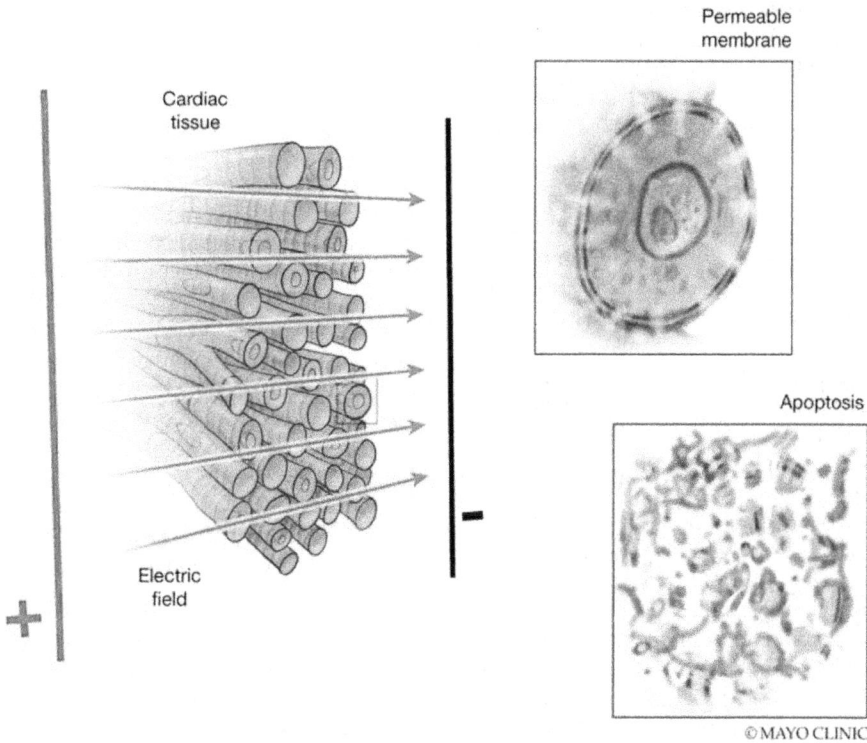

© MAYO CLINIC

Fig. 1. Mechanism of electroporation. Delivery of a high voltage PEF results in pore formation and increased cell membrane permeability. These changes may be reversible with a return to normal cell function or irreversible with progression to cell death. (*Data from* Ezzeddine FM, Asirvatham SJ, Nguyen DT. Pulsed Field Ablation: A Comprehensive Update. *J Clin Med* 2024, 13, 5191. https://doi.org/10.3390/jcm13175191.)

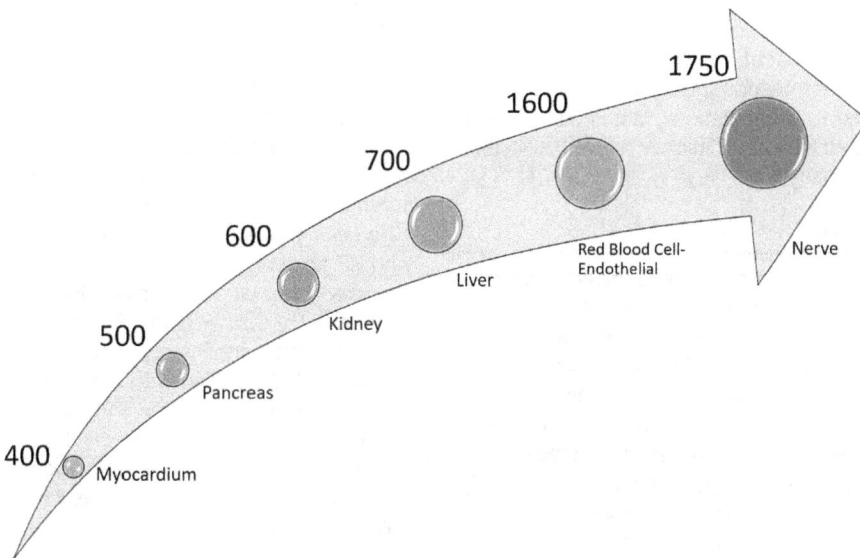

Fig. 2. Electroporation thresholds across different tissue types. The scale illustrates the required energy (voltage/cm) for irreversible electroporation, with lower thresholds seen in myocardium (400 V/cm) and progressively higher thresholds in nerve tissue (1750 V/cm). These differences in tissue susceptibility are critical for optimizing IRE procedures in various organs, ensuring selective and effective treatment. (*Data from* Kos B, et al. Determination of lethal electric field threshold for pulsed field ablation in ex vivo perfused porcine and human hearts. Front Cardiovasc Med 2023;10:1160231.)

The ADVENT trial demonstrated a similar and favorable safety profile.[10] This was further reinforced by the recent MANIFEST-17 K study evaluating the safety and efficacy of PFA in 17,642 patients with AF across 106 centers reporting major complications in only 1% of patients.

Esophagus

Several studies have highlighted the advantages of PFA in avoiding esophageal injuries. None of the animal models using PFA showed lumen stenosis, ulcers, epithelial damages, or fistulas.[19] Evidence from acute canine experiments by Zyl and colleagues, using histologic analysis of the esophagus following the targeting of 5 epicardial ganglionated plexi (GP) with saline-irrigated PEF, showed complete preservation of the esophagus.[34] Similar results were obtained by Song and colleagues, where no micropathological esophageal changes were observed 4 weeks after monophasic or bipolar IRE.[35] Additionally, the EU-PORIA registry reported the absence of atrio-esophageal fistula or symptomatic esophageal injuries among the 1,233 involved patients.[9] Cardiac magnetic resonance (CMR) imaging provided robust anatomic and functional evidence before and after ablation. Cochet and colleagues demonstrated through CMR imaging acute esophageal lower gadolinium enhancement in 43% of patients treated with thermal ablation, while the esophagus was completely spared from such damage using PFA.[36] Moreover, the study by Kirstein and colleagues also provided insight into the impact of PFA on intraluminal esophageal temperature change. Although a dose-dependent esophageal temperature rise was reported to be statistically significant, it was not associated with any clinically relevant esophageal thermal injury.[37]

Phrenic Nerve

Phrenic nerve injury is a well-recognized complication of thermal ablation techniques, often resulting in diaphragmatic paresis and patient discomfort. Conversely, reports on the effects of electroporation on nerves are mixed, with some studies indicating minimal impact while others document transient injury followed by recovery within 7 weeks.[38–40] Neuronal regeneration post-ablation potentially reflect the basis of phrenic nerve preservation during PFA.[38] In vivo experimental studies demonstrated preservation of endoneurium architecture despite histologic nerve damage, which reflects the potential for axonal regeneration.[39,40] Van Driel and colleagues demonstrated preserved phrenic nerve function and intact histologic structure following electroporation at energy levels sufficient to create

myocardial lesions.[7] Howard and colleagues investigated the acute and chronic effects of PFA dosing on phrenic nerve function in a porcine model. Using accelerometers and continuous pacing, they demonstrated a dose-dependent phrenic nerve response, with catheter proximity to the nerve serving as a key predictor.[41] Guo and colleagues evaluated the effects of PFA on the autonomic nervous system and found no changes in serum nerve injury biomarkers pre- or post-ablation. Additionally, no cases of phrenic nerve paresis or palsy were observed.[42] A recent systematic review and meta-analysis conducted by Amin and colleagues, which included 2255 patients, reported a 62% reduced risk of developing phrenic nerve palsy in patients undergoing PFA versus thermal ablation, with a risk ratio of 0.38 (95% CI [0.15, 0.98], $P=.05$).[32] Similarly, the MANIFEST-17 K study reinforced this safety profile with no reports of persistent phrenic nerve injury among the 17,642 included patients.[26]

Pulmonary Veins

PV stenosis is a well-known complication of thermal ablation. Narrowing of the PVs occurs as a result of fibrosis of necrotic myocardium, intimal thickening, thrombus formation, endocardial contraction, and elastic lamina proliferation, all of which are secondary to thermal injury.[43] In contrast, PFA induces less chronic fibrosis than thermal ablation, likely due to its unique healing process, which preserves tissue compliance and may mitigate the risk of pulmonary vein narrowing following AF ablation. This effect is further attributed to its non-thermal mechanism. In a study conducted on porcine PVs, circular electroporation did not result in PV stenosis or narrowing whereas RF ablation did.[6] Howard and colleagues presented the first quantitative comparison using computed tomography angiography of PVs. Measurements taken pre-ablation and at 2, 4, 6, 8 and 12-weeks post-ablation showed severe stenosis with RF ablation compared to PFA.[44] A secondary analysis of the randomized ADVENT trial found no change in PV caliber with PFA. In fact, the aggregate reduction in PV cross-sectional area was smaller with PFA than with thermal ablation, and nearly 50% of PFA-treated PVs showed no diameter decrease, compared to an 80% decrease in RF-treated PVs. This further corroborates previous observational studies that reported the absence of pulmonary vein narrowing with this technique.[45]

Heart Conduction System

The impact of PFA on the conduction system is limited, with only 2 studies conducted to date. The first study by Livia and colleagues investigated the use of IRE as a potential ablative modality of

Purkinje/fascicular fibers in a canine heart ex vivo.[46] They demonstrated that IRE can ablate the Purkinje fibers in a dose-dependent manner while providing a safety advantage by reducing collateral damage, whereas His bundle could not be ablated at any energy delivery up to 2500V.

In another study, Sugrue and colleagues successfully delivered PEF on Purkinje fibers with limited damage to the underlying myocardium, however, electrical isolation of His bundle was also not achieved.[47]

With the current evidence, PFA might seem a more attractive to conduction system ablation because of the limited damage to underlying myocardial tissue. On the other hand, His bundle ablation was not achieved in these 2 studies. More studies are needed to further expand on the feasibility of His bundle IRE ablation. Until then, RFA will still be the preferred modality for His bundle ablation.

Intrinsic Cardiac Autonomic Nervous System

The intrinsic cardiac autonomic nervous system (ICANS) is a highly complex neural network that resides mostly in the atria and plays an important role in the development and maintenance of AF. ICANS are often inadvertently targeted during thermal AF catheter ablation given its anatomic proximity to the PVs antras. In contrast, due to its cardioselectivity, PFA may not affect the ICANS; however, the evidence remains scarce. In fact, a study by Stojadinović and colleagues utilized extracardiac vagal stimulation to compare the effects of PFA and irrigated RF-guided PVI on the sinus and atrioventricular nodes. They showed that RF ablation significantly attenuated the response to vagal stimulation, whereas this effect was much less pronounced after PFA ablation, with responses rapidly returning to baseline.[48] The authors concluded that cardiac vagal function is preserved in patients treated with PFA. Another recent study by Tohoku-and colleagues evaluated the impact of PFA or CB ablation on ICANS in patients undergoing PV isolation for paroxysmal AF (PFA: 54 patients, CB: 43 patients).[49] The serum S100 B protein was evaluated as a marker of ablation-related ICANS injury. The study found that S100 B increased in both groups, PFA and CB, yet the magnitude of change was at least 4-fold higher in CB compared with PFA.[49] In another study assessing the impact of PFA on GP during conventional pulmonary vein isolation (PVI), PFA did not ablate the GP (as documented by no change in resting heart at 3 month post-ablation) in contrary to RF and CB where 90% of GPs where ablated.[50] This further confirms the absence of bystander injury

to the ICANS by PFA. Further studies are still needed to assess whether the absence of bystander ICANS injury with PFA may affect procedural success. However, early clinical experience with PFA suggests it is unlikely to have a negative impact.

EFFICACY

Efficacy in AF ablation is defined as freedom from AF at 1 year without using antiarrhythmic drugs (or the rate of AF recurrence at 1 year). Reddy and colleagues (2018) evaluated the first clinical use of PFA in the treatment of AF.[51] The study demonstrated a rapid, safe, and tissue-selective AF ablation with short procedure time. Further studies supported the efficacy and safety profile of PFA in treating AF. The IMPULSE (a safety and feasibility study of the IOWA Approach endocardial ablation system to treat AF) and PEFCAT (a safety and feasibility study of the FARAPULSE endocardial ablation system to treat paroxysmal AF) trials results were published in 2019, highlighting the durability and safety of PFA.[52] With waveform refinement, the PVI durability at 3-months was 100 % and freedom from AF recurrence was 87% at 12 months.[52] The 1-year outcomes from the IMPULSE, PEFCAT, and PEFCAT II trials evaluating the FARAPULSE PFA system for paroxysmal AF demonstrated arrhythmia-free survival rates of 78.5 ± 3.8% in the overall cohort and 84.5 ± 5.4% in the optimized biphasic PFA waveform group, aligning with prior studies and reinforcing the durability of PFA for PVI.[53] Further studies highlighted the ability to form durable lesions while selectively isolating cardiac tissues for safe and effective ablation results.[54,55]

The PULSED AF study (pulsed field ablation to irreversibly electroporate tissue and treat AF), a prospective, global multicenter, nonrandomized, paired single-arm trial conducted in patients with paroxysmal and persistent AF, demonstrated that the freedom from arrhythmia recurrence was 66.2% for patients with paroxysmal AF and 55.1% for those with persistent AF at 1 year. The study also evaluated the efficacy of PVI and achieved 100% successful isolation with no majoradverse events.[11] This was further supported by Futing and colleagues[56], who reported the first real-world experience of PFA in 30 patients with paroxysmal AF. PVI was achieved in all patients, with a median procedure time of 116 minutes.[56]

Multiple meta-analyses have shown that PFA is associated with shorter procedure times yet longer fluoroscopy durations.[33,57] A recent meta-analysis by Azzi and colleagues, including 18 studies with 4,998 patients, found that PFA had a significantly shorter procedural duration than thermal ablation (mean difference: −21.68 minutes), while fluoroscopy time was slightly longer (mean difference: +4.53 minutes).[33] The meta anlaysis found that PFA had a higher first-pass isolation rate (OR: 6.82, 95% CI 1.37–34.01) and a lower treatment failure rate (OR: 0.83, 95% CI 0.70–0.98). However, when assessing PVI success, results were statistically insignificant (OR: 1.62, 95% CI 0.21–12.36),[33] findings that align with the meta-analysis by Atlaas and colleagues and the ADVENT trial. The ADVENT trial,[10] a landmark randomized controlled trial, established the noninferiority of PFA to conventional thermal ablation in both efficacy and safety. At 1-year follow-up, 73.3% of PFA-treated patients and 71.3% of those undergoing thermal ablation achieved the primary efficacy endpoint, defined as freedom from initial procedural failure, atrial tachyarrhythmias beyond the 3-month blanking period, antiarrhythmic drug use, cardioversion, or repeat ablation.Notably, PFA was associated with a shorter procedure time (105.8 ± 29.4 minutes) compared to thermal ablation (123.1 ± 42.1 minutes), though fluoroscopy duration was slightly longer, a finding consistent with prior studies. These results further reinforce PFA's role as a durable and efficient strategy for pulmonary vein isolation in patients with atrial fibrillation.

SUMMARY

PFA has emerged as promising novel modality in the field of cardiac electrophysiology, representing a paradigm shift in arrhythmia management. Unlike conventional thermal methods, PFA relies on the mechanisms of reversible and irreversible electroporation, enabling precise myocardial cell targeting while preserving the integrity of collateral organs. Early studies underscore its efficacy, demonstrating durable pulmonary vein isolation and favorable safety profiles. However, variability in lesion durability and formation across studies signals the need for continued research to optimize ablation parameters and further elucidate long-term outcomes. As PFA technology advances, it holds the potential to significantly refine the current approach to cardiac ablation, offering a safer and more effective alternative to traditional thermal techniques.

CLINICS CARE POINTS

- Pulsed Field Ablation (PFA) uses electroporation to selectively ablate cardiomyocytes, reducing collateral damage to nearby structures such as the phrenic nerve and esophagus.

- Clinical trials demonstrate that PFA offers a safe and effective alternative to thermal ablation with shorter procedure time and comparable outcomes.

- Although early studies show promising long-term safety, ongoing research aims to refine parameters to enhance PFA lesion durability further.

DISCLOSURE

The authors have nothing to disclose. This study was not funded.

REFERENCES

1. Arbelo E, Dagres N. The 2020 ESC atrial fibrillation guidelines for atrial fibrillation catheter ablation, CABANA, and EAST. Europace 2022;24(Suppl 2): ii3–7.
2. du Fay de Lavallaz J, Badertscher P, Ghannam M, et al. Severe periprocedural complications after ablation for atrial fibrillation: an international collaborative individual patient data registry. JACC Clin Electrophysiol 2024;10(7 Pt 1):1353–64.
3. Benali K, Khairy P, Hammache N, et al. Procedure-related complications of catheter ablation for atrial fibrillation. J Am Coll Cardiol 2023;81(21):2089–99.
4. Matos CD, Hoyos C, Miranda-Arboleda AF, et al. Pulsed field ablation of atrial fibrillation: a comprehensive review. Rev Cardiovasc Med 2023;24(11):337.
5. Kueffer T, Stettler R, Maurhofer J, et al. Pulsed-field vs cryoballoon vs radiofrequency ablation: outcomes after pulmonary vein isolation in patients with persistent atrial fibrillation. Heart Rhythm 2024;21(8):1227–35.
6. van Driel VJ, Neven KGEJ, van Wessel H, et al. Pulmonary vein stenosis after catheter ablation: electroporation versus radiofrequency. Circ Arrhythm Electrophysiol 2014;7(4):734–8.
7. van Driel VJ, Neven K, van Wessel H, et al. Low vulnerability of the right phrenic nerve to electroporation ablation. Heart Rhythm 2015;12(8):1838–44.
8. Wittkampf FH, van Driel VJ, van Wessel H, et al. Myocardial lesion depth with circular electroporation ablation. Circ Arrhythm Electrophysiol 2012;5(3): 581–6.
9. Schmidt B, Bordignon S, Neven K, et al. EUropean real-world outcomes with Pulsed field ablatiOn in patients with symptomatic atRIAl fibrillation: lessons from the multi-centre EU-PORIA registry. Europace 2023;25(7):euad185.
10. Reddy VY, Lehmann JW, Gerstenfeld EP, et al. A randomized controlled trial of pulsed field ablation versus standard-of-care ablation for paroxysmal atrial fibrillation: the ADVENT trial rationale and design. Heart Rhythm 2023;4(5):317–28.

11. Verma A, Boersma L, Haines DE, et al. First-in-Human experience and acute procedural outcomes using a novel pulsed field ablation system: the PULSED AF pilot trial. Circ Arrhythm Electrophysiol 2022;15(1): e010168.

12. Maor E, Sugrue A, Witt C, et al. Pulsed electric fields for cardiac ablation and beyond: a state-of-the-art review. Heart Rhythm O2 2019;16(7):1112–20.

13. Ezzeddine FM, Asirvatham SJ, Nguyen DT. Pulsed field ablation: a comprehensive update. J Clin Med 2024;13(17):5191.

14. Chun KJ, Miklavčič D, Vlachos K, et al. State-of-the-art pulsed field ablation for cardiac arrhythmias: ongoing evolution and future perspective. Europace 2024;26(6).

15. Tokman M, Lee JH, Levine ZA, et al. Electric field-driven water dipoles: nanoscale architecture of electroporation. PLoS One 2013;8(4):e61111.

16. Tabaja C, Younis A, Hussein AA, et al. Catheter-based electroporation: a novel technique for catheter ablation of cardiac arrhythmias. JACC Clin Electrophysiol 2023;9(9):2008–23.

17. Batista Napotnik T, Polajžer T, Miklavčič D. Cell death due to electroporation - a review. Bioelectrochemistry 2021;141:107871.

18. Maor E, Ivorra A, Rubinsky B. Non thermal irreversible electroporation: novel technology for vascular smooth muscle cells ablation. PLoS One 2009;4(3): e4757.

19. Pierucci N, Mariani MV, Laviola D, et al. Pulsed field energy in atrial fibrillation ablation: from physical principles to clinical applications. J Clin Med 2024;13(10): 2980.

20. Kos B, Mattison L, Ramirez D, et al. Determination of lethal electric field threshold for pulsed field ablation in ex vivo perfused porcine and human hearts. Front Cardiovasc Med 2023;10:1160231.

21. Hunter DW, Kostecki G, Fish JM, et al. In vitro cell selectivity of reversible and irreversible: electroporation in cardiac tissue. Circ Arrhythm Electrophysiol 2021;14(4):e008817.

22. Baena-Montes JM, O'Halloran T, Clarke C, et al. Electroporation parameters for human cardiomyocyte ablation in vitro. J Cardiovasc Dev Dis 2022; 9(8):240.

23. Davalos RV, Mir IL, Rubinsky B. Tissue ablation with irreversible electroporation. Ann Biomed Eng 2005; 33(2):223–31.

24. Younis A, Santangeli P, Garrott K, et al. Impact of contact force on pulsed field ablation outcomes using focal point catheter. Circ Arrhythm Electrophysiol 2024;17(6):e012723.

25. Verma A, Zhong P, Castellvi Q, et al. Thermal profiles for focal pulsed electric field ablation. JACC Clin Electrophysiol 2023;9(9):1854–63.

26. Ekanem E, Neuzil P, Reichlin T, et al. Safety of pulsed field ablation in more than 17,000 patients with atrial fibrillation in the MANIFEST-17K study. Nat Med 2024;30(7):2020–9.

27. Witt CM, Sugrue A, Padmanabhan D, et al. Intrapulmonary vein ablation without stenosis: a novel balloon-based direct current electroporation approach. J Am Heart Assoc 2018;7(14):e009575.

28. Neven K, van Es R, van Driel V, et al. Acute and long-term effects of full-power electroporation ablation directly on the porcine esophagus. Circ Arrhythm Electrophysiol 2017;10(5):e004672.

29. du Pré BC, van Driel VJ, van Wessel H, et al. Minimal coronary artery damage by myocardial electroporation ablation. Europace 2013;15(1):144–9.

30. Rudolph I, Mastella G, Bernlochner I, et al. Efficacy and safety of pulsed field ablation compared to cryoballoon ablation in the treatment of atrial fibrillation: a meta-analysis. Eur Heart J Open 2024;4(3): oeae044.

31. van de Kar MRD, Slingerland SR, van Steenbergen GJ, et al. Pulsed field versus cryoballoon ablation for atrial fibrillation: a real-world observational study on procedural outcomes and efficacy. Neth Heart J 2024; 32(4):167–72.

32. Amin AM, Nazir A, Abuelazm MT, et al. Efficacy and safety of pulsed-field versus conventional thermal ablation for atrial fibrillation: a systematic review and meta-analysis. J Arrhythm 2024;40(5):1059–74.

33. de Campos M, Moraes VRY, Daher RF, et al. Pulsed-field ablation versus thermal ablation for atrial fibrillation: a meta-analysis. Heart Rhythm O2 2024; 5(6):385–95.

34. van Zyl M, Khabsa M, Tri JA, et al. Open-chest pulsed electric field ablation of cardiac ganglionated plexi in acute canine models. J Innov Card Rhythm Manag 2022;13(7):5061–9.

35. Song Y, Yang L, He J, et al. Ultra-microhistological study of nonthermal irreversible electroporation on the esophagus. Heart Rhythm 2023;20(3):343–51.

36. Cochet H, Nakatani Y, Sridi-Cheniti S, et al. Pulsed field ablation selectively spares the oesophagus during pulmonary vein isolation for atrial fibrillation. Europace 2021;23(9):1391–9.

37. Kirstein B, Heeger CH, Vogler J, et al. Impact of pulsed field ablation on intraluminal esophageal temperature. J Cardiovasc Electrophysiol 2024;35(1): 78–85.

38. Chang D, Arbogast A, Chinyere IR. Pulsed field ablation and neurocardiology: inert to efferents or delayed destruction? Rev Cardiovasc Med 2024; 25(3):106.

39. Schoellnast H, Monette S, Ezell PC, et al. Acute and subacute effects of irreversible electroporation on nerves: experimental study in a pig model. Radiology 2011;260(2):421–7.

40. Schoellnast H, Monette S, Ezell PC, et al. The delayed effects of irreversible electroporation ablation on nerves. Eur Radiol 2013;23(2):375–80.

41. Howard B, Haines DE, Verma A, et al. Characterization of phrenic nerve response to pulsed field ablation. Circ Arrhythm Electrophysiol 2022;15(6):e010127.

42. Guo F, Wang J, Deng Q, et al. Effects of pulsed field ablation on autonomic nervous system in paroxysmal atrial fibrillation: a pilot study. Heart Rhythm 2023;20(3):329–38.

43. Pürerfellner H, Martinek M. Pulmonary vein stenosis following catheter ablation of atrial fibrillation. Curr Opin Cardiol 2005;20(6):484–90.

44. Howard B, Haines DE, Verma A, et al. Reduction in pulmonary vein stenosis and collateral damage with pulsed field ablation compared with radiofrequency ablation in a canine model. Circ Arrhythm Electrophysiol 2020;13(9):e008337.

45. Mansour M, Gerstenfeld EP, Patel C, et al. Pulmonary vein narrowing after pulsed field versus thermal ablation. Europace 2024;26(2).

46. Livia C, Sugrue A, Witt T, et al. Elimination of Purkinje fibers by electroporation reduces ventricular fibrillation vulnerability. J Am Heart Assoc 2018;7(15):e009070.

47. Sugrue A, Vaidya VR, Livia C, et al. Feasibility of selective cardiac ventricular electroporation. PLoS One 2020;15(2):e0229214.

48. Stojadinović P, Wichterle D, Peichl P, et al. Autonomic changes are more durable after radiofrequency than pulsed electric field pulmonary vein ablation. JACC Clin Electrophysiol 2022;8(7):895–904.

49. Tohoku S, Schmidt B, Schaack D, et al. Impact of pulsed-field ablation on intrinsic cardiac autonomic nervous system after pulmonary vein isolation. JACC Clin Electrophysiol 2023;9(9):1864–75.

50. Musikantow DR, Reddy VY, Skalsky I, et al. Targeted ablation of epicardial ganglionated plexi during cardiac surgery with pulsed field electroporation (NEURAL AF). J Interv Card Electrophysiol 2023. https://doi.org/10.1007/s10840-023-01615-8.

51. Reddy VY, Koruth J, Jais P, et al. Ablation of atrial fibrillation with pulsed electric fields: an ultra-rapid, tissue-selective modality for cardiac ablation. JACC Clin Electrophysiol 2018;4(8):987–95.

52. Reddy VY, Neuzil P, Koruth JS, et al. Pulsed field ablation for pulmonary vein isolation in atrial fibrillation. J Am Coll Cardiol 2019;74(3):315–26.

53. Reddy VY, Dukkipati SR, Neuzil P, et al. Pulsed field ablation of paroxysmal atrial fibrillation: 1-year outcomes of IMPULSE, PEFCAT, and PEFCAT II. JACC Clin Electrophysiol 2021;7(5):614–27.

54. Schiavone M, Solimene F, Moltrasio M, et al. Pulsed field ablation technology for pulmonary vein and left atrial posterior wall isolation in patients with persistent atrial fibrillation. J Cardiovasc Electrophysiol 2024;35(6):1101–11.

55. Reddy VY, Anic A, Koruth J, et al. Pulsed field ablation in patients with persistent atrial fibrillation. J Am Coll Cardiol 2020;76(9):1068–80.

56. Füting A, Reinsch N, Höwel D, et al. First experience with pulsed field ablation as routine treatment for paroxysmal atrial fibrillation. Europace 2022;24(7):1084–92.

57. Aldaas OM, Malladi C, Han FT, et al. Pulsed field ablation versus thermal energy ablation for atrial fibrillation: a systematic review and meta-analysis of procedural efficiency, safety, and efficacy. J Interv Card Electrophysiol 2024;67(3):639–48.

Extrapulmonary Vein Areas with Pulsed Field Ablation
Is the Transition Completed?

Vincenzo Mirco La Fazia, MD[a], Carola Gianni, MD[a], Giuseppe Stifano, MD[b], Sanghamitra Mohanty, MD[a], Gaetano Chiricolo, MD[b], J. David Burkhardt, MD[a], Amin Al-Ahmad, MD[a], Andrea Natale, MD[b,c],*

KEYWORDS

• Atrial fibrillation • Catheter ablation • Pulsed field ablation • Extrapulmonary vein trigger

KEY POINTS

- *Importance of nonpulmonary vein (non-PV) triggers*: Non-PV triggers contribute to the recurrence of atrial fibrillation following catheter ablation.
- *Safety of pulsed field ablation (PFA):* it has been shown to provide better safety outcomes than thermal energy sources when targeting non-PV triggers.
- *Efficacy of PFA in non-PV trigger ablation*: While PVisolation is well established, more data are needed to understand how to ablate effectively extra-PV areas.

INTRODUCTION

Atrial fibrillation (AF) is the most common arrhythmia worldwide, which is estimated to affect approximately 33 million individuals worldwide.[1] AF significantly impacts both mortality and morbidity, leading to a recognized increase in the risk of thromboembolic events and heart failure.[2,3] Catheter ablation (CA) prevents AF recurrences, decreases AF burden, and improves quality of life in symptomatic paroxysmal or persistent AF.[4–10]

The 2024 European Society of Cardiology (ESC) guidelines on AF recommend CA for patients with paroxysmal or persistent AF who are resistant to or intolerant of antiarrhythmic drug therapy. Notably, CA is now recommended as a first-line option within a shared decision-making framework for rhythm control in patients with paroxysmal AF, further emphasizing its role in improving patient outcomes. A specific focus is placed on the role of CA in patients with AF and left ventricular systolic dysfunction to enhance left ventricular function.[11] These recommendations are shared also in the 2024 European Heart Rhythm Association (EHRA) consensus on CA.[12]

Two decades ago, a landmark study established that the pulmonary veins (PVs) are the most frequent trigger source of AF, leading to the emergence of pulmonary vein isolation (PVI) as the cornerstone of CA for AF.[13]

The aim of this review is to examine the evidence and ablation strategies for non-PV triggers originating from the following sites: the posterior wall (PW) of the left atrium (LA), the left atrial appendage (LAA), the coronary sinus (CS), the superior vena cava (SVC), and the left superior vena cava (LSVC) and others.

[a] Department of Clinical Cardiac Electrophysiology, Texas Cardiac Arrhythmia Institute, St David's Medical Center, 3000 North Interstate Highway 35 Suite 700, Austin, TX 78705, USA; [b] Division of Cardiology, Department of Biomedicine and Prevention, Policlinico Tor Vergata, Roma 00133, Italy; [c] Texas Cardiac Arrhythmia Institute, St David's Medical Center, 3000 North Interstate Highway 35 Suite 700, Austin, TX 78705, USA
* Corresponding author. Texas Cardiac Arrhythmia Institute, St David's Medical Center, 3000 North Interstate Highway 35 Suite 700, Austin, TX 78705.
E-mail address: dr.natale@gmail.com

Card Electrophysiol Clin 17 (2025) 155–166
https://doi.org/10.1016/j.ccep.2025.02.004
1877-9182/25/© 2025 Elsevier Inc. All rights reserved, including those for text and data mining, AI training, and similar technologies.

BEYOND PULMONARY VEINS

Non-PV triggers are ectopic beats that initiate AF, originating from areas other than the PVs. They typically cluster in specific regions, including the left atrial PW, other thoracic veins, such as the SVC, CS, and vein of Marshall (VOM), the crista terminalis (CT), interatrial septum (IAS), and the LAA. These structures contain myocardial cells capable of automatic depolarization and serve as substrates for micro-re-entry due to their rapid conduction, functioning as independent triggers for AF.[14–16]

The prevalence of non-PV triggers varies across studies, largely influenced by the protocols for their induction and the criteria used to define "significant" triggers. Studies using low-dose or stepwise increasing doses of isoproterenol tend to report a lower incidence of non-PV triggers, and some only consider triggers significant if they reliably initiate AF.[17,18] However, when performing ablation under deep sedation or general anesthesia, high-dose isoproterenol is necessary to induce non-PV triggers, making even isolated premature atrial contractions and nonsustained atrial tachycardias clinically relevant.

A prospective study involving approximately 2100 patients demonstrated that AF initiation from non-PV trigger sources occurred in about 11% of patients with persistent and long-standing persistent AF referred for CA.[17] The idea that AF recurrences can arise from non-PV trigger sites in patients with isolated PVs during repeat procedures was further supported by another study of around 500 patients with AF with a follow-up of a decade.[19,20] More recently, our group showed that in a population with persistent AF, non-PV triggers

could be identified in 70% of cases, and their elimination significantly improved clinical outcomes.[10]

Non-PV triggers can be observed in a high percentage of patients with AF, being more prevalent among those with nonparoxysmal AF, female gender, obesity, sleep apnea, older age, low left ventricular ejection fraction, severe left atrial scarring, hypertrophic cardiomyopathy, and previous heart surgery. In these cohorts, targeting non-PV triggers during the initial procedure is essential.[21–29]

Considering the results from these studies, the consensus states that if a reproducible focal trigger initiating AF is identified outside the PV ostia during an ablation procedure, the ablation of this focal trigger is beneficial.

OUR EXPERIENCE IN ABLATING NONPULMONARY VEIN TRIGGER

Ablation of non-PV triggers can be empirical or performed after induction using high-dose isoproterenol (an infusion of 20–30 mg/min for 10–15 minutes, with adequate pressure support).

In our laboratory, mapping of non-PV triggers is guided by multiple catheters positioned along both the right and left atria: a 10 pole circular mapping catheter in the left superior PV recording far-field LAA activity (to avoid mechanical ectopies), an ablation catheter in the right superior PV recording far-field IAS activity, and a 20 pole linear catheter with electrodes spanning from the SVC to the right atrium/CT and the CS. With this catheter setup, when focal ectopic atrial activity is observed, the activation sequence is compared to that of sinus rhythm, allowing for quick identification of the area of origin.[16]

In our laboratory, every patient, including those with paroxysmal AF, undergoes empirical PVI, left atrial PW isolation, and SVC isolation. In patients with a history indicative of a higher prevalence of non-PV triggers, we also perform empirical CS isolation and extend left atrial ablation along the septum (anterior to the right PV antra) and the inferior wall of the LA down to the CS, addressing IAS and additional left atrial PW triggers. Empirical LAA isolation during the first procedure is usually reserved for patients with long-standing persistent AF, who commonly display severe scarring in the PV and left atrial PW.

BEYOND THERMAL ABLATION: PULSED FIELD ABLATION

Pulsed field ablation (PFA) is a novel, largely nonthermal ablation modality based on the process of irreversible electroporation. This mechanism is often described as nonthermal and cardiac tissue selective. In the 1980s, direct current shock was used for the ablation of cardiac arrhythmias, but due to significant complications such as arcing and barotrauma associated with these early technologies, PFA was no longer clinically pursued.[30] However, in the last decade, preclinical studies have demonstrated that modern PFA has the potential to create tissue-selective ablation lesions using short, high-energy electrical pulses that induce cell death while avoiding the side effects related to thermal energy sources.[31–34]

Parameters such as pulse amplitude, pulse width, number of pulses, polarity (biphasic or monophasic), and pulse cycle, as well as catheter shape, geometry, and the distance of the tissue or cells from the catheter or electrodes, significantly influence the creation of effective lesions. This is particularly important because the electric field diminishes rapidly with distance from the electrode or catheter.[35–38]

Various catheter platforms have been developed and can be categorized into 2 types: single-shot devices, designed specifically for PVI, and point-by-point devices.

First in-human trials of PFA demonstrated safe and efficient AF ablation procedures, achieving high rates of both immediate PVI and durability on invasive remapping, resulting in low rates of arrhythmia recurrence.[39,40]

A recent study comparing PFA with radiofrequency and cryoablation in 1572 patients demonstrated significantly shorter procedural along with a higher first-pass PVI rate with PFA, and a significantly lower number of PV reconnections at the time of repeat ablation. However, long-term survival from arrhythmia and complications were similar among the 3 groups.[41]

Extensive ablation of non-PV area with RF led to augmented risk of left stiff atrial syndrome with increase in pulmonary pressure. A recent study demonstrated that, during follow-up, mean pulmonary artery pressure increased in all patients who underwent RF ablation, whereas in the majority of patients with PFA (89.3%), it remained stable.[42]

POSTERIOR WALL

The LA PW, from an embryologic, anatomic, and electrophysiological perspective, is considered an extension of the PVs.[43]

In patients with AF, the PW undergoes progressive remodeling over time. This concept is supported by microscopic evidence, which shows greater lymphonuclear and fatty infiltration, along with increased fibrosis in patients with persistent AF.[44–46]

Despite the growing evidence that effective PW isolation (PWI) leads to better outcomes in patients with persistent AF, this strategy has not been widely adopted, and there is no standard consensus on how to achieve PWI.[47–52] The recent CAPLA trial failed to demonstrate procedural success, defined as freedom from any arrhythmia lasting more than 30 seconds without antiarrhythmic medication after a single procedure. However, this study has important limitations: a small sample size and a patient population primarily composed of those with early persistent AF and the strategy for PWI employed in the study involved a posterior box with power settings between 25 and 40 W, which may not have been sufficient, as indicated by the high rate of reconnection in the PW (75%) at 3 years follow-up.

In our opinion, the best strategy to achieve durable PWI is through debulking with the radiofrequency catheter moving on the PW until complete abolition on potential (power 48–50 W for 10–15 seconds). However, this requires expertise in catheter manipulation and avoiding overheating of the esophagus (**Fig. 1**). This approach seems more feasible with PFA.

Anatomic thickness, epicardial fat, and Bachmann's bundle, make achieving durable LAPW isolation particularly challenging during thermal ablation procedures. In our experience, the pentaspline PFA catheter is used to ablate directly the PW in flower configuration under fluoro and intracardiac echocardiography (ICE) guidance. The shape and flexibility of the splines allowed broad coverage of the PW with limited facile repositioning (**Fig. 2**).

A recent analysis demonstrated that PFA is superior to RF in achieving transmural PWI, as assessed through mapping of both the endocardial and epicardial surfaces.[53] PFA offers several advantages over RF ablation. First, PFA demonstrates a favorable safety profile regarding the esophagus, with no esophageal lesions detected in a study where PFA was performed adjacent to the esophagus. Second, the use of a pentaspline PFA catheter in a flower configuration allows for rapid ablation of the entire surface of the posterior LA, taking less than 10 minutes in the study, thereby making the procedure less time-consuming. Third, PFA may achieve enhanced transmural penetration in areas rich in adipose and fibrous tissue, such as the left atrial PW and the overlying septopulmonary bundle.[54]

The premarket trial (PersAFOne) demonstrated the feasibility and durability of PFA lesions on the PW.[55] This single-arm study enrolled 25 patients and utilized a pentaspline single-shot catheter for PVI and PWI, with remapping conducted after 2 to 3 months. No reconnections were observed

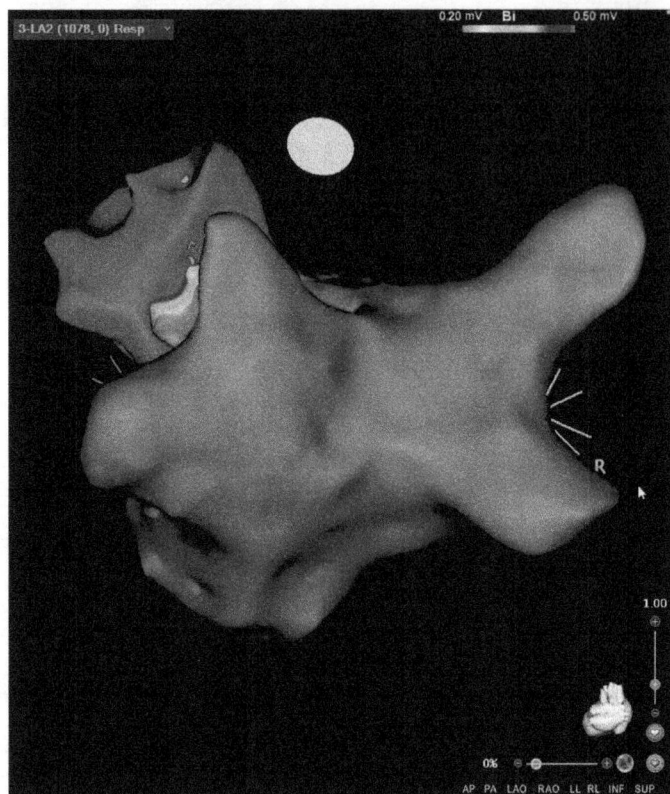

Fig. 1. Voltage map post pulsed field ablation in a patient with persistent AF showing complete isolation of the PVs and the entire PW including the bottom part below the PVs (*central part*: between the 4PVs; *inferior part*: below the *line* joining the inferior borders of the inferior pulmonary vein-encircling lesions to the coronary sinus).

during the remapping of the PW. Additionally, postprocedural endoscopy revealed no damage to the esophageal mucosa.

A recent prospective trial involving 215 patients confirmed these promising results.[56] After a median follow-up period of 7.3 months post-PWI, among the 26 patients who underwent remapping for recurrence, 85% maintained persistent PWI, with only 4 patients experiencing significant lesion regression of more than 10 mm.

In the observational registry (MANIFEST-PF) examining the first postapproval clinical use of PFA for treating persistent AF, the addition of PW ablation did not improve freedom from atrial arrhythmia at 12 months.[57] The primary effectiveness outcome showed a freedom from atrial arrhythmia recurrence rate of 73.1% for PVI alone and 66.4% for PVI plus LAPW ablation at the 12 month follow-up.

The PIFPAF-PFA study (NCT05986526) aims to clarify the existing gap about the effectiveness of PWI in achieving high arrhythmia-free survival. This prospective, open-label trial will include 206 participants and will compare PVI only with PVI plus PWI using PFA. Randomization will occur after assessing myocardial scarring via 3 dimensional electroanatomic mapping. The primary endpoint is the recurrence of atrial arrhythmias within 12 months, monitored by an implantable cardiac device, with an estimated completion date of July 2028.

Superior Vena Cava

SVC is a significant site for the initiation of non-PV triggers.[58,59] Embryologically, it originates from the right sinus horn, which is the origin also of the sinoatrial node, making it capable of spontaneous firing.[60] SVC isolation has been shown to improve outcomes when added to PVI in patients with either documented SVC triggers or as an empirical strategy in both paroxysmal and nonparoxysmal AF.[61,62]

When ablating the SVC with RF, it is crucial to avoid injury to the phrenic nerve and the sinus node. Phrenic nerve mapping is performed at high output pacing (20 mA) after reversing paralytic agents during general anesthesia. In up to 10% of patients, complete isolation of the SVC may not be achievable due to the risk of phrenic nerve injury. PFA seems to overcome this issue.

A recent study published by Ollitrault evaluated the safety and feasibility of SVC isolation with PFA.[63] In their cohort of 105 patients, SVC isolation was achieved in all cases utilizing both the flower and basket configurations of the Farawave catheter, under fluoro guidance. They reported

A

B

C

D

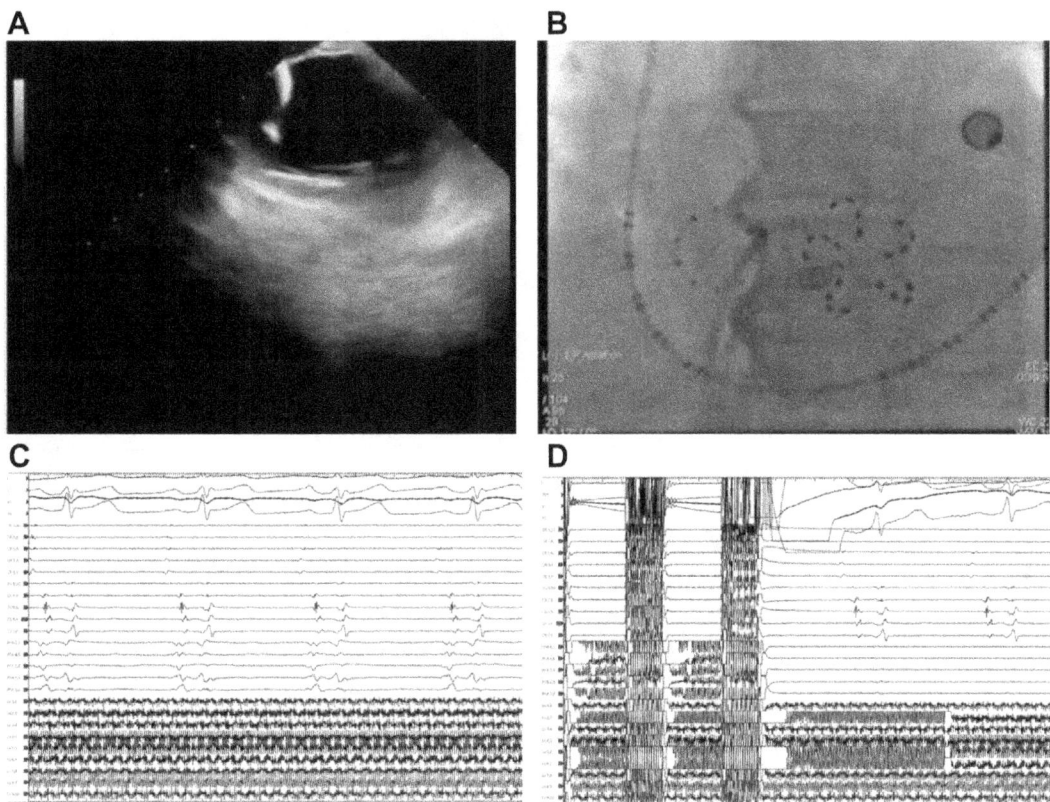

Fig. 2. The pentaspline catheter in flower configuration with good contact on PW visualized by ICE (*A*) and fluoroscopy (*B*). Electrogram (EGM) recorded with the ablation catheter before (*C*) and after (*D*) isolation of PW.

64% incidence of transient phrenic nerve injury, which resolved by the end of the procedure.

In our experience, this rate is lower and can be explained by a different approach: we began employing the basket configuration only after observing a prolapse of one petal in the right atrium. Furthermore, the use of ICE is crucial, as it allows visualization of the junction between the right atrium and the SVC to prevent a lower position of the catheter (**Fig. 3**).

The presence of cardiac implantable electronic devices (CIEDs) was considered a potential issue during PFA due to the risk of electromagnetic interference. In particular, there may be a risk of oversensing resulting in pacing inhibition or inappropriate therapy, mode switching. Therefore, the presence of a CIED was an exclusion criterion in the large PFA-randomized trials like PEFCAT and IMPULSE.[40]

The PFA in CIEDs trial enrolled 20 consecutive patients with pacemakers, defibrillators, and resynchronization devices.[64] No pacemaker inhibition was observed in patients who were pacemaker-dependent. There was no dislodgment of leads, and pre-PFA and post-PFA interrogation of the devices showed no significant changes in the parameters or functions of the CIED.

Another ex vivo study involving CIEDs obtained from recent interventions, such as upgrade procedures or system removals, connected the CIED to leads positioned in a saline bath.[65] The PFA catheter was positioned less than 5 cm from the lead tip and less than 15 cm from the generator. PFA was then applied to create a total of 45 lesions before the CIED was reinterrogated, showing no resulting malfunction or damage to the CIEDs or leads.

CORONARY SINUS

Myocardial connections of varying numbers and morphology have been demonstrated between the CS and the LA on necropsied hearts.[66]

Myocardial connections of varying numbers and morphologies have been demonstrated between the CS and the LA in necropsied hearts.[67] This muscular sleeve can potentially serve as an ectopic trigger or may be part of a re-entrant circuit for AF. Thus, disconnecting the CS from the LA would reduce the inducibility of AF.[68] Given the presence of myocardial sleeves, CS isolation

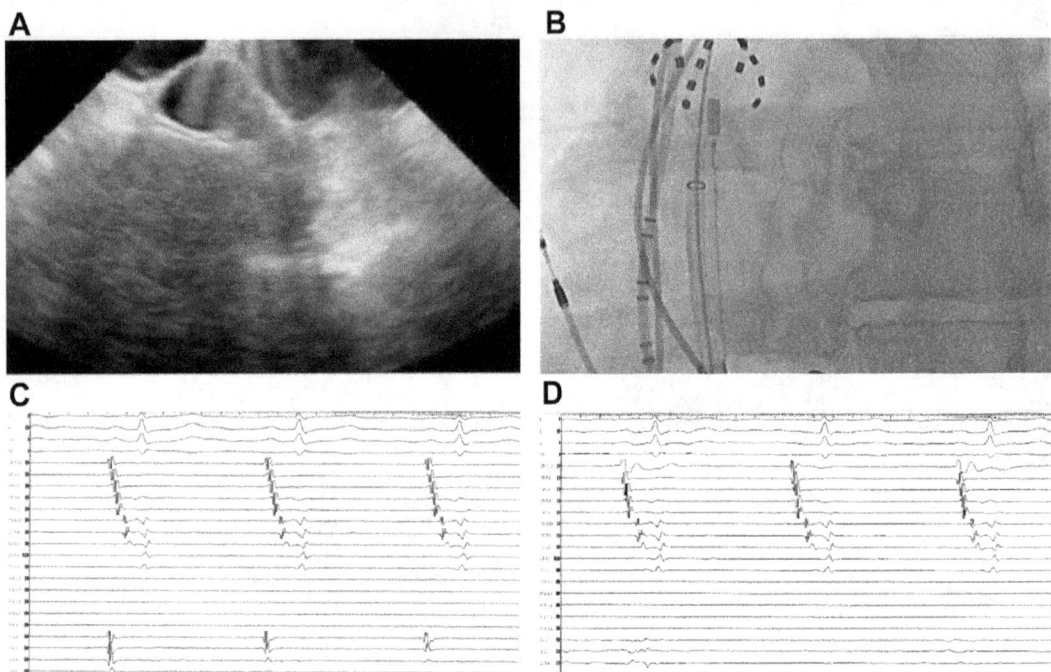

Fig. 3. The pentaspline catheter in basket configuration at the junction RA/SVC at the lower border of right pulmonary artery visualized by ICE (*A*) and fluoroscopy (*B*). EGM before (*C*) and after (*D*) isolation of SVC.

is often challenging and requires ablation both endocardially and epicardially with RF.

Our strategy for achieving complete isolation of the CS involves starting the ablation at the lower part of the PW along the CS. We divide the CS into 3 sections: distal, mid, and proximal. For each site, we deliver 3 to 4 lesion sets until the atrial electrogram disappears on the 10 poles of the duodecapolar catheter inside the CS (**Fig. 4**).

In our experience, during the waiting period, CS often regains conduction, necessitating additional application to achieve acute isolation. While more data are needed regarding persistent CS isolation, our preliminary findings indicate that in patients who underwent redo procedures, the CS typically showed reconnection. This may be attributed to the considerable distance between the endocardium of the LA, where PFA is delivered, and the CS. Another contributing factor to the high rate of reconnection could be the inadequate contact achieved by the pentaspline catheter, which was initially designed for PVI.

A prior study assessing feasibility of PFA for atrial tachycardia, which enrolled 28 patients, demonstrated that all mitral lines created by PFA were acutely blocked, except for one patient who required epicardial radiofrequency ablation within the CS.[69]

The low efficacy of the PFA pentaspline catheter in achieving mitral line isolation was confirmed by

Kueffer and colleagues.[70] In this study, RF ablation was required in 50% of patients to achieve block along the mitral line.

Timing is crucial for assessing mitral isthmus block, as demonstrated by Boveda and colleagues.[71] In this study involving 45 patients undergoing PVI plus PWI and mitral line, the latter was acutely blocked in all patients. However, after a 20 minute waiting period, block regression was observed in 6 patients. During PFA, coronary spasm of circumflex artery occurred in 2 patients. Special care must be taken during ablation in this area because of its proximity to the coronary artery. However, the risk of vasospasm can be mitigated through the preventive administration of nitrates.[72]

LEFT ATRIAL APPENDAGE

Non-PV triggers can originate from the LAA, with their prevalence increasing in patients with nonparoxysmal AF.[73,74] Empirical LAA isolation can be considered a first-line approach for patients with long-standing persistent AF.[75,76] Isolation of the LAA can be performed using techniques similar to those used for PVI, although it presents more challenges due to the considerable variability in LAA ostial anatomy.

The BELIEF trial, a randomized study aimed at assessing the benefits of empiric LAA isolation in patients with long-standing persistent AF, reported

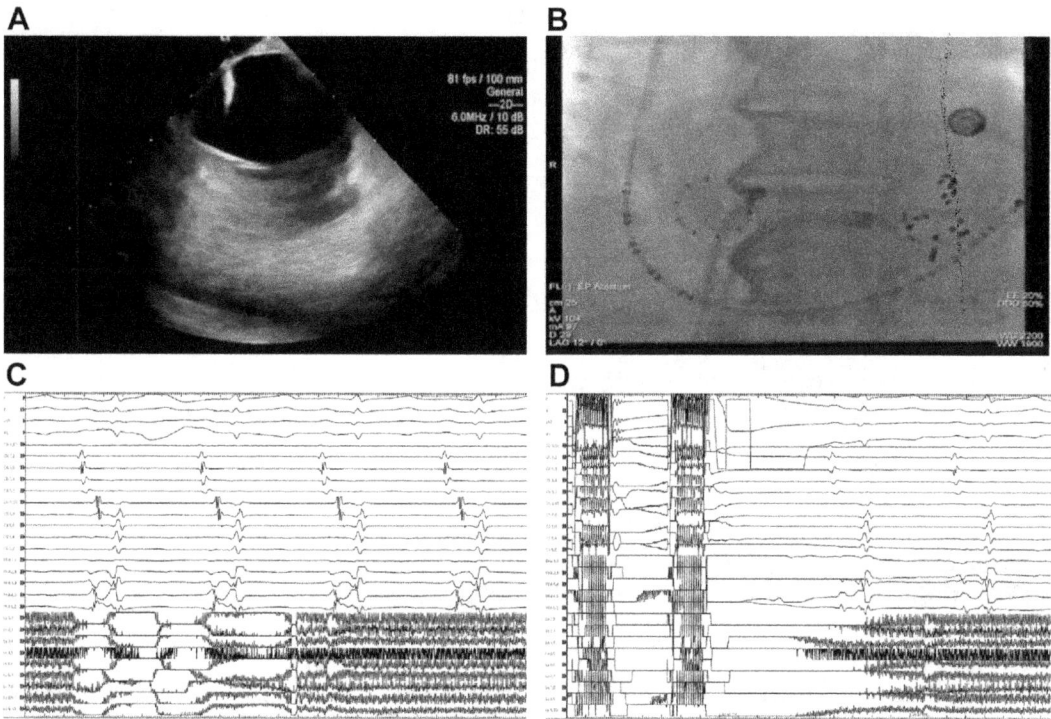

Fig. 4. The pentaspline catheter in flower configuration in the perimitral area visualized by ICE (*A*) and fluoroscopy (*B*). EGM before (*C*) and after (*D*) CS isolation.

improved freedom from atrial arrhythmias.[76] Additionally, 2 meta-analyses involving approximately 2000 patients with persistent AF and long-standing persistent atrial fibrillation (LSPAF) demonstrated the incremental benefits of left atrial appendage electrical isolation (LAAEI) when added to PVI.[76,77] However, LAA mechanical function can be impaired after isolation. Therefore, it is crucial to continue long-term anticoagulation or consider LAA occlusion following isolation, even in patients who maintain sinus rhythm.[78]

Our approach to achieving LAA isolation involves positioning the pentaspline catheter 1 cm inside the LAA and maneuvering it around the ostium to ensure complete coverage (**Fig. 5**). Acute isolation is often observed and confirmed with an adenosine bolus injection. While the reconnection rate appears to be high, these reconnections are generally small, requiring only a minor delivery of RF energy to achieve effective isolation.

Coronary spasms may occur also during LAA isolation. However, in our experience, we have not observed any changes in the ST segment during ablation, even in the absence of nitrate administration.

There are only a few documented cases of LAA isolation using PFA.

Simultaneous LAA isolation and occlusion were achieved using a novel device that integrates PFA electrodes into the LAA occluder (E-SeaLA, Hangzhou Dinova EP Technology Co., Ltd).[79] A custom 14F deflectable delivery sheath was used to position the device at the LAA ostium, where it was adjusted to the appropriate position before deployment to occlude the LAA. Subsequently, PFA applications were delivered in a biphasic-bipolar waveform through the device's electrodes to the LAA orifice/neck region, utilizing sequences of microsecond-scale pulses ranging from 1400 V to 1800 V; the total PFA duration to isolate the LAA was 12 seconds. Coronary angiography performed before and 7 minutes after PFA revealed no evidence of arterial spasm.

Audiat and colleagues[80] reported a case in which LAA isolation was achieved despite the presence of an occluder (Amplatzer, Abbott Medical inc) in the LAA. The flower configuration was initially used to target the antrum of the left superior PV. However, multiple attempts to deliver PFA were immediately halted by the Farapulse (Boston Scientific) system due to overlap between the electrodes of the PFA catheter and the disk of the Amulet device, which extended beyond the posterolateral ridge.

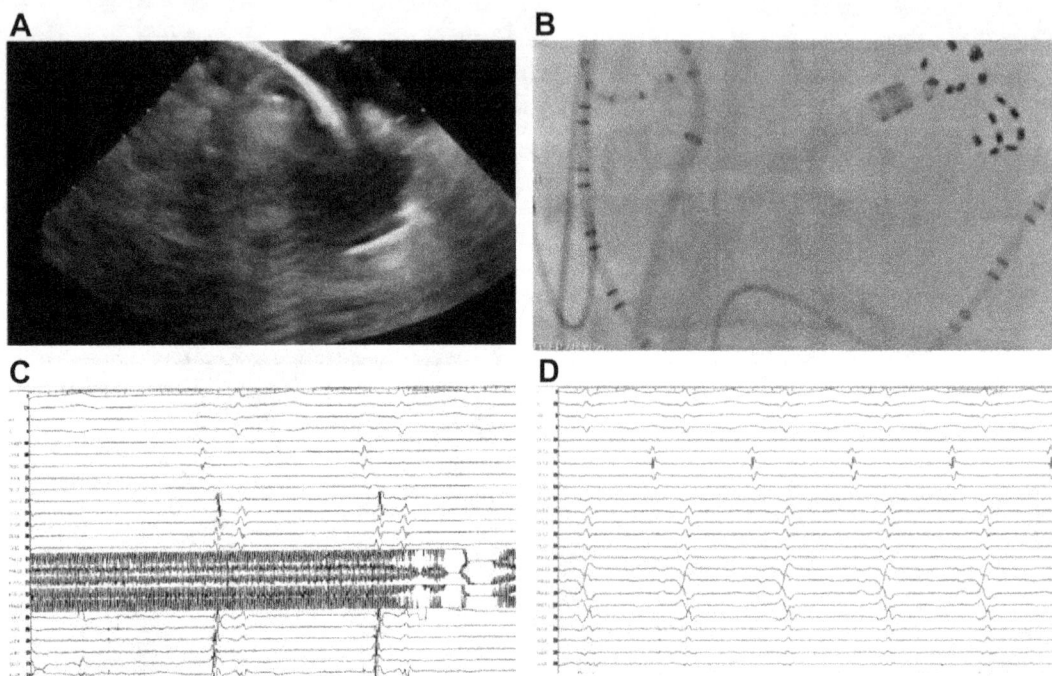

Fig. 5. The pentaspline catheter in flower configuration at the LAA ostium visualized by ICE (*A*) and fluoroscopy (*B*). EGM before (*C*) and after (*D*) LAA isolation.

PERSISTENT LEFT SUPERIOR VENA CAVA

Persistent PLSVC occurs in patients with a persistent left superior cardinal vein, which normally regresses to the VOM in most individuals.[81,82] Given its arrhythmogenic potential, isolation of the PLSVC should be performed as a first-line treatment.

In a case report, Combes and colleagues[83] described the isolation of PLSVC using the Faradrive catheter in a basket configuration, requiring 20 applications to achieve complete isolation. The ablation was performed with the infusion of nitrates, and no instances of ST change were noted.

SUMMARY

PFA has emerged as an innovative technology capable of selectively targeting myocardial tissue, thereby reducing risks associated with thermal energy. As with PVI, the main limitation of non-PV trigger ablation is its durability. A successful procedure depends on the creation of lasting transmural ablation lesions, ensuring that no viable tissue remains. Further data are required to confirm the efficacy of PFA in ablating areas beyond the PVs.

CLINICS CARE POINTS

- *Recognize the role of non-PV triggers*: Clinicians should be aware that non-PV triggers significantly contribute to the recurrence of AF after CA. Comprehensive mapping and assessment of these triggers are essential for effective treatment.

- *Implement PFA techniques*: PFA should be considered as a preferred technique for non-PV trigger ablation due to its safety profile and ability to create tissue-selective lesions, minimizing collateral damage to surrounding structures.

- *Focus on durability*: While PFA has shown promising acute efficacy, clinicians must remain vigilant regarding the durability of non-PV trigger isolation especially in critical area like CS and LAA.

- *Incorporate empirical strategies*: In patients with a high likelihood of non-PV triggers, isolation of there should be driven by the response to high dose of isoproterenol or might be empirical during the initial ablation procedure to enhance success rates.

DISCLOSURE

Dr A. Natale is a consultant for Biosense Webster, Stereotaxis, and Abbott Medical, and has received speaker honoraria/travel from Medtronic, Atricure, Biotronik, and Janssen. All other authors have reported that they have no relationships relevant to the contents of this article to disclose.

REFERENCES

1. Chugh SS, Havmoeller R, Narayanan K, et al. Worldwide epidemiology of atrial fibrillation: a global burden of disease 2010 study. Circulation 2014; 129(8):837–47.
2. Elsheikh S, Hill A, Irving G, et al. Atrial fibrillation and stroke: state-of-the-art and future directions. Curr Probl Cardiol 2024;49(1 Pt C):102181.
3. La Fazia VM, Pierucci N, Mohanty S, et al. Atrial fibrillation ablation in heart failure with preserved ejection fraction. Card Electrophysiol Clin 2024. https://doi.org/10.1016/j.ccep.2024.08.006.
4. Calkins H, Reynolds MR, Spector P, et al. Treatment of atrial fibrillation with antiarrhythmic drugs or radiofrequency ablation: two systematic literature reviews and meta-analyses. Circ Arrhythm Electrophysiol 2009;2:349–61.
5. Jais P, Cauchemez B, Macle L, et al. Catheter ablation versus antiarrhythmic drugs for atrial fibrillation: the A4 study. Circulation 2008;118:2498–505.
6. Packer DL, Kowal RC, Wheelan KR, et al. Cryoballoon ablation of pulmonary veins for paroxysmal atrial fibrillation: first results of the North American Arctic Front (STOP AF) pivotal trial. J Am Coll Cardiol 2013;61:1713–23.
7. Poole JE, Bahnson TD, Monahan KH, et al. Recurrence of atrial fibrillation after catheter ablation or antiarrhythmic drug therapy in the CABANA trial. J Am Coll Cardiol 2020;75:3105–18.
8. Mont L, Bisbal F, Hernandez-Madrid A, et al. Catheter ablation vs. antiarrhythmic drug treatment of persistent atrial fibrillation: a multicentre, randomized, controlled trial (SARA study). Eur Heart J 2014;35:501–7.
9. Scherr D, Khairy P, Miyazaki S, et al. Five-year outcome of catheter ablation of persistent atrial fibrillation using termination of atrial fibrillation as a procedural endpoint. Circ Arrhythm Electrophysiol 2015;8:18–24.
10. La Fazia VM, Massaro G, Mohanty S, et al. Improvement of erectile dysfunction after atrial fibrillation ablation: a medication dependency analysis. JACC Clin Electrophysiol 2024. https://doi.org/10.1016/j.jacep.2024.08.002.
11. Van Gelder IC, Rienstra M, Bunting KV, et al. 2024 ESC Guidelines for the management of atrial fibrillation developed in collaboration with the European Association for Cardio-Thoracic Surgery (EACTS). Eur Heart J 2024;45(36):3314–414.
12. Tzeis S, Gerstenfeld EP, Kalman J, et al. 2024 European heart rhythm association/heart rhythm society/Asia Pacific heart rhythm society/Latin American heart rhythm society expert consensus statement on catheter and surgical ablation of atrial fibrillation. Heart Rhythm 2024;21(9):e31–149.
13. Haïssaguerre M, Jaïs P, Shah DC, et al. Spontaneous initiation of atrial fibrillation by ectopic beats originating in the pulmonary veins. N Engl J Med 1998;339(10):659–66.
14. Blom NA, Gittenberger-de Groot AC, DeRuiter MC, et al. Development of the cardiac conduction tissue in human em- bryos using HNK-1 antigen expression: possible relevance for understanding of abnormal atrial automaticity. Circulation 1999;99:800–6.
15. Simone CV, Noheria A, Lachman N, et al. Myocardium of the superior vena cava, coronary sinus, vein of marshall, and the pulmonary vein ostia: gross anatomic studies in 620 hearts. J Cardiovasc Electrophysiol 2012;23:1304–9.
16. Gianni C, Mohanty S, Trivedi C, et al. Novel concepts and approaches in ablation of atrial fibrillation: the role of non-pulmonary vein triggers. Europace 2018;20(10):1566–76.
17. Santangeli P, Zado ES, Hutchinson MD, et al. Prevalence and distribution of focal triggers in persistent and long-standing persistent atrial fibrillation. Heart Rhythm 2016;13(2):374–82.
18. Santangeli P, Marchlinski FE. Techniques for provocation, localization and ablation of nonpulmonary vein triggers for atrial fibrillation. Heart Rhythm 2017;14: 1087–96.
19. Gokoglan Y, Mohanty S, Gunes MF, et al. Pulmonary vein antrum isolation in patients with paroxysmal atrial fibrillation: more than a decade of follow-up. Circ Arrhythm Electrophysiol 2016;9(5):e003660.
20. Della Rocca DG, Di Biase L, Mohanty S, et al. Targeting non-pulmonary vein triggers in persistent atrial fibrillation: results from a prospective, multicentre, observational registry. Europace 2021;23(12):1939–49.
21. Patel D, Mohanty P, Di Biase L, et al. Outcomes and complications of catheter ablation for atrial fibrillation in females. Heart Rhythm 2010;7:167–72.
22. Mohanty S, Mohanty P, Di Biase L, et al. Impact of metabolic syndrome on procedural outcomes in patients with atrial fibrillation undergoing catheter ablation. J Am Coll Cardiol 2012;59:1295–301.
23. Patel D, Mohanty P, Di Biase L, et al. Safety and efficacy of pulmonary vein antral isolation in patients with obstructive sleep apnea: the impact of continuous positive airway pressure. Circ Arrhythm Electrophysiol 2010;3:445–51.
24. Santangeli P, Di Biase L, Mohanty P, et al. Catheter ablation of atrial fibrillation in octogenarians: safety and outcomes. J Cardiovasc Electrophysiol 2012; 23:687–93.
25. Zhao Y, Di Biase L, Trivedi C, et al. Importance of non-pulmonary vein triggers ablation to achieve long-term freedom from paroxysmal atrial fibrillation in patients with low ejection fraction. Heart Rhythm 2016;13:141–9.
26. Verma A, Wazni OM, Marrouche NF, et al. Pre- existent left atrial scarring in patients undergoing pulmonary vein antrum isola- tion. J Am Coll Cardiol 2005; 45:285–92.

27. Santangeli P, Di Biase L, Themistoclakis S, et al. Catheter ablation of atrial fibrillation in hypertrophic cardiomyopathy long-term outcomes and mechanisms of arrhythmia recurrence. Circ Arrhythm Electrophysiol 2013;6:1089–94.

28. Bai R, Di Biase L, Mohanty P, et al. Catheter ab- lation of atrial fibrillation in patients with mechanical mitral valve: long-term out- come of single procedure of pulmonary vein antrum isolation with or without non-pulmonary vein trigger ablation. J Cardiovasc Electrophysiol 2014;25:824–33.

29. La Fazia VM, Pierucci N, Mohanty S, et al. Catheter ablation approach and outcome in HIV+ patients with recurrent atrial fibrillation. J Cardiovasc Electrophysiol 2023;34(12):2527–34.

30. Gallagher JJ, Svenson RH, Kasell JH, et al. Catheter technique for closed-chest ablation of the atrioventricular conduction system. N Engl J Med 1982;306:194–200.

31. Wittkampf FHM, van Driel VJ, van Wessel H, et al. Myocardial lesion depth with circular electroporation ablation. Circ Arrhythm Electrophysiol 2012;5:581–6.

32. van Driel VJHM, Neven K, van Wessel H, et al. Low vulnerability of the right phrenic nerve to electroporation ablation. Heart Rhythm 2015;12:1838–44.

33. van Driel VJHM, Neven KGEJ, van Wessel H, et al. Pulmonary vein stenosis after catheter ablation: electroporation versus radiofrequency. Circ Arrhythm Electrophysiol 2014;7:734–8.

34. Verma A, Asivatham SJ, Deneke T, et al. Primer on pulsed electrical field ablation: understanding the benefits and limitations. Circ Arrhythm Electrophysiol 2021;14:e010086.

35. Verma A, Haines DE, Boersma LV, et al. Pulsed field ablation for the treatment of atrial fibrillation: PULSED AF pivotal trial. Circulation 2023;147:1422–32.

36. Peng W, Polajžer T, Yao C, et al. Dynamics of cell death due to electroporation using different pulse parameters as revealed by different viability assays. Ann Biomed Eng 2024;52:22–35.

37. Davalos RV, Mir LM, Rubinsky B. Tissue ablation with irreversible electroporation. Ann Biomed Eng 2005;33:223–31.

38. Kinosita K Jr, Tsong TY. Voltage-induced pore formation and hemolysis of human erythrocytes. Biochim Biophys Acta 1977;471:227–42.

39. Reddy VY, Gerstenfeld EP, Natale A, et al. Pulsed field or conventional thermal ablation for paroxysmal atrial fibrillation. N Engl J Med 2023;389:1660–71.

40. Reddy VY, Dukkipati SR, Neuzil P, et al. Pulsed field ablation of paroxysmal atrial fibrillation: 1-year outcomes of IMPULSE, PEFCAT, and PEFCAT II. JACC Clin Electrophysiol 2021;7:614–27.

41. Della Rocca DG, Marcon L, Magnocavallo M, et al. Pulsed electric field, cryoballoon, and radiofrequency for paroxysmal atrial fibrillation ablation: a propensity score-matched comparison. Europace 2023;26(1):euae016.

42. Mohanty S, Della Rocca DG, Torlapati PG, et al. Pulsed-field ablation does not worsen baseline pulmonary hypertension following prior radiofrequency ablations. JACC Clin Electrophysiol 2024;10(3):477–86.

43. Abdulla R, Blew GA, Holterman MJ. Cardiovascular embryology. Pediatr Cardiol 2004;25(3):191–200.

44. Rohr S. Arrhythmogenic implications of fibroblast-myocyte interactions. Circ Arrhythm Electrophysiol 2012;5(2):442–52.

45. Wilber DJ. Fibroblasts, focal triggers, and persistent atrial fibrillation: is there a connection? Circ Arrhythm Electrophysiol 2012;5(2):249–51.

46. Platonov PG, Mitrofanova LB, Orshanskaya V, et al. Structural abnormalities in atrial walls are associated with presence and persistency of atrial fibrillation but not with age. J Am Coll Cardiol 2011;58(21):2225–32.

47. Bai R, Di Biase L, Mohanty P, et al. Proven isolation of the pulmonary vein antrum with or without left atrial posterior wall isolation in patients with persistent atrial fibrillation. Heart Rhythm 2016;13(1):132–40.

48. He X, Zhou Y, Chen Y, et al. Left atrial posterior wall isolation reduces the recurrence of atrial fibrillation: a meta-analysis. J Interv Card Electrophysiol 2016;46(3):267–74.

49. Sanders P, Hocini M, Jais P, et al. Complete isolation of the pulmonary veins and posterior left atrium in chronic atrial fibrillation. Long-term clinical outcome. Eur Heart J 2007;28(15):1862–71.

50. Kim JS, Shin SY, Na JO, et al. Does isolation of the left atrial posterior wall improve clinical outcomes af- ter radiofrequency catheter ablation for persistent atrial fibrillation?: a prospective randomized clinical trial. Int J Cardiol 2015;181:277–83.

51. McLellan AJA, Prabhu S, Voskoboinik A, et al. Isolation of the posterior left atrium for patients with persistent atrial fibrillation: routine adenosine challenge for dormant posterior left atrial conduction im- proves long-term outcome. Europace 2017;19(12):1958–66.

52. Kistler PM, Chieng D, Sugumar H, et al. Effect of catheter ablation using pulmonary vein isolation with vs without posterior left atrial wall isolation on atrial arrhythmia recurrence in patients with persistent atrial fibrillation: the CAPLA randomized clinical trial. JAMA 2023;329(2):127–35.

53. Solimene F, Compagnucci P, Tondo C, et al. Direct epicardial validation of posterior wall electroporation in persistent atrial fibrillation. JACC Clin Electrophysiol 2024;10(6):1200–2.

54. Pambrun T, Duchateau J, Delgove A, et al. Epicardial course of the septopulmonary bundle: anatomical considerations and clinical implications for roof line completion. Heart Rhythm 2021;18(3):349–57.

55. Reddy VY, Anic A, Koruth J, et al. Pulsed field ablation in patients with persistent atrial fibrillation. J Am Coll Cardiol 2020;76(9):1068–80.

56. Kueffer T, Tanner H, Madaffari A, et al. Posterior wall ablation by pulsed-field ablation: procedural safety, efficacy, and findings on redo procedures. Europace 2023;26(1):euae006.

57. Turagam MK, Neuzil P, Schmidt B, et al. Safety and effectiveness of pulsed field ablation to treat atrial fibrillation: one-year outcomes from the MANIFEST-PF registry. Circulation 2023;148(1):35–46.

58. Arruda M, Mlcochova H, Prasad SK, et al. Electrical isolation of the superior vena cava: an adjunctive strategy to pulmonary vein antrum isolation improving the outcome of AF ablation. J Cardiovasc Electrophysiol 2007;18(12):1261–6.

59. Tsai CF, Tai CT, Hsieh MH, et al. Initiation of atrial fibrillation by ectopic beats originating from the superior vena cava: electrophysiological characteristics and results of radiofrequency ablation. Circulation 2000;102(1):67–74.

60. Huang BH, Wu MH, Tsao HM, et al. Morphology of the thoracic veins and left atrium in paroxysmal atrial fibrillation initiated by superior caval vein ectopy. J Cardiovasc Electrophysiol 2005;16(4):411–7.

61. Ejima K, Kato K, Iwanami Y, et al. Impact of an empiric isolation of the superior vena cava in addition to circumferential pulmonary vein isolation on the outcome of paroxysmal atrial fibrillation ablation. Am J Cardiol 2015;116(11):1711–6.

62. Corrado A, Bonso A, Madalosso M, et al. Impact of systematic isolation of superior vena cava in addition to pulmonary vein antrum isolation on the outcome of paroxysmal, persistent, and permanent atrial fibrillation ablation: results from a randomized study. J Cardiovasc Electrophysiol 2010;21(1):1–5.

63. Ollitrault P, Chaumont C, Font J, et al. Superior vena cava isolation using a pentaspline pulsed-field ablation catheter: feasibility and safety in patients undergoing atrial fibrillation catheter ablation. Europace 2024;26(7):euae160.

64. Chen S, Chun JKR, Bordignon S, et al. Pulsed field ablation-based pulmonary vein isolation in atrial fibrillation patients with cardiac implantable electronic devices: practical approach and device interrogation (PFA in CIEDs). J Interv Card Electrophysiol 2023;66(8):1929–38.

65. Lennerz C, O'Connor M, Schaarschmidt C, et al. Pulsed field ablation in patients with cardiac implantable electronic devices: an ex vivo assessment of safety. J Interv Card Electrophysiol 2024. https://doi.org/10.1007/s10840-024-01758-2.

66. Chauvin M, Shah DC, Haissaguerre M, et al. The anatomic basis of connections between the coronary sinus musculature and the left atrium in humans. Circulation 2000;101(6):647–52.

67. Morita H, Zipes DP, Morita ST, et al. Isolation of canine coronary sinus musculature from the atria by radiofrequency catheter ablation prevents induction of atrial fibrillation. Circ Arrhythm Electrophysiol 2014;7(6):1181–8.

68. Yin X, Zhao Z, Gao L, et al. Frequency gradient within coronary sinus predicts the long-term outcome of persistent atrial fibrillation catheter ablation. J Am Heart Assoc 2017;6(3) [pii: e004869].

69. Gunawardene MA, Harloff T, Jularic M, et al. Contemporary catheter ablation of complex atrial tachycardias after prior atrial fibrillation ablation: pulsed field vs. radiofrequency current energy ablation guided by high-density mapping. Europace 2024;26(4):euae072.

70. Kueffer T, Seiler J, Madaffari A, et al. Pulsed-field ablation for the treatment of left atrial reentry tachycardia. J Interv Card Electrophysiol 2023;66(6):1431–40.

71. Davong B, Adeliño R, Delasnerie H, et al. Pulsed-field ablation on mitral isthmus in persistent atrial fibrillation: preliminary data on efficacy and safety. JACC Clin Electrophysiol 2023;9(7 Pt 2):1070–81.

72. Malyshev Y, Neuzil P, Petru J, et al. Nitroglycerin to ameliorate coronary artery spasm during focal pulsed-field ablation for atrial fibrillation. JACC Clin Electrophysiol 2024;10(5):885–96.

73. Hocini M, Shah AJ, Nault I, et al. Localized reentry within the left atrial appendage: arrhythmogenic role in patients undergoing ablation of persistent atrial fibrillation. Heart Rhythm 2011;8:1853–61.

74. Romero J, Natale A. Di Biase L Left atrial appendage empirical electrical isolation for persistent atrial fibrillation: time for a change in practice. Europace 2017;19:699–702.

75. Di Biase L, Burkhardt JD, Mohanty P, et al. Left atrial appendage isolation in patients with longstanding persistent AF undergoing catheter ablation: BELIEF trial. J Am Coll Cardiol 2016;68:1929–40.

76. Romero J, Michaud GF, Avendano R, et al. Benefit of left atrial appendage electrical isolation for persistent and long-standing persistent atrial fibrillation: a systematic review and meta-analysis. Europace 2018. https://doi.org/10.1093/europace/eux372 [EPUB ahead of print: 12 January 2018].

77. Friedman DJ, Black-Maier EW, Barnett AS, et al. Left atrial appendage electrical isolation for treatment of recurrent atrial fibrillation: a meta-analysis. JACC Clin Electrophysiol 2018;4(1):112–20.

78. Mohanty S, Torlapati PG, La Fazia VM, et al. Best anticoagulation strategy with and without appendage occlusion for stroke-prophylaxis in postablation atrial fibrillation patients with cardiac amyloidosis. J Cardiovasc Electrophysiol 2024;35(7):1422–8.

79. Tang M, Wang X, Reddy VY. Simultaneous pulsed field ablation and mechanical closure of left atrial appendage using a novel device. JACC Case Rep 2023;22:101963.

80. Audiat C, Della Rocca DG, de Asmundis C, et al. Interference from lobe-and-disk left atrial appendage occluder affecting left superior pulmonary vein pulsed field ablation. Heart Rhythm 2024;21(8): 1240–1.

81. Dearstine M, Taylor W, Kerut EK. Persistent left superior vena cava: chest x-ray and echocardiographic findings. Echocardiography 2000;17(5): 453–65.

82. Turagam MK, Atoui M, Atkins D, et al. Persistent left superior vena cava as an arrhythmogenic source in atrial fibrillation: results from a multicenter experienceence. J Interv Card Electrophysiol 2019;54(2):93–100.

83. Menè R, Sousonis V, Combes S, et al. Pulsed field ablation of a persistent left superior vena cava in recurrent paroxysmal atrial fibrillation and its effect on the mitral isthmus: a case report. HeartRhythm Case Rep 2023;10(1):6–10.

Pulsed Field Ablation Versus Thermal Energy Ablation for Atrial Fibrillation

Kishan Padalia, MD[a], Wendy S. Tzou, MD[b],*

KEYWORDS

- Atrial fibrillation • Catheter ablation • Ablation biophysics • Radiofrequency ablation • Cryoablation
- Pulsed field ablation

KEY POINTS

- Pulsed field ablation, in commercially available formulations, is as effective as thermal ablation in controlling atrial fibrillation.
- Pulsed field ablation has myocardial selectivity and distinct ablation mechanism, which may reduce risks of phrenic nerve or esophageal injury and pulmonary vein stenosis.
- Pulsed field ablation may reduce overall procedure time, although often at the cost of increased fluoroscopy use, compared to thermal ablation.
- Pulsed field ablation incurs risks of coronary vasospasm and acute kidney injury from hemolysis, which must be considered and proactively managed.

INTRODUCTION

For more than 2 decades, catheter ablation for atrial fibrillation (AF) has been predominantly performed with either radiofrequency or cryothermal energy. These energies cause nonselective tissue injury mediated by thermal conduction of heat or cold, respectively. In the last several years, pulsed field ablation (PFA) has emerged as a theoretically nonthermal energy alternative, utilizing electrical field applications to cause myocyte-specific, irreversible electroporation (**Fig. 1**). PFA has been used to effectively and safely achieve control of AF through pulmonary vein (PV) isolation as well as adjunctive non-PV ablation. In the following sections, the authors review and compare the biophysics of radiofrequency and cryothermal ablation and discuss comparative outcomes between thermal and PFA for AF.

BIOPHYSICS
Radiofrequency Ablation

Radiofrequency ablation (RFA) for cardiac arrhythmias was first introduced in 1985.[1] Standard RFA utilizes alternating electrical current delivered from an electrode tip directly into myocardium (**Fig. 2**). The circuit is completed via a dispersive grounding patch on the body surface. The electromagnetic energy applied to tissue is transformed into thermal energy through resistive heating.[2] Resistive heat production is proportional to current density that distributes radially and decreases rapidly with distance from the active electrode. Therefore, resistive heating only affects tissue in direct contact with the catheter tip. The majority of RFA lesion volume results from passive, conductive heating to deeper, adjacent tissue. Assuming fixed convective cooling from regional blood flow and stable catheter–tissue contact, the total RFA

[a] Division of Cardiology, Department of Medicine, University of Colorado, Anschutz Medical Campus, Aurora, CO 80045, USA; [b] Division of Cardiology, Department of Medicine, Electrophysiology Section, Cardiac Electrophysiology, University of Colorado School of Medicine, 12401 East 17th Avenue, MS B-132, Aurora, CO 80045, USA
* Corresponding author.
E-mail address: WENDY.TZOU@CUANSCHUTZ.EDU

Card Electrophysiol Clin 17 (2025) 167–181
https://doi.org/10.1016/j.ccep.2025.02.005
1877-9182/25/© 2025 Elsevier Inc. All rights are reserved, including those for text and data mining, AI training, and similar technologies.

Abbreviations

AF	atrial fibrillation
LAA	left atrial appendage
PFA	pulsed field ablation
PV	pulmonary vein
PW	posterior wall
RFA	radiofrequency ablation

lesion size is determined by total current delivery.[3] Total current delivery, in turn, depends on electrode size and local tissue impedance and can be controlled by altering power and duration of ablation (**Fig. 3**).[4] Determination of effective current delivery is guided by temperature recorded near the electrode–tissue interface, which is a surrogate for temperature of myocardium beyond the tip-tissue interface. Effective, irreversible RFA lesions form when myocardium is heated to a temperature of 50°C or greater.[5] However, avoiding excessive heating is critical, given risk of adverse events. Formation of char or coagulum on the catheter tip, which limits electrode and lesion size, is substantially reduced with open irrigation during RFA. However, steam pops, which are often audible tissue eruptions from boiling of water within heated tissue, may still occur and result in perforations or increased thrombogenicity. Importantly, injury from thermal conduction is not specific to cardiac tissue. RFA in the left atrium can harm adjacent noncardiac structures, including the esophagus and phrenic nerve.[6] Advances in catheter design, including open-irrigation, contact-force-sensing, and integration of thermocouples within catheter tips, have been important to improve safety and outcomes of RFA for AF.[7–9] These advances have also facilitated use of high-power, short-duration RFA for AF, which produces wider and shallower lesions. In atrial tissue, this usually provides sufficient depth to achieve transmurality with decreased risk of collateral damage to adjacent organs.[10,11]

Cryothermal Ablation

Similar to RFA, lesion formation with cryoablation occurs using thermal conduction. However, convective cooling and progressive hypothermia at the catheter–tissue interface produce different cellular effects and injury patterns (**Fig. 4**).[12,13] As cooling is applied, cardiac myocyte metabolism slows with progressively dysfunctional ion channels and increasingly acidic pH. These effects from cooling prior to freezing are reversible. Ice crystals begin to form in the extracellular and intracellular space below −15°C and −40°C, respectively. This process results in both mechanical disruption of the cell membrane and biochemical changes in intracellular osmotic and diffusion gradients, which lead to cell membrane lysis and impairment of critical intracellular channels, enzymes, and lipoproteins. Microvascular destruction also occurs resulting in significant ischemic cellular injury. The combination of these effects results in significant cellular dysfunction and, ultimately, death. After freezing application ceases, thawing occurs with tissue passively returning to body temperature. A hyperemic microvascular response ensues with enlargement and coalescence of ice crystals propagating cellular injury with subsequent hemorrhage and inflammation. In the following weeks, the lesion matures with apoptosis and fibrosis extending to the periphery of the frozen tissue. Compared to RFA, this typically creates more sharply demarcated lesions with less disruption of structural tissue integrity.[12]

Cryoballoon systems were specifically designed to achieve "one-shot" PV isolation. Pressurized nitric oxide is delivered to the distal aspect of the inner balloon.[12] There, it evaporates into a gas and can

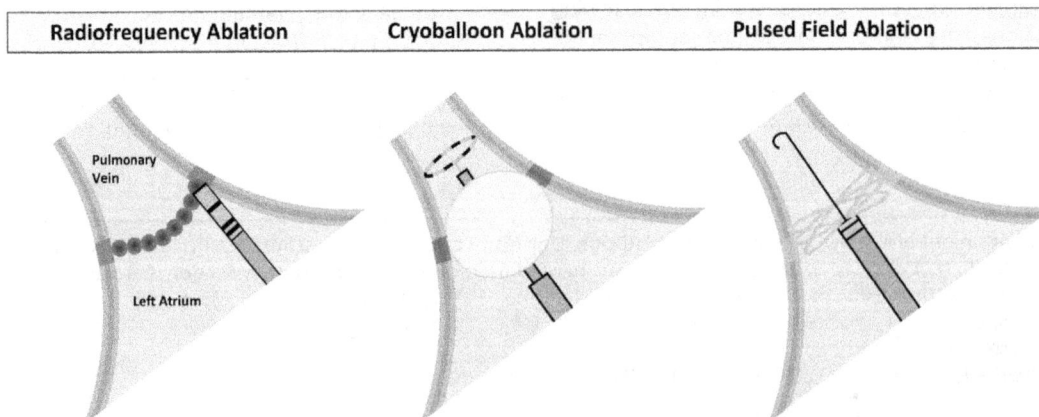

Radiofrequency Ablation	Cryoballoon Ablation	Pulsed Field Ablation

Pulmonary Vein

Left Atrium

Fig. 1. Energy modalities available for catheter ablation of atrial fibrillation.

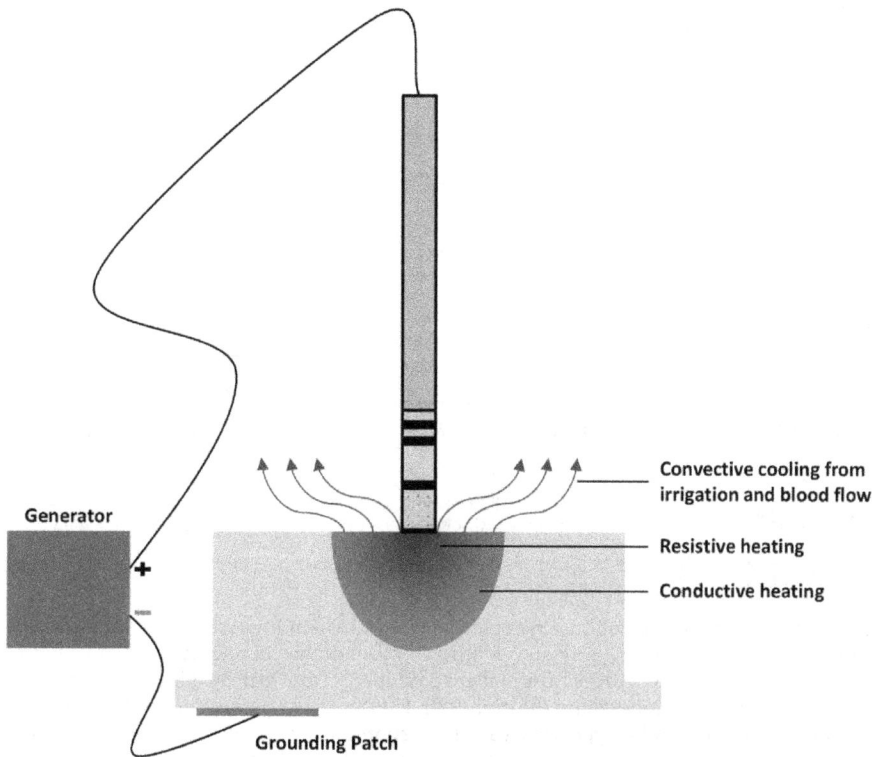

Fig. 2. Biophysics of heating from radiofrequency ablation. Alternating electrical current is delivered from the catheter tip into myocardial tissue and then to a dispersive electrode on the body surface. The image shows regions of myocardial tissue undergoing resistive heating near the catheter tip and conductive heat heating away from the catheter tip. Convective cooling at the catheter tip occurs from both the local blood pool and continuous irrigation.

achieve a temperature of $-80°C$, absorbing heat from surrounding tissue prior to returning to the console. Conductive cooling spreads radially from the balloon with magnitude of cooling decreasing from $0.7°C$ per second at 1 mm to $0.2°C$ per second at 5 mm.[14] The optimal zone of freezing is contingent on effective cryorefrigerent delivery and the relative size, orientation, and contact of

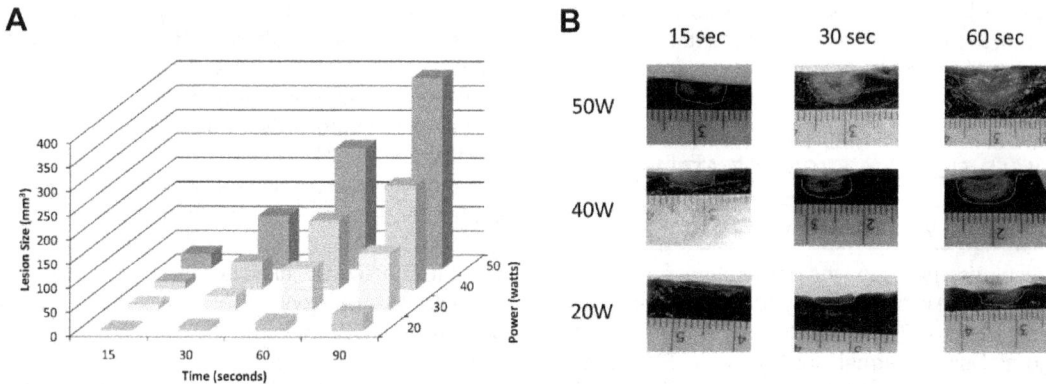

Fig. 3. Ablation volumes for varying degrees of power and duration in an ex vivo model with representative ablation lesions. (*A*) Greater power delivery and longer radiofrequency ablation time increase ablation lesion size. Compared with a proportional change in radiofrequency duration, the same proportional increase in power delivery produces a significantly larger lesion volume. (*B*) Representative ablation lesions are shown at 20W, 40W, and 50W for various durations. (*From* Ryan T. Borne et al., Longer Duration Versus Increasing Power During Radiofrequency Ablation Yields Different Ablation Lesion Characteristics, JACC: Clinical Electrophysiology, 4 (7), 2018, 902-908, https://doi.org/10.1016/j.jacep.2018.03.020.)

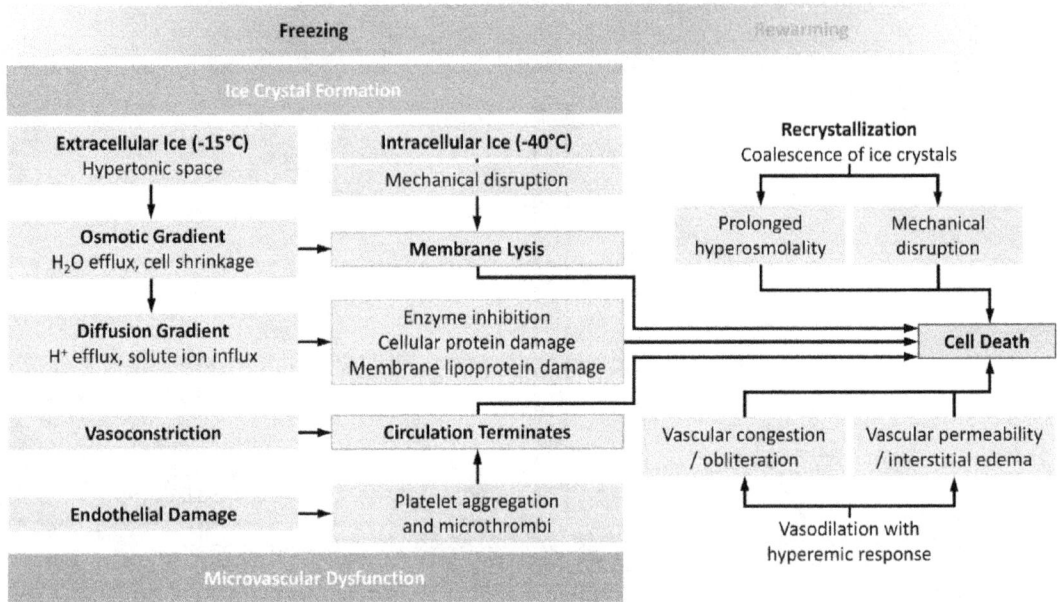

Fig. 4. Lesion formation with cryoablation. Cryoablation causes cellular injury through multiple pathways. During the freezing phase, formation of ice crystals leads to both mechanical and osmotic stress with subsequent membrane lysis and impairment of critical intracellular components (*top left*). Simultaneously, there is significant ischemic injury from microcirculatory failure (*bottom left*). Further injury occurs during the rewarming phase, as ice crystals coalesce (*top right*) and a hyperemic vascular response leads to inflammation and hemorrhage (*bottom right*). (*From* Jason G. Andrade et al., Cryoballoon Ablation as Initial Treatment for Atrial Fibrillation: JACC State-of-the-Art Review, Journal of the American College of Cardiology, 78 (9), 2021, 914-930, https://doi.org/10.1016/j.jacc.2021.06.038.)

the cryoballoon with the ostium of the PV. Durable, lesion formation is associated with decreased time to isolation, balloon temperature nadir, duration of thaw times, and degree of PV occlusion.[15] Contemporary cryoballoon systems have refined cryorefrigerant delivery and balloon shape and compliance to provide a more consistent zone of freezing with multiple balloon angulations.[16] This has allowed for more reliable creation of wide, antral lesions for a range of different pulmonary venous anatomies.[17]

CLINICAL OUTCOMES OF THERMAL VERSUS PULSED-FIELD ABLATION FOR ATRIAL FIBRILLATION
Pulmonary Vein Isolation

PV isolation has been the cornerstone for AF ablation since Haissaguerre and colleagues' initial description of PV trigger RFA more than 25 years ago.[18] Using thermal energy, focal PV ablation and ostial PV isolation incur increased risk of PV stenosis and may not eliminate all PV-related AF triggers.[19,20] These findings lead to the adoption of wide, antral, and circumferential isolation of the bilateral PVs as the standard of care.[21] Randomized and observational studies demonstrate that the success of PV isolation in preventing

recurrence of AF greater than 30 seconds at 1 year is inversely proportional to the persistence of AF (**Table 1**), ranging from approximately 60 to 80%, 40% to 60%, and 20% to 40% for paroxysmal, persistent, and long-standing persistent AF, respectively.[22–25] PV isolation is more effective than medical therapy in both drug-refractory and treatment-naïve patients with AF.[26,27] In particular, patients with coexisting systolic heart failure appear to derive the most clinical benefit from AF catheter ablation with significant improvements in mortality, heart failure events, and cardiac function.[28–30]

Randomized clinical trials demonstrate approximately equivalent rates of success in catheter ablation for AF regardless of energy modality. The FIRE AND ICE clinical trial randomized 762 patients with paroxysmal AF to PV isolation with cryoballoon (CBA) versus RFA. There was no significant difference in freedom from recurrent atrial arrhythmias at 1 year (64% vs 65%). On average, CBA was 17 minutes shorter but required 5 more minutes of fluoroscopy compared to RFA. CBA was less dependent on operator skill and dexterity with single-shot PV isolation in most cases obviating the need for significant catheter manipulation, and freeze-mediated adhesion facilitating

Table 1
Efficacy of pulmonary vein isolation with thermal versus pulsed field ablation in key randomized controlled trials

Authors, Year	Study Population	Intervention	Control	Outcomes
Radiofrequency Ablation				
Krittayaphong et al,[70] 2003	30 patients with drug-refractory PeAF	RFA PVI	Amiodarone	1 y freedom from AF 79% vs 40% (P = .018)
Wazni et al,[71] 2005	70 patients with drug naïve PAF or PeAF	RFA PVI	AAD	1 y freedom from AF recurrence 87% vs 37% (P<.001) and hospitalization 9% vs 54% (P<.001).
Stabile et al,[72] 2006	137 patients with drug-refractory PAF or PeAF	RFA PVI + MI + AAD	AAD	1 y freedom from AA 56% vs 9% (P<.001)
Oral et al,[73] 2006	146 patients with PeAF	RFA PVI	Amiodarone + DCCV	1 y freedom from AA 74% vs 58% (P = .05)
Pappone et al,[74] 2006	198 patients with drug-refractory PAF	RFA PVI	AAD	1 y freedom from AA 86% vs 22% (P<.001)
Jaïs et al,[75] 2008	112 patients with drug-refractory PAF	RFA PVI	AAD	1 y freedom from AF 89% vs 23% (P<.001)
Forleo et al,[76] 2009	70 patients with T2DM + pAF or PeAF	RFA PVI	AAD	1 y freedom from AF 80% vs 43% (P = .001) and hospitalization 9% vs 34% (P = .01)
Wilber et al,[77] 2010	167 patients with drug-refractory PAF	RFA PVI	AAD	9 mo freedom from AF 66% vs 16% (P<.001)
MacDonald et al,[78] 2011	41 patients with PeAF with LVEF ≤35%	RFA PVI	± Digoxin	At mean 10 mo follow-up, freedom from AF 50% vs 0%. No difference in LVEF
Cosedis et al,[79] 2012	294 patients with drug-naïve PAF	RFA PVI	AAD	2 y freedom from AF 85% vs 71% (P = .004) and burden of AF 9% vs 18% (P = .007)
Mont et al,[80] 2014	146 patients with drug-refractory PeAF	RFA PVI	AAD	1 y freedom from AA 70% vs 44% (P = .002)
Morillo et al,[81] 2014	127 patients with drug-naïve PAF	RFA PVI	AAD	2 y freedom from AA 46% vs 28% (P = .02)
Di Biase et al,[30] 2016	203 patients with PeAF, ICD, and LVEF ≤40%	RFA PVI + PWI	Amiodarone	2 y freedom from AF 70% vs 34% (P<.001), hospitalization 31% vs 57% (P<.001), and mortality 8% vs 18% (P = .037)
Prabhu et al,[82] 2017	68 patients with PeAF and LVEF ≤45%	RFA PVI + PWI	Rate control	6 mo improvement in LVEF 18% vs 4% (P<.001)
Marrouche et al,[28] 2018	363 patients with PAF or PeAF and LVEF ≤35%	RFA PVI	Rate control or AAD	At median 38 mo follow-up, composite of death or HF hospitalization 29% vs 45% (P = .007) and death alone 13% vs 25% (P = .01)

(continued on next page)

Table 1
(continued)

Authors, Year	Study Population	Intervention	Control	Outcomes
Packer et al,[27] 2019	2204 patients with PAF or PeAF	RFA/CBA PVI	Rate control or AAD	At median 4 y follow-up, composite of death, stroke, major bleeding, or cardiac arrest 8% vs 9% (*P* = .3); freedom from AF recurrence 50% vs 31% (*P*<.001).
Kuck et al,[83] 2021	255 patients with drug-refractory PAF	RFA PVI	AAD	3 y progression from PAF to PeAF 2% vs 18% (*P*<.001)
Parkash et al,[84] 2022	411 patients with PAF or PeAF with HF	RFA PVI	Rate control	At median 37 mo follow-up, composite of death or HF event 23% vs 33% (*P* = .066)
Sohns et al,[29] 2023	194 patients with end-stage HF with LVEF ≤35%	RFA PVI	Rate control or AAD	At median 18 mo follow-up, composite of death, LVAD, or heart transplant 8% vs 30% (*P*<.001), death alone 6% vs 20%
Cryoballoon Ablation				
Packer et al,[85] 2013	245 patients with drug-refractory PAF or PeAF	CBA PVI	AAD	1 y freedom from AF 70% vs 7% (*P*<.001)
Kuck et al,[66] 2016	762 patients with drug-refractory PAF	CBA PVI	RFA PVI	1 y freedom from AA 65% vs 64% (*P*<.001 for non-inferiority) and primary safety end-point 10% vs 13% (*P* = .24)
Andrade et al,[86] 2020	303 patients with drug-naïve PAF	CBA PVI	AAD	1 y freedom from AA 57% vs 32% (*P*<.001). At 3 y follow-up, freedom from AA 44% vs 23%, hospitalizations 5% vs 17%
Wazni et al,[87] 2020	203 patients with drug-naïve PAF	CBA PVI	AAD	1 y freedom from AA 75% vs 45% (*P*<.001)
Kuniss et al,[88] 2021	218 patients with drug-naïve PAF	CBA PVI	AAD	1 y freedom from AA 82% vs 68% (*P* = .01)
Dulai et al,[89] 2024	126 patients with PAF and PeAF	CBA PVI	Sham ± DCCV	6 mo reduction in AF burden 60% vs 35% (*P*<.001) and AFEQT survey score 77 vs 58 (*P*<.05)
Pulsed Field Ablation				
Reddy et al,[32] 2023	607 patients with drug-refractory PAF	PFA PVI	RFA or CBA PVI	1 y freedom from AA 73% vs 71% (posterior probability of non-inferiority >0.999)
Anter et al,[90] 2024	420 patients with drug-refractory PeAF	PFA + RFA PVI ± PWI	RFA PVI ± PWI	1 y freedom from AA 74 vs 66% (*P*<.001 for non-inferiority)

Abbreviations: AA, atrial arrhythmia; AAD, anti-arrhythmic drug; AF, atrial fibrillation; AFEQT, Atrial Fibrillation Effect on Quality-Of-Life Questionnaire; CBA, cryoballoon ablation; DCCV, direct current cardioversion; GDMT, goal-directed medical therapy; HF, heart failure; ICD, implantable cardiac defibrillator; LVAD, left ventricular assist device; LVEF, left ventricular ejection fraction; MI, mitral isthmus; PAF, paroxysmal atrial fibrillation; PeAF, persistent atrial fibrillation; PFA, pulsed field ablation; PVI, pulmonary vein isolation; RFA, radiofrequency ablation; T2DM, Type 2 diabetes mellitus.

catheter stability in the remaining instances. Accordingly, in contrast to RFA, CBA outcomes are similar in both high-volume and low-volume centers.[31]

PFA for AF was initially reported in clinical studies in 2018. The ADVENT clinical trial randomized 607 patients with paroxysmal AF to PV isolation with PFA versus thermal ablation (**Table 2**).[32] There was no significant difference in freedom from recurrent atrial arrhythmia at 1 year (73% vs 71%). However, in a sub-analysis, the number of patients with an overall AF burden less than 0.1% was significantly higher following PFA than thermal ablation (82% vs 75%).[33] On average, PFA was 20 minutes shorter but required 7 more minutes of fluoroscopy versus thermal ablation. Incorporation of electroanatomic mapping with future PFA platforms should decrease fluoroscopy times and hopefully will decrease current cost, in the future. Similar to CBA, operator experience and procedural volume do not appear to significantly impact outcomes with PFA compared to RFA.[34]

Adjunctive Non-pulmonary Vein Ablation

PV isolation alone is only modestly effective in patients with persistent and long-standing persistent AF. Accordingly, adjunctive non-PV ablation has been investigated in these patients to improve efficacy (**Table 3**). RFA affords greater flexibility and precision in creating adjunctive, non-PV lesions than currently commercially available PFA or CBA catheters. This is particularly true when focal or linear lesions may be more appropriate, including for adjunctive ablation of atrial flutter and focal supraventricular tachycardias, especially atrioventricular nodal reentrant tachycardia. Approximately, 10% of patients with persistent AF have focal triggers outside the PV with common sites including the crista terminalis, mitral annulus, superior vena cava, the left atrial posterior wall (PW), and the left atrial appendage (LAA).[35] Although comprehensive identification and ablation of non-PV AF triggers have not been evaluated in randomized trials, observational data suggest that doing so can significantly decrease AF recurrence.[36]

Table 2
Clinical and procedural differences among radiofrequency, cryoballoon, and pulsed field pulmonary vein isolation for paroxysmal atrial fibrillation in a comparative randomized clinical trial

	Radiofrequency	Cryoballoon	Pulsed Field
Primary Mechanism of Tissue Injury	Thermal	Thermal	Non-thermal
Efficacy of Pulmonary Vein Isolation			
Acute procedural success	99.4%	99.3%	99.2%
1 y freedom from arrhythmia	69.2%	73.6%	73.1%
Atrial arrhythmia burden <0.1%[a]	74.1%	75.8%	81.9%
Complications			
Overall	2.4%	1.5%	2.3%
Serious	2.4%	0.0%	2.0%
Technical Aspects			
Learning curve	High	Low	Low
Procedure time (minutes)[a]	126	120	106
Left atrial dwell time (minutes)[a]	88	79	59
Total ablation time (minutes)[a]	54	45	29
Fluoroscopy time (minutes)[a]	12	16	21
Feasibility of Adjunctive Techniques			
Focal non-PV trigger ablation	High	Low	Low
Posterior wall isolation	High	Moderate	High
Left atrial appendage isolation	High	High	Unknown
Hybrid epicardial ablation	High	Unknown	Unknown
Ganglionated plexus modification	High	Unknown	Low

[a] Statistically significant difference among groups.
Data from Reddy VY, Gerstenfeld EP, Natale A, et al. Pulsed field or conventional thermal ablation for paroxysmal atrial fibrillation. N Engl J Med 2023;389(18):1660–71. https://doi.org/10.1056/NEJMoa2307291; and Reddy VY, Mansour M, Calkins H, et al. Pulsed field vs conventional thermal ablation for paroxysmal atrial fibrillation: recurrent atrial arrhythmia burden. J Am Coll Cardiol 2024;84(1):61–74. https://doi.org/10.1016/j.jacc.2024.05.001.

Table 3
Efficacy of adjunctive non-pulmonary vein ablation for atrial fibrillation in key clinical studies

Authors, Year	Study Type	Study Population	Intervention	Control	Outcomes
Focal Non-PV Ablation					
Narayan et al,[91] 2012	Observational	92 patients with PAF or PeAF	RFA PVI + focal impulse and rotor modulation	RFA PVI	At median 9 mo follow-up, freedom from AF 82% vs 45% (P<.001)
Verma et al,[37] 2015	Randomized	589 patients with PeAF	Arm 1: RFA PVI + fractionated EGMs Arm 2: RFA PVI + LA roof, MI lines	RFA PVI	1.5 y freedom from AF 49% vs 46% vs 59% (P = .15)
Vogler et al,[39] 2015	Randomized	205 patients with PeAF	RFA PVI + fractionated EGMs + step-wise linear RFA of LA, CS, and RA	RFA PVI	1 y freedom from AA 58% vs 61% (P = .71)
Hayashi et al,[36] 2015	Observational	59 patients with PAF and non-PV triggers	RFA PVI + non-PV triggers	RFA PVI	At mean 27 mo follow-up, freedom from AF 91% vs 32% (P<.001)
Marrouche et al,[38] 2022	Randomized	843 patients PeAF	RFA or CBA PVI + MRI-guided atrial fibrosis	RFA or CBA PVI	1.5 mo freedom from AA 57% vs 54% (P = .63)
Posterior Wall Isolation					
Kim et al,[41] 2015	Randomized	120 patients with PeAF	RFA PVI + LA linear + PWI	RFA PVI + LA linear	1 y freedom from AF 83% vs 63% (P = .02)
Lee et al,[92] 2019	Randomized	217 patients with PeAF	RFA PVI + PWI	RFA PVI	At mean 16 mo follow-up, freedom from AF 74% vs 76% (P = .78)
Aryana et al,[43] 2021	Randomized	110 patients with PeAF and LSPeAF	CBA/RFA PVI + PWI	CBA/RFA PVI	1 y freedom from AF 75% vs 55% (P = .028)
Kistler et al,[42] 2023	Randomized	338 patients with PeAF	RFA PVI + PWI	RFA PVI	1 y freedom from AA 52% vs 54% (P = .98)
Turagam et al,[46] 2024	Observational	547 patients with PeAF	PFA PVI + PWI	PFA PVI	1 y freedom from AA 66% vs 73% (P = .68)

Left Atrial Appendage Isolation

Study	Type	Patients	Intervention	Comparison	Outcome
Di Biase et al,[52] 2016	Randomized	173 patients with LSPeAF	RFA PVI + PWI + SVCI + LA linear + non-PV triggers + LAAI	RFA PVI + PWI + SVCI + LA linear + non-PV triggers	1 y freedom from AA 56% vs 28% (P = .001)
Yorgun et al,[53] 2017	Observational	100 patients with PeAF	CB PVI + LAAI	CBA PVI	1 y freedom from AA 86% vs 67% (P<.001)

Hybrid Epicardial Ablation

Study	Type	Patients	Intervention	Comparison	Outcome
DeLurgio et al,[47] 2020	Randomized	153 patients with PeAF and LSPeAF	Epicardial and Endocardial RFA PVI + PWI	Endocardial RFA PVI + LA roof	1 y freedom from AA 68% vs 50% (P = .036)
Doll et al,[48] 2023	Randomized	154 patients with PeAF and LSPeAF	Epicardial and Endocardial RFA PVI + PWI + LA lines + LAA exclusion	Endocardial RFA PVI ± adjunctive ablation	1 y freedom from AA 72% vs 39% (P<.001)
Heijden et al,[49] 2023	Randomized	41 patients with LSPeAF	Epicardial and Endocardial RFA PVI + PWI + LAA exclusion	Endocardial RFA PVI + PWI ± LA linear ablation	1 y freedom from AA 89% vs 41% (P = .002)

Ganglionated Plexus Modification

Study	Type	Patients	Intervention	Comparison	Outcome
Katritsis et al,[56] 2013	Randomized	242 patients with PAF	Arm 1: RFA PVI + LA GP Arm 2: RFA LA GP	RFA PVI	2 y freedom from AA 74% vs 48% vs 56% (P = .004)
Driessen et al,[57] 2016	Randomized	240 patients with PAF and PeAF	Epicardial RFA PVI ± Dallas lesion set + GPs	Epicardial RFA PVI ± Dallas lesion set	1 y freedom from AF 71% vs 68% (P = .70)
Sandler et al,[58] 2021	Randomized	67 patients with PAF	RFA ectopy-triggering GP	RFA PVI	1 y freedom from AA 49% vs 61% (P = .27)

Abbreviations: AA, atrial arrhythmia; AF, atrial fibrillation; CBA, cryoballoon; CS, coronary sinus; EGM, electrocardiogram; GP, ganglionated plexi; LA, left atrium; LAAI, left atrial appendage isolation; LSPeAF, long-standing persistent atrial fibrillation; PAF, paroxysmal atrial fibrillation; PeAF, persistent atrial fibrillation; PFA, pulsed field ablation; PV, pulmonary vein; PVI, pulmonary vein isolation; PWI, posterior wall isolation; RA, right atrium; RFA, radiofrequency ablation; SVCI, superior vena cava isolation.

Data from Turagam MK, Neuzil P, Schmidt B, et al. Impact of left atrial posterior wall ablation during pulsed-field ablation for persistent atrial fibrillation. JACC Clin Electrophysiol 2024;10(5):900–12. https://doi.org/10.1016/j.jacep.2024.01.017.

Table 4
Safety of radiofrequency, cryoballoon, and pulsed field ablation for atrial fibrillation in contemporary registries

	Real-AF[62]	Cryo AF Global[63]	NCDR[64]	MANIFEST-17K[65]
Demographic				
Ablation Energy	Radiofrequency	Cryothermal	Thermal	Pulsed field
Years of Enrollment	2018–2022	2016–2020	2016–2020	2022–2023
Patients	2470	2922	76,219	17,642
Age (years, mean)	65	61	66	64
Female	44%	36%	35%	35%
Safety				
Overall complications	1.90%	-	2.50%	4.19%
Major complications	-	3.40%	-	0.98%
Arrhythmia	-	1.60%	-	-
Vascular	0.50%	0.70%	0.80%	2.50%
Pericarditis	0.50%	0.20%	-	0.17%
Effusion/Tamponade	0.20%	0.40%	0.44%	0.69%
Pulmonary vein stenosis	0.12%	0%	-	0%
Phrenic nerve injury	0.08%	0.50%	0.02%	0.06%
Esophageal injury	0.08%	0.03%	-	0%
Stroke/transient ischemic attack	0%	0.20%	0.11%	0.24%
Coronary vasospasm	-	-	-	0.14%
Hemolysis renal failure	-	-	-	0.04%
Death	0%	0.03%	0.05%	0.03%

Data from Refs.[62–65]

Several clinical trials have investigated the utility of adjunctive substrate modification compared to PV isolation alone. Areas of complex, fractionated electrograms or atrial fibrosis detected by cardiac magnetic resonance imaging may represent abnormal atrial substrate that is helping initiate or maintain AF; however, RFA targeting these areas has not improved outcomes.[37,38] Similarly, creating multiple linear left atrial lesions with RFA to mimic atrial debulking achieved in surgical Cox-Maze procedures also has not consistently improved clinical outcomes.[37,39]

The posterior left atrium has similar embryologic origins to PVs and is prone to interstitial fibrosis making it a potential source of both AF triggers and substrate for maintenance.[40] However, catheter-based PW isolation has demonstrated inconsistent incremental benefit compared to PV isolation alone.[41,42] This inconsistency is, in large part, due to inherent challenges in safely creating durable, transmural lesions using thermal energy sources endocardially without risking esophageal injury.[42,43] Further, atrial tissue in the PW, particularly at the roof, is thick and surrounded by epicardial fat, often with epicardial connections that are difficult to disrupt endocardially.[44,45] Although PFA has been very successful in achieving acute PW isolation with substantially less concern for esophageal injury, a recent analysis of the Manifest-PF Registry demonstrated no clinical benefit compared to PV isolation alone (see **Table 3**).[46]

The comparative success of surgical ablation involving the PW in patients with persistent AF supports the need to create transmural lesions in this area to improve clinical outcomes. Hybrid epicardial and endocardial RFA with both PV and PW isolation is more effective than endocardial PV isolation alone.[47] Additional exclusion of the LAA also appears to add incremental benefit.[48,49] The LAA can be a common source of non-PV triggers with extensive pectinate muscles and heterogenous fiber orientation also facilitating reentry and AF maintenance.[50,51] LAA isolation can be accomplished effectively with all of the energy modalities, although reports of improved clinical outcomes compared to PV isolation alone have only been published using thermal ablation to date.[52,53] Notably, LAA isolation has been associated with a higher incidence of cardiac perforation and stroke in some cohorts.[51,54] The increased risk of stroke highlights the importance of uninterrupted anticoagulation or LAA occlusion following LAA isolation.

The intrinsic cardiac autonomic nervous system is made up of interconnected ganglionated plexi. Hyperactivity in the 4 major ganglionated plexi that innervate PV myocardial sleeves may contribute to AF initiation and maintenance.[55] RFA of these ganglionated plexi has demonstrated variable incremental benefit compared to PV isolation alone, likely underscoring the mechanistic variability of AF and importance of patient selection.[56–58] CBA affects the left atrial ganglionated plexi but has not been evaluated in clinical studies due to its limited versatility in mapping and ablation.[59] In contrast to thermal ablation, PFA has minimal effect on ganglionated plexi given its tissue selectivity.[60]

Complications

The rate of procedural complications from AF catheter ablation has dramatically improved with refinements in ablation technique, catheter technology, and operator experience. A meta-analysis of randomized controlled trials of thermal ablation for AF from 2012 to 2022 demonstrated significant improvement in rates of complications overtime.[61] The overall and major complication rate in the last 5 years was 3.8% and 1.9%, respectively.[61] Analogously, contemporary registry data have demonstrated similarly low rate of complications (**Table 4**).[62–65] The overall rate of major complications is similar between thermal energy sources and PFA, with notable except that CBA confers higher risk of phrenic nerve injury compared to either of the other modalities, and there have been no reports to date of esophageal injury, persistent phrenic nerve injury, or significant PV stenosis with PFA.[32,65,66]

Notably, PFA does cause some heating, and there is potential for thermal injury with higher energy applications and stacked lesions, which may account for reports of transient phrenic nerve injury.[65] The risk attributable to individual PFA platforms, with highly variable and proprietary electric field strengths and pulse characteristics, remains to be seen. Two unique complications of PFA are coronary artery vasospasm and acute renal failure from hemolysis. Coronary vasospasm is predominantly subclinical and can be attenuated with nitroglycerin, but clinical studies assessing the long-term risk of coronary stenosis are needed.[67] Acute kidney injury from hemolysis is closely related to the number of PFA applications and can be attenuated with post-ablation hydration.[68,69]

SUMMARY

Radiofrequency, cryothermal, and pulsed-field energies have been approximately equally effective in achieving durable PV isolation and freedom from recurrent atrial arrhythmias in patients with AF. The learning curve for CBA or PFA in AF ablations tends to be less than that for RFA. PFA, using currently available platforms, is associated with the greatest efficiency in terms of procedure and left atrial dwell times, whereas RFA incurs the least fluoroscopy exposure. RFA allows the greatest versatility for mapping and ablation, especially of focal, non-PV areas. CBA appears to have a higher risk of persistent phrenic nerve injury than either RFA or PFA. The tissue selectivity and mechanism of cellular injury of PFA appear to reduce the risks of esophageal injury, persistent phrenic nerve injury, or PV stenosis that are rarely observed with thermal ablation. However, PFA confers unique risks of coronary vasospasm and acute renal failure from hemolysis that require additional studies to assess long-term consequences.

CLINICS CARE POINTS

- PFA can effectively and efficiently control AF in most patients, but current platforms lack the versatility of radiofrequency energy, especially in ablating non-PV areas for which more focal lesions may be more beneficial.

- The overall risk of collateral injury to pericardiac structures with currently available PFA platforms appears low, although risk with future platforms employing highly variable catheter designs and energy delivery characteristics remains to be seen.

- Coronary vasospasm and hemolysis-induced kidney injury are additional risk considerations to mitigate when utilizing PFA.

DISCLOSURES

Dr W.S. Tzou has served on Advisory Board, as Consultant, or received research funding or speaker honoraria from Abbott, American Heart Association, American College of Cardiology, Bayer, Biosense Webster, Biotronik, Boston Scientific, Kardium, Medtronic, and Varian. Dr K. Padalia has no relevant disclosures.

REFERENCES

1. Huang SK, Bharati S, Graham AR, et al. Closed chest catheter desiccation of the atrioventricular junction using radiofrequency energy–a new method of catheter ablation. J Am Coll Cardiol 1987;9(2): 349–58.
2. Haemmerich D. Biophysics of radiofrequency ablation. Crit Rev Biomed Eng 2010;38(1):53–63.

3. Bourier F, Ramirez FD, Martin CA, et al. Impedance, power, and current in radiofrequency ablation: insights from technical, ex vivo, and clinical studies. J Cardiovasc Electrophysiol 2020;31(11):2836–45.

4. Borne RT, Sauer WH, Zipse MM, et al. Longer duration versus increasing power during radiofrequency ablation yields different ablation lesion characteristics. JACC Clin Electrophysiol 2018;4(7):902–8.

5. Haines DE. The biophysics of radiofrequency catheter ablation in the heart: the importance of temperature monitoring. Pacing Clin Electrophysiol 1993; 16(3 Pt 2):586–91.

6. Cappato R, Ali H. Surveys and registries on catheter ablation of atrial fibrillation: fifteen years of history. Circ Arrhythm Electrophysiol 2021;14(1):e008073.

7. Dorwarth U, Fiek M, Remp T, et al. Radiofrequency catheter ablation: different cooled and noncooled electrode systems induce specific lesion geometries and adverse effects profiles. Pacing Clin Electrophysiol 2003;26(7 Pt 1):1438–45.

8. Afzal MR, Chatta J, Samanta A, et al. Use of contact force sensing technology during radiofrequency ablation reduces recurrence of atrial fibrillation: a systematic review and meta-analysis. Heart Rhythm 2015;12(9):1990–6.

9. Nakagawa H, Yamanashi WS, Pitha JV, et al. Comparison of in vivo tissue temperature profile and lesion geometry for radiofrequency ablation with a saline-irrigated electrode versus temperature control in a canine thigh muscle preparation. Circulation 1995; 91(8):2264–73.

10. Leshem E, Zilberman I, Tschabrunn CM, et al. High-power and short-duration ablation for pulmonary vein isolation: biophysical characterization. JACC Clin Electrophysiol 2018;4(4):467–79.

11. Ravi V, Poudyal A, Abid QU, et al. High-power short duration vs. conventional radiofrequency ablation of atrial fibrillation: a systematic review and meta-analysis. Europace 2021;23(5):710–21.

12. Andrade JG, Dubuc M, Guerra PG, et al. The biophysics and biomechanics of cryoballoon ablation. Pacing Clin Electrophysiol 2012;35(9):1162–8.

13. Andrade JG, Wazni OM, Kuniss M, et al. Cryoballoon ablation as initial treatment for atrial fibrillation: JACC state-of-the-art review. J Am Coll Cardiol 2021;78(9): 914–30.

14. Takami M, Misiri J, Lehmann HI, et al. Spatial and time-course thermodynamics during pulmonary vein isolation using the second-generation cryoballoon in a canine in vivo model. Circ Arrhythm Electrophysiol 2015;8(1):186–92.

15. Aryana A, Mugnai G, Singh SM, et al. Procedural and biophysical indicators of durable pulmonary vein isolation during cryoballoon ablation of atrial fibrillation. Heart Rhythm 2016;13(2):424–32.

16. Straube F, Dorwarth U, Schmidt M, et al. Comparison of the first and second cryoballoon: high-volume single-center safety and efficacy analysis. Circ Arrhythm Electrophysiol 2014;7(2):293–9.

17. Kenigsberg DN, Martin N, Lim HW, et al. Quantification of the cryoablation zone demarcated by pre- and post-procedural electroanatomic mapping in patients with atrial fibrillation using the 28-mm second-generation cryoballoon. Heart Rhythm 2015;12(2):283–90.

18. Haïssaguerre M, Jaïs P, Shah DC, et al. Spontaneous initiation of atrial fibrillation by ectopic beats originating in the pulmonary veins. N Engl J Med 1998;339(10):659–66.

19. Chen SA, Hsieh MH, Tai CT, et al. Initiation of atrial fibrillation by ectopic beats originating from the pulmonary veins: electrophysiological characteristics, pharmacological responses, and effects of radiofrequency ablation. Circulation 1999;100(18):1879–86.

20. Pappone C, Rosanio S, Oreto G, et al. Circumferential radiofrequency ablation of pulmonary vein ostia: a new anatomic approach for curing atrial fibrillation. Circulation 2000;102(21):2619–28.

21. Proietti R, Santangeli P, Di Biase L, et al. Comparative effectiveness of wide antral versus ostial pulmonary vein isolation: a systematic review and meta-analysis. Circ Arrhythm Electrophysiol 2014;7(1):39–45.

22. Clarnette JA, Brooks AG, Mahajan R, et al. Outcomes of persistent and long-standing persistent atrial fibrillation ablation: a systematic review and meta-analysis. Europace 2018;20(Fi_3):f366–76.

23. Imberti JF, Ding WY, Kotalczyk A, et al. Catheter ablation as first-line treatment for paroxysmal atrial fibrillation: a systematic review and meta-analysis. Heart 2021;107(20):1630–6.

24. Brooks AG, Stiles MK, Laborderie J, et al. Outcomes of long-standing persistent atrial fibrillation ablation: a systematic review. Heart Rhythm 2010;7(6):835–46.

25. Michaud GF, Stevenson WG. Atrial fibrillation. N Engl J Med 2021;384(4):353–61.

26. Turagam MK, Musikantow D, Whang W, et al. Assessment of catheter ablation or antiarrhythmic drugs for first-line therapy of atrial fibrillation: a meta-analysis of randomized clinical trials. JAMA Cardiol 2021; 6(6):697–705.

27. Packer DL, Mark DB, Robb RA, et al. Effect of catheter ablation vs antiarrhythmic drug therapy on mortality, stroke, bleeding, and cardiac arrest among patients with atrial fibrillation: the CABANA randomized clinical trial. JAMA 2019;321(13):1261–74.

28. Marrouche NF, Brachmann J, Andresen D, et al. Catheter ablation for atrial fibrillation with heart failure. N Engl J Med 2018;378(5):417–27.

29. Sohns C, Fox H, Marrouche NF, et al. Catheter ablation in end-stage heart failure with atrial fibrillation. N Engl J Med 2023;389(15):1380–9.

30. Di Biase L, Mohanty P, Mohanty S, et al. Ablation versus amiodarone for treatment of persistent atrial fibrillation in patients with congestive heart failure and an implanted device: results from the AATAC

multicenter randomized trial. Circulation 2016;133(17): 1637–44.

31. Providencia R, Defaye P, Lambiase PD, et al. Results from a multicentre comparison of cryoballoon vs. radiofrequency ablation for paroxysmal atrial fibrillation: is cryoablation more reproducible? Europace 2017;19(1):48–57.

32. Reddy VY, Gerstenfeld EP, Natale A, et al. Pulsed field or conventional thermal ablation for paroxysmal atrial fibrillation. N Engl J Med 2023;389(18):1660–71.

33. Reddy VY, Mansour M, Calkins H, et al. Pulsed field vs conventional thermal ablation for paroxysmal atrial fibrillation: recurrent atrial arrhythmia burden. J Am Coll Cardiol 2024;84(1):61–74.

34. Turagam MK, Neuzil P, Schmidt B, et al. Safety and effectiveness of pulsed field ablation to treat atrial fibrillation: one-year outcomes from the MANIFEST-PF Registry. Circulation 2023;148(1):35–46.

35. Santangeli P, Zado ES, Hutchinson MD, et al. Prevalence and distribution of focal triggers in persistent and long-standing persistent atrial fibrillation. Heart Rhythm 2016;13(2):374–82.

36. Hayashi K, An Y, Nagashima M, et al. Importance of nonpulmonary vein foci in catheter ablation for paroxysmal atrial fibrillation. Heart Rhythm 2015;12(9): 1918–24.

37. Verma A, Jiang CY, Betts TR, et al. Approaches to catheter ablation for persistent atrial fibrillation. N Engl J Med 2015;372(19):1812–22.

38. Marrouche NF, Wazni O, McGann C, et al. Effect of MRI-guided fibrosis ablation vs conventional catheter ablation on atrial arrhythmia recurrence in patients with persistent atrial fibrillation: the DECAAF II Randomized Clinical Trial. JAMA 2022;327(23): 2296–305.

39. Vogler J, Willems S, Sultan A, et al. Pulmonary vein isolation versus defragmentation: the CHASE-AF Clinical Trial. J Am Coll Cardiol 2015;66(24):2743–52.

40. Benito EM, Cabanelas N, Nuñez-Garcia M, et al. Preferential regional distribution of atrial fibrosis in posterior wall around left inferior pulmonary vein as identified by late gadolinium enhancement cardiac magnetic resonance in patients with atrial fibrillation. Europace 2018;20(12):1959–65.

41. Kim JS, Shin SY, Na JO, et al. Does isolation of the left atrial posterior wall improve clinical outcomes after radiofrequency catheter ablation for persistent atrial fibrillation?: a prospective randomized clinical trial. Int J Cardiol 2015;181:277–83.

42. Kistler PM, Chieng D, Sugumar H, et al. Effect of catheter ablation using pulmonary vein isolation with vs without posterior left atrial wall isolation on atrial arrhythmia recurrence in patients with persistent atrial fibrillation: the CAPLA Randomized Clinical Trial. JAMA 2023;329(2):127–35.

43. Aryana A, Allen SL, Pujara DK, et al. Concomitant pulmonary vein and posterior wall isolation using cryoballoon with adjunct radiofrequency in persistent atrial fibrillation. JACC Clin Electrophysiol 2021;7(2): 187–96.

44. Ho SY, Cabrera JA, Sanchez-Quintana D. Left atrial anatomy revisited. Circ Arrhythm Electrophysiol 2012; 5(1):220–8.

45. Barrio-Lopez MT, Sanchez-Quintana D, Garcia-Martinez J, et al. Epicardial connections involving pulmonary veins: the prevalence, predictors, and implications for ablation outcome. Circ Arrhythm Electrophysiol 2020;13(1):e007544.

46. Turagam MK, Neuzil P, Schmidt B, et al. Impact of left atrial posterior wall ablation during pulsed-field ablation for persistent atrial fibrillation. JACC Clin Electrophysiol 2024;10(5):900–12.

47. DeLurgio DB, Crossen KJ, Gill J, et al. Hybrid convergent procedure for the treatment of persistent and long-standing persistent atrial fibrillation: results of CONVERGE Clinical Trial. Circ Arrhythm Electrophysiol 2020;13(12):e009288.

48. Doll N, Weimar T, Kosior DA, et al. Efficacy and safety of hybrid epicardial and endocardial ablation versus endocardial ablation in patients with persistent and longstanding persistent atrial fibrillation: a randomised, controlled trial. EClinicalMedicine 2023;61: 102052.

49. van der Heijden CAJ, Weberndörfer V, Vroomen M, et al. Hybrid ablation versus repeated catheter ablation in persistent atrial fibrillation: a randomized controlled trial. JACC Clin Electrophysiol 2023;9(7 Pt 2):1013–23.

50. Krul SP, Berger WR, Smit NW, et al. Atrial fibrosis and conduction slowing in the left atrial appendage of patients undergoing thoracoscopic surgical pulmonary vein isolation for atrial fibrillation. Circ Arrhythm Electrophysiol 2015;8(2):288–95.

51. Di Biase L, Burkhardt JD, Mohanty P, et al. Left atrial appendage: an underrecognized trigger site of atrial fibrillation. Circulation 2010;122(2):109–18.

52. Di Biase L, Burkhardt JD, Mohanty P, et al. Left atrial appendage isolation in patients with longstanding persistent AF undergoing catheter ablation: BELIEF Trial. J Am Coll Cardiol 2016;68(18):1929–40.

53. Yorgun H, Canpolat U, Kocyigit D, et al. Left atrial appendage isolation in addition to pulmonary vein isolation in persistent atrial fibrillation: one-year clinical outcome after cryoballoon-based ablation. Europace 2017;19(5):758–68.

54. Kim YG, Shim J, Oh SK, et al. Electrical isolation of the left atrial appendage increases the risk of ischemic stroke and transient ischemic attack regardless of postisolation flow velocity. Heart Rhythm 2018; 15(12):1746–53.

55. Stavrakis S, Nakagawa H, Po SS, et al. The role of the autonomic ganglia in atrial fibrillation. JACC Clin Electrophysiol 2015;1(1–2):1–13.

56. Katritsis DG, Giazitzoglou E, Zografos T, et al. Rapid pulmonary vein isolation combined with autonomic

ganglia modification: a randomized study. Heart Rhythm 2011;8(5):672–8.

57. Driessen AHG, Berger WR, Krul SPJ, et al. Ganglion plexus ablation in advanced atrial fibrillation: the AFACT Study. J Am Coll Cardiol 2016;68(11):1155–65.

58. Sandler B, Kim MY, Sikkel MB, et al. Targeting the ectopy-triggering ganglionated plexuses without pulmonary vein isolation prevents atrial fibrillation. J Cardiovasc Electrophysiol 2021;32(2):235–44.

59. Garabelli P, Stavrakis S, Kenney JFA, et al. Effect of 28-mm cryoballoon ablation on major atrial ganglionated plexi. JACC Clin Electrophysiol 2018;4(6):831–8.

60. Gerstenfeld EP, Mansour M, Whang W, et al. Autonomic effects of pulsed field vs thermal ablation for treating atrial fibrillation: subanalysis of ADVENT. JACC Clin Electrophysiol 2024;10(7 Pt 2):1634–44.

61. Benali K, Khairy P, Hammache N, et al. Procedure-related complications of catheter ablation for atrial fibrillation. J Am Coll Cardiol 2023;81(21):2089–99.

62. Osorio J, Miranda-Arboleda AF, Velasco A, et al. Real-world data of radiofrequency catheter ablation in paroxysmal atrial fibrillation: short- and long-term clinical outcomes from the prospective multicenter REAL-AF Registry. Heart Rhythm 2024. https://doi.org/10.1016/j.hrthm.2024.04.090.

63. Chun KRJ, Okumura K, Scazzuso F, et al. Safety and efficacy of cryoballoon ablation for the treatment of paroxysmal and persistent AF in a real-world global setting: results from the Cryo AF Global Registry. J Arrhythm 2021;37(2):356–67.

64. Hsu JC, Darden D, Du C, et al. Initial findings from the national cardiovascular data registry of atrial fibrillation ablation procedures. J Am Coll Cardiol 2023;81(9):867–78.

65. Ekanem E, Neuzil P, Reichlin T, et al. Safety of pulsed field ablation in more than 17,000 patients with atrial fibrillation in the MANIFEST-17K study. Nat Med 2024;30(7):2020–9.

66. Kuck KH, Brugada J, Fürnkranz A, et al. Cryoballoon or radiofrequency ablation for paroxysmal atrial fibrillation. N Engl J Med 2016;374(23):2235–45.

67. Reddy VY, Petru J, Funasako M, et al. Coronary arterial spasm during pulsed field ablation to treat atrial fibrillation. Circulation 2022;146(24):1808–19.

68. Popa MA, Venier S, Menè R, et al. Characterization and clinical significance of hemolysis after pulsed field ablation for atrial fibrillation: results of a multicenter analysis. Circ Arrhythm Electrophysiol 2024;17(10):e012732.

69. Mohanty S, Casella M, Compagnucci P, et al. Acute kidney injury resulting from hemoglobinuria after pulsed-field ablation in atrial fibrillation: is it preventable? JACC Clin Electrophysiol 2024;10(4):709–15.

70. Krittayaphong R, Raungrattanaamporn O, Bhuripanyo K, et al. A randomized clinical trial of the efficacy of radiofrequency catheter ablation and amiodarone in the treatment of symptomatic atrial fibrillation. J Med Assoc Thai 2003;86(Suppl 1):S8–16.

71. Wazni OM, Marrouche NF, Martin DO, et al. Radiofrequency ablation vs antiarrhythmic drugs as first-line treatment of symptomatic atrial fibrillation: a randomized trial. JAMA 2005;293(21):2634–40.

72. Stabile G, Bertaglia E, Senatore G, et al. Catheter ablation treatment in patients with drug-refractory atrial fibrillation: a prospective, multi-centre, randomized, controlled study (Catheter Ablation for the Cure of Atrial Fibrillation Study). Eur Heart J 2006;27(2):216–21.

73. Oral H, Pappone C, Chugh A, et al. Circumferential pulmonary-vein ablation for chronic atrial fibrillation. N Engl J Med 2006;354(9):934–41.

74. Pappone C, Augello G, Sala S, et al. A randomized trial of circumferential pulmonary vein ablation versus antiarrhythmic drug therapy in paroxysmal atrial fibrillation: the APAF Study. J Am Coll Cardiol 2006;48(11):2340–7.

75. Jaïs P, Cauchemez B, Macle L, et al. Catheter ablation versus antiarrhythmic drugs for atrial fibrillation: the A4 study. Circulation 2008;118(24):2498–505.

76. Forleo GB, Mantica M, De Luca L, et al. Catheter ablation of atrial fibrillation in patients with diabetes mellitus type 2: results from a randomized study comparing pulmonary vein isolation versus antiarrhythmic drug therapy. J Cardiovasc Electrophysiol 2009;20(1):22–8.

77. Wilber DJ, Pappone C, Neuzil P, et al. Comparison of antiarrhythmic drug therapy and radiofrequency catheter ablation in patients with paroxysmal atrial fibrillation: a randomized controlled trial. JAMA 2010;303(4):333–40.

78. MacDonald MR, Connelly DT, Hawkins NM, et al. Radiofrequency ablation for persistent atrial fibrillation in patients with advanced heart failure and severe left ventricular systolic dysfunction: a randomised controlled trial. Heart 2011;97(9):740–7.

79. Cosedis Nielsen J, Johannessen A, Raatikainen P, et al. Radiofrequency ablation as initial therapy in paroxysmal atrial fibrillation. N Engl J Med 2012;367(17):1587–95.

80. Mont L, Bisbal F, Hernández-Madrid A, et al. Catheter ablation vs. antiarrhythmic drug treatment of persistent atrial fibrillation: a multicentre, randomized, controlled trial (SARA study). Eur Heart J 2014;35(8):501–7.

81. Morillo CA, Verma A, Connolly SJ, et al. Radiofrequency ablation vs antiarrhythmic drugs as first-line treatment of paroxysmal atrial fibrillation (RAAFT-2): a randomized trial. JAMA 2014;311(7):692–700.

82. Prabhu S, Taylor AJ, Costello BT, et al. Catheter ablation versus medical rate control in atrial fibrillation and systolic dysfunction: the CAMERA-MRI Study. J Am Coll Cardiol 2017;70(16):1949–61.

83. Kuck KH, Lebedev DS, Mikhaylov EN, et al. Catheter ablation or medical therapy to delay progression of

atrial fibrillation: the randomized controlled atrial fibrillation progression trial (ATTEST). Europace 2021; 23(3):362–9.

84. Parkash R, Wells GA, Rouleau J, et al. Randomized ablation-based rhythm-control versus rate-control trial in patients with heart failure and atrial fibrillation: results from the RAFT-AF trial. Circulation 2022; 145(23):1693–704.

85. Packer DL, Kowal RC, Wheelan KR, et al. Cryoballoon ablation of pulmonary veins for paroxysmal atrial fibrillation: first results of the North American Arctic Front (STOP AF) pivotal trial. J Am Coll Cardiol 2013;61(16):1713–23.

86. Andrade JG, Wells GA, Deyell MW, et al. Cryoablation or drug therapy for initial treatment of atrial fibrillation. N Engl J Med 2021;384(4):305–15.

87. Wazni OM, Dandamudi G, Sood N, et al. Cryoballoon ablation as initial therapy for atrial fibrillation. N Engl J Med 2021;384(4):316–24.

88. Kuniss M, Pavlovic N, Velagic V, et al. Cryoballoon ablation vs. antiarrhythmic drugs: first-line therapy for patients with paroxysmal atrial fibrillation. Europace 2021;23(7):1033–41.

89. Dulai R, Sulke N, Freemantle N, et al. Pulmonary vein isolation vs sham intervention in symptomatic atrial fibrillation: the SHAM-PVI randomized clinical trial. JAMA 2024. https://doi.org/10.1001/jama.2024.17921.

90. Anter E, Mansour M, Nair DG, et al. Dual-energy lattice-tip ablation system for persistent atrial fibrillation: a randomized trial. Nat Med 2024;30(8):2303–10.

91. Narayan SM, Krummen DE, Shivkumar K, et al. Treatment of atrial fibrillation by the ablation of localized sources: CONFIRM (conventional ablation for atrial fibrillation with or without focal impulse and rotor modulation) trial. J Am Coll Cardiol 2012;60(7):628–36.

92. Lee JM, Shim J, Park J, et al. The electrical isolation of the left atrial posterior wall in catheter ablation of persistent atrial fibrillation. JACC Clin Electrophysiol 2019;5(11):1253–61.

Efficiency of Pulsed Field Ablation for Atrial Fibrillation

Alexandra Steyer, MD[a], Kyoung-Ryul Julian Chun, MD[a,b], D. Schaack, MD[a], Boris Schmidt, MD, FHRS[a,c],*

KEYWORDS

• PFA • Efficiency • Durability • Remapping

KEY POINTS

• Ablation results of current, first generation pulsed field ablation (PFA) catheters are associated with high durability rates and similar clinical outcomes in terms of freedom from arrhythmias.
• In the past, improved pulmonay vein isolation (PVI) durability was suggested. A lack of large, prospective or randomised trials however, hinder comprehensive analysis of overall PFA efficacy.
• PFA appears to deliver comparable effectiveness to particularly cryoballon with however, shorter procedure times and robust saffety profile, making it a compelling technology.

BACKGROUND

Pulsed field ablation (PFA) has recently emerged as a viable energy source for catheter ablation particularly of atrial fibrillation (AF).[1,2] The development of new catheters and optimization of pulse parameters have increasingly spurred the interest surrounding this technology.[2] Electroporation is created by applying a local high voltage, nanosecond pulsed electric field across a cellular membrane with transient membrane destabilization and cell death.[3] Early in vitro and animal models supported the notion of a greater cardiomyocyte susceptibility.[4,5] Followingly, consecutive clinical trials could demonstrate subsidiary esophageal injury and the apparent absence of nontransient phrenic nerve palsy.[6–8] The overall safety and noninferiority of this energy source for pulmonary vein isolation (PVI) compared to previously established thermal methods has been demonstrated in several trials.[6,9,10]

Further refinements of PFA technology, approval of multiple novel catheters and growing availability of outcome data have enabled first deductions on the performance of this energy source for PVI. Regarding general therapeutic efficacy, PFA should be considered in terms of lesion durability and freedom from arrhythmia. Furthermore, comparison of PFA to preexisting ablation methods and in different temporal AF patterns is necessary to contextualize the current placement of this technology.[8] The need for further development of efficient PVI approaches is strengthened by increasing AF incidence, overburdened health care systems, and an aging population with growing life expectancy and hence a larger lifetime risk of AF.[11]

LESION DURABILITY
Single-Shot Pulsed Field Ablation

In an attempt to understand and accordingly improve PFA lesion durability remapping studies

a Department of Cardiology, Cardioangiologisches Centrum Bethanien, Wilhelm-Epstein Str. 4, Frankfurt/Main 60431, Germany; b Clinic for Rhythmologie, University Hospital Lübeck, Schleswig-Holstein, Ratzberger Allee 160, 23538 Lübeck, Germany; c Department of Cardiology, University Hospital Frankfurt, Theodor-Stern-Kai 7, 60596 Frankfurt, Germany
* Corresponding author.
E-mail address: b.schmidt@ccb.de
Twitter: @borisschmidt5

Card Electrophysiol Clin 17 (2025) 183–190
https://doi.org/10.1016/j.ccep.2025.02.006
1877-9182/25/© 2025 Elsevier Inc. All rights are reserved, including those for text and data mining, AI training, and similar technologies.

were initiated. In a first-in-human trial using a pentaspline PFA catheter with an optimized waveform durable PVI was demonstrated 93.0 ± 30.1 days after the index procedure in 96% of pulmonary veins (PVs). This resulted in complete electrical PVI of all PVs in 84.1% of patients.[10] Since then, most data on PVI durability emerged from remapping during repeat procedures for recurrent arrhythmia. Furthermore, the nonstandardized dosing and mode of PFA application in terms of pulse parameters and catheter configuration in most premarket trials warrants consideration when interpreting ensuing durability data. Subanalyses from repeat procedures after pentaspline PFA PVI in patients with recurrent arrhythmia within a large European registry showed durable PVI in 54/149 (36%) patients and 72% of PVs.[12,13] These divergent findings may be attributed to selection bias due to performing repeat procedures only when clinically indicated in patients with documented recurrent atrial arrhythmia. Furthermore, the latter trial performed repeat procedures exclusively outside of the blanking period (median of 226 days, interquartile range [IQR] 157–292) and included all AF patients irrespective of temporal AF classification. These observations are largely comparable to other trials reporting on repeat ablation procedures.[6,13–16] An overview of PVI durability from relevant trials including data from repeat procedures can be seen in **Fig. 1**. A targeted remapping study performed in patients receiving repeat ablation due to recurrent atrial arrhythmia after PVI via PFA reported an overall PV reconnection in 9/99 (9.1%) PVs and durable PVI in 19/25 (76%) of patients.[16] A dominant proportion (16/25 patients) however, presented with atrial tachycardia (AT) and thus an overall greater number of durable PVI. Most reconnections were attributed to gaps in the left superior pulmonary vein (LSPV) and were associated with the use of the 35 mm rather than the 31 mm FARAWAVE catheter. As for recurrent AT, the posterior wall was identified as the most common critical isthmus with localized reentry particularly between previous PVI lesions. In terms of additive linear lesions using the same catheter, the PerAF trial, reported durable left atrial

posterior wall (LAPW) ablation and cavotricuspid isthmus (CTI) ablation in 21/22 and 9/12 3 months after the index procedure in patients with persistent AF.[17] Linear LAPW ablation was performed using a pentaspline catheter whereas CTI was achieved via a focal PFA application. Concerning the comparison of PVI durability rates after index PFA and thermal ablation, a single center observational study with 145 patients undergoing repeat procedures reported of significantly less PV reconnections after pentaspline PFA (19.1% vs 27.5% and 34.8% of PVs for PFA, fourth-generation cryoballoon and radiofrequency [RF] ablation respectively).[18] These findings were contrary to the only randomized trial comparing PFA with thermal ablation, showing no divergent PVI durability in a small group of 34/607 patients receiving a repeat procedure.[6] The finalized results from a prospective remapping trial comparing both RF and PFA in persistent AF patients with compulsory repeat procedures irrespective of arrhythmia recurrence are currently being awaited.[19] The InspIRE trial implementing a different, variable-loop PFA catheter (Inspire Biosense Webster), showed a greater number of reconnections in 69.2% (27/39) of PVs; however, only a minor patient group receiving PFA with the optimized waveform underwent repeat procedure (10/186).[20] Using yet another ablation system with a novel spherical multielectrode array catheter (Globe PF, Kardium), Turagam and colleagues recently showed 100% PVI durability in a small sample of mandated remapping procedures after application of an optimized 3 PF-pulses per PV.[21] Overall, it must be said that data on durability from repeat procedures after PFA is limited, particularly in the case of systematic remapping. Furthermore, most available data on durability stems from repeat procedures after ablation with the FARAPULSE system (Boston Scientific).

Data from Focal Pulsed Field Ablation Catheters

A first in-human trial using a centrally irrigated spherical lattice catheter with the ability to toggle between PFA and RF-ablation could show durable PVI in 97% of PVs (n = 124) receiving the most optimized waveform and mandated remapping.[22] This trial enrolled a greater proportion of patients with persistent AF (108/178) and allowed for additional linear lesions if indicated by the operator. Both a combined RF/PFA and a purely PFA approach were employed, demonstrating comparable results in terms of PVI durability at remapping. Recently, early results from the use of another lattice-tip catheter with a larger diameter (34 mm compared to 9 mm with the Sphere-9 catheter,

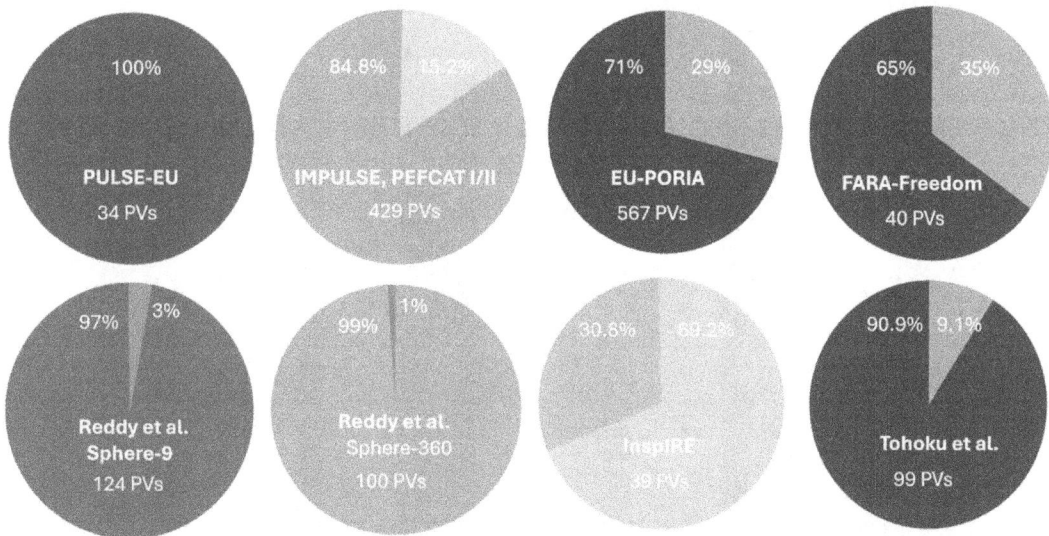

Fig. 1. An overview of PVI durability and PV reconnection from trials including data from repeat procedures. The top row includes data from a subgroup in FARA-Freedom and a subanalysis of the EU-PORIA as well as systematic remapping findings from the pooled IMPULSE, PEFCAT I/II trials (*lighter blue*). All trials implementing the FARA-PULSE Boston Scientific ablation system are shown in blue; the remapping trials are shown in dark blue. The other colored pie charts refer to approval trials using the following devices: Globe PF Kardium (*purple*), Inspire Biosense Webster (*green*), Affera Sphere 9, and Sphere0-360 Medtronic (*red shades*). Underneath the trial titles (if available) or first author names the number of assessed PVs per trial can be seen. The number of durable PVI (shown in percentages) is shown in the dark blue pie chart wedge. The number PV reconnections (shown in percentages) are shown in the lighter blue wedge. (*Data from* Kueffer T, Bordignon S, Neven K, et al. Durability of pulmonary vein isolation using pulsed-field ablation. JACC Clin Electrophysiol 2024;10(4):698–708. https://doi.org/10.1016/j.jacep.2023.11.026.)

both Medtronic) could show similar PVI durability rates.[23] The prospective, multicenter Sphere-360 study demonstrated lesion durability in 99% of PVs 87.8 ± 71.1 days after PVI with an optimized waveform (PULSE 3) in a subgroup of patients receiving mandated remapping procedure.

ARRHYTHMIA-FREE SURVIVAL
Prospective Studies

Foundational analyses of 12-month results from the pooled IMPULSE, PEFCAT, and PEFCAT II trials implementing the FARAWAVE pentaspline catheter and PFA-system demonstrated an overall arrhythmia-free survival of 78.5%.[10] Noteworthy in this multicenter study was the remapping and consequent reablation at the 2-month to 3-month mark as well as an adapted ablation protocol after optimization of PFA waveform for roughly half of the cohort. Nonetheless, comparable findings could be shown by predominantly European trials since these initial results.[9,10,12–14,20,24,25] Arrhythmia-free survival rates at 1-year post ablation appear to be in the realms of 66.2% to 81.6% and 55.1% to 71.5% for paroxysmal and persistent AF respectively (**Fig. 2**). A recent study using the same

ablations system could show freedom from a composite primary effectiveness endpoint in 66.6% of subjects.[12] The implemented composite endpoint including the use of anti-arrhythmic drugs (AAD) after the initial blanking period as well as diligent weekly electrocardiography (ECG) monitoring with good compliance, are perhaps illustrative of the lower effectiveness compared to foregoing trials. Similarly, the PULSED-AF pivotal study employing the pulse select ablation system included any amiodarone use during the blanking period if not established before ablation.[9] PULSED-AF examined equal proportions of paroxysmal and persistent AF and interestingly displayed similar effectiveness to FARA-freedom with the comparable intensity of rhythm monitoring. To date, the trend has been toward the use of arrhythmia-free survival as an endpoint when failing to observe greater than 30s atrial arrhythmia for deduction of treatment success. Lately, the dichotomous definition of arrhythmia recurrence has been challenged by data showing improved quality of life and reduced health care utilization simply by reducing AF burden.[26] A recent ADVENT substudy could show residual arrhythmia burden of lesser than 0.1% post-PFA PVI in 78.4% of patients

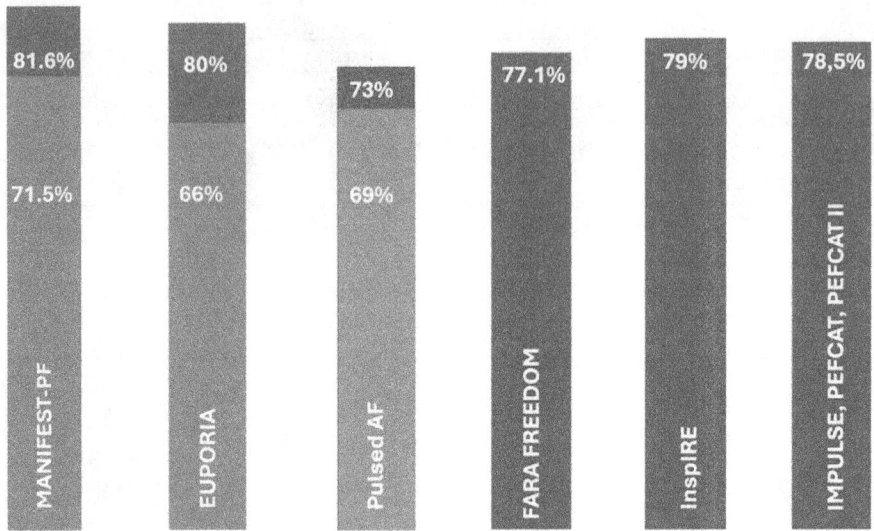

Fig. 2. An overview of arrhythmia-free survival (patient numbers shown in percentages of the study cohort) from outcome trials with a 12-month follow-up. The red bars indicate registry-based trials. In bars containing 2 differently segments, patients were distinguished according to their temporal pattern (paroxysmal and persistent AF).

with an accordingly lesser need for adjunctive therapies and greater improvement in quality of life.[27] It seems likely that the use of more holistic endpoints such as arrhythmia burden may prove more appropriate for the evaluation of general procedural efficiency in the future.

Registries

EU-PORIA and MANIFEST-PF, 2 large registry studies, each with over 1000 patients could show higher arrhythmia-free survival rates.[12,24] The limitations of retrospective analyses of registries as well as the lenient and inter-center variable rhythm monitoring during follow-up impede direct comparison of these trials. Furthermore, the above-mentioned prospective multicentric studies included only patients with failed Class I/III AAD and in the case of FARA-Freedom and Impulse/PEFCAT I/II excluded patients with persistent AF. Both mentioned registries implemented an all-comers approach with consecutive enrollment, ultimately resulting in a distribution of paroxysmal and persistent AF in 65/33% and 60/37%. EUPORIA reported prior Class I/III AAD use in only 55% of the population, perhaps suggesting a different stage of disease in a relevant portion of enrolled patients.

OVERALL PERFORMANCE AND COMPARISON TO THERMAL ENERGIES

Thus far, the general efficacy of PFA in terms of arrhythmia recurrence and lesion durability appears largely comparable to established thermal PVI

methods.[6,18,25,28,29] A direct comparison of PFA and thermal ablation in a randomized, single-blind trial, could prove noninferiority of pentaspline PFA regarding the primary efficacy endpoint.[6] The composite endpoint being defined as the recurrence of arrhythmia, procedural failure, or necessity of clinical intervention in terms of AAD use, cardioversion, or repeat ablation. Similarly, a 400-patient large retrospective analysis showed no significant difference in terms of recurrence rate with PFA or cryoballoon at 12 months.[25] Interestingly, both Urbanek and colleagues and a multicentric retrospective study using propensity score matching to compare PFA with thermal ablation could observe more spontaneous conversion with PFA.[18,25] In comparison to RF-Ablation, the SPHERE-PER AF trial using a novel centrally irrigate point-by-point lattice-tip catheter (Sphere 9, Medtronic) could overserve no significant difference of composite effectiveness endpoint with PFA rather than standard of care RF in patients with persistent AF in Kaplan-Meier analyses (73.5% and 65.2% respectively).[30] Freedom from arrhythmia recurrence, AAD use, cardioversion, or necessary repeat procedure post blanking were considered within the primary effectiveness analyses. A notably greater number of additive linear ablations were performed in the treatment group compared to the RF group with however no proof of resulting heterogeneity in treatment effect. This catheter possesses a larger lesion footprint with a resulting improved current distribution due to its compressible lattice-tip construction and hence the ability to create more contiguous lesions and reduce the risk of gaps

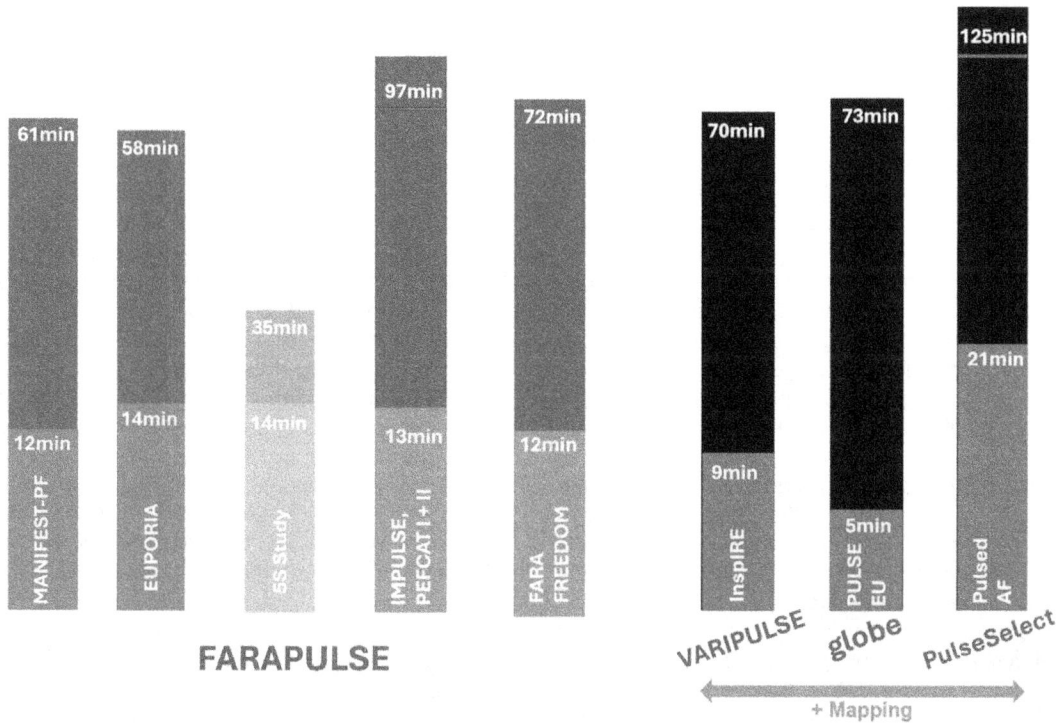

Fig. 3. An overview of procedural times (the bottom component of the bar) and the fluoroscopy time (top component of the bar) from relevant PFA trials for PVI. The red bars indicate registry trials. The green bar is exemplary of a streamlined, minimalist PFA strategy. The adjoining lighter blue bars show data from 2 prospective trials. The first 5 bars include the use of the FARAPULSE ablation system. The darker blue bars to the right-hand side employ use of more recently available PFA ablation devices; The corresponding names can be found underneath each of the bars. Furthermore, additive mapping was performed in these trials as shown by the arrow underneath the bars. The red lines on 2 of the bars demonstrate the addition of a 20-min intraprocedural waiting period to exclude PV reconnection. The data shown for the 5S study refers to the optimized phase II part of the trial. Similarly, the data from the following feasibility studies IMPULSE, PEFCAT I/II, InspIRE, PULSE-EU refer to the procedures after protocol optimization. Data from patients with both paroxysmal and persistent AF is available only for the registry trials, the 5S Study and the PULSE-EU trial. All numbers refer to the median except for the figures from IMPULSE/PEFACTI/II, FARA-Freedom, InspIRE as well as for the procedure time from the PULSE-EU trial. For the sake of a simpler overview no standard deviations or ranges were shown. (*Data from* Refs.[8,12,14,24])

compared to previous focal ablation devices. A small patient group of 26/420 received repeat ablation in this trial with the findings of durable PVI in 66.7% vs. 48.4% for PFA via the Sphere 9 catheter, there was however no report on the observations from the linear ablations. The ability to perform mapping and switch between PFA and RF-ablation with one catheter makes this novel ablation system interesting also in terms of procedural efficiency.[2] A further consideration when comparing efficacy to established thermal PVI is the inclusion of operator learning curves in most cornerstone PFA efficacy trials. A recent EUPORIA subanalysis showed that general operator experience was less effectual than specific foregoing cryoballoon experience for lesion durability.[13] The effectiveness of PFA may increase further as operator experience in technique and dosing develops

and further energy-specific and catheter advancements transpire.

PROCEDURAL EFFICIENCY AND WORK-FLOW OPTIMIZATION

After acute PVI, irreversible electroporation is usually performed with the center-specific and catheter-specific, variable number of consolidative applications. The omission of the postablation thawing process typical for cryoballoon ablation or the need for electroanatomic mapping and point-by-point ablation with RF-ablation have enabled shorter procedure times with PFA.[31] Most published large, multicenter data comprises the use of the FARAPULSE due to being the first PFA ablation system to receive Conformité Européenne (CE)-Mark in 2021.[6,12,14,24] This multielectrode catheter with easily changeable spline configuration delivers a sequence of 5 waveforms within 2.5 seconds of active ablation. Conventionally, 1 pair of applications is delivered in 1 configuration and 1 position before the catheter is rotated slightly and the second pair of applications are delivered. After configuration change, this process is repeated leaving a total of 8 standard applications per PV.[6] In total 20 seconds of ablation with the addition of a short waiting period between each application for generator recharge, in which the position and configuration can be adjusted. For PVI alone fluoroscopic guidance is usually sufficient, enabling the omission of introducing a mapping catheter and hence a second transseptal puncture. The elimination of electroanatomic mapping was able to progressively reduce the procedural time from a median of 43 to 35 minutes in the 5S study.[8] This trial examined a streamlined approach to PVI, with an initial validation phase using paired electroanatomic mapping in the first 25 enrolled patients and an adjoining phase 2 with a single-catheter approach and an increased ablation voltage to 2.0 V. Electrograms from the ablation catheter were shown sufficient to deduce PVI after comparison to baseline recordings from a spiral mapping catheter. Furthermore, no imaging was performed before ablation to screen for variable PV anatomy. The initial PEFCAT I & II/IMPULSE feasibility study included a 20-min waiting period and consequently a longer average procedure duration of 97 minutes.[10] Since then, successive trials using the same catheter could show a procedure time ranging around an hour (**Fig. 3**[8,12,14,24]). Comparable procedure times could also be shown for more recently available Inspire (Biosense Webster) and PulseSelect (Medtronic) PFA catheters.[9,20,21] The incorporation of electroanatomical mapping systems with these novel catheters led to an observed reduction in fluoroscopy time.[9,31] Although the elimination of mapping was generally shown to streamline PVI, additive electroanatomic guidance may be beneficial in improving lesion quality and workflow in patients with complex PV anatomies.[8,32] Other factors worthy of consideration when evaluating general procedural efficiency are the use of deep sedation rather than general anesthesia and vascular management. Deep sedation has been shown to provide a good safety profile with the potential benefit of less intensive preprocedural patient preparation and quicker postprocedural recovery.[8,33] Shortening procedure times seems particularly relevant in improving safety for multimorbid or frail patients. Regarding access site management, the use of vascular closure devices with potentially enhanced postprocedural efficiency due to reduction of vascular complications and quicker patient ambulation may be considered after cost-effectiveness analyses.[34]

SUMMARY AND OUTLOOK

Ablation results of current, first generation PFA catheters are associated with high durability rates and similar clinical outcomes in terms of freedom from arrhythmias. Some studies suggest a trend toward improved PVI durability and reduced AF burden. It is reasonable to expect that future technological improvements such as full three-dimensional (3D) integration, markers of catheter to tissue contact, and better understanding of dosing will further improve ablation outcomes.

Ongoing prospective randomized multicenter trials are investigating the role of PFA for first-line ablation of patients with persistent AF. Moreover, PFA offers the possibility to rechallenge ablation strategies outside PVI such as posterior wall isolation, linear ablation, and many more.

Although the performance of PFA in terms of treatment effectiveness appears largely comparable to particularly cryoballoon PVI, a relevant reduction in procedural time subsidized by a good safety profile has continued to make this technology attractive. The growing experience with this energy source and the accelerating availability of PFA ablation devices with innovative design features with further optimization of waveform protocols and catheter maneuverability may enhance lesion quality in the future. Accordingly, the accessibility and approval of more ablation systems require more diversified and systematic remapping studies. There is also a need for more standardized rhythm monitoring in outcome studies to appreciate differences in treatment effects when employing different catheters and different ablation strategies or adapted workflows.

Currently, there is a dominance of data from approval studies for novel PFA devices and studies implementing the FARAPULSE with a lack of large prospective or randomized, long-term trials, which ultimately hinder comprehensive analysis of overall PFA efficacy for PVI. Furthermore, this piece focuses largely on PVI with single-shot devices, whether additive linear ablations in terms of 'PVI +' approaches improve the general efficacy of this energy source needs further methodical examination in the future. Similarly, more comparative data on PFA and thermal ablation for persistent and long-standing persistent AF is required to draw conclusions on the effectiveness of PFA in this patient subset in which the ideal ablation strategy remains unclear.

CLINICS CARE POINTS

- Reduction in procedural times and good safety features contribute to the general efficiency of Pulsed field ablation (PFA) for the treatment of atrial fibrillation.
- A lack of large, systematic long-term, remapping trials challenges comprehensive analysis of overall PFA efficacy in terms of lesion durability and freedom from arrhythmia.
- Real-world data on the effectiveness of PFA after further development of novel catheters with waveform-optimization is currently being awaited.

DISCLOSURES

K-R.J. Chun and B. Schmidt belong to the advisory board and receive nonrelevant speaker fees and research grants from BSCI, Medtronic, and Abbott.

REFERENCES

1. Reddy VY, Koruth J, Jais P, et al. Ablation of atrial fibrillation with pulsed electric fields. JACC Clin Electrophysiol 2018;4(8):987–95.
2. Chun KRJ, Miklavčič D, Vlachos K, et al. State-of-the-art pulsed field ablation for cardiac arrhythmias: ongoing evolution and future perspective. Europace 2024;26(6). https://doi.org/10.1093/europace/euae134.
3. Sugrue A, Maor E, Del-Carpio Munoz F, et al. Cardiac ablation with pulsed electric fields: principles and biophysics. EP Europace 2022;24(8):1213–22.
4. Koruth J, Kawamura I, Dukkipati SR, et al. Preclinical assessment of the feasibility, safety and lesion durability of a novel "single-shot" pulsed field ablation catheter for pulmonary vein isolation. EP Europace 2023;25(4):1369–78.
5. Koruth JS, Kuroki K, Kawamura I, et al. Pulsed field ablation versus radiofrequency ablation. Circ Arrhythm Electrophysiol 2020;13(3). https://doi.org/10.1161/circep.119.008303.
6. Reddy VY, Gerstenfeld EP, Natale A, et al. Pulsed field or conventional thermal ablation for paroxysmal atrial fibrillation. N Engl J Med 2023. https://doi.org/10.1056/nejmoa2307291.
7. Ekanem E, Neuzil P, Reichlin T, et al. Safety of pulsed field ablation in more than 17,000 patients with atrial fibrillation in the MANIFEST-17K study. Nat Med 2024;1–10. https://doi.org/10.1038/s41591-024-03114-3.
8. Schmidt B, Bordignon S, Tohoku S, et al. 5S study: safe and simple single shot pulmonary vein isolation with pulsed field ablation using sedation. Circ Arrhythm Electrophysiol 2022;15(6). https://doi.org/10.1161/circep.121.010817.
9. Verma A, Haines DE, Boersma LV, et al. Pulsed field ablation for the treatment of atrial fibrillation: PULSED AF pivotal trial. Circulation 2023;147(19). https://doi.org/10.1161/circulationaha.123.063988.
10. Reddy VY, Dukkipati SR, Neuzil P, et al. Pulsed field ablation of paroxysmal atrial fibrillation: 1-year outcomes of IMPULSE, PEFCAT, and PEFCAT II. JACC Clin Electrophysiol 2021;7(5):614–27.
11. Van IC, Rienstra M, Bunting KV, et al. 2024 ESC Guidelines for the management of atrial fibrillation developed in collaboration with the European Association for Cardio-Thoracic Surgery (EACTS). Eur Heart J 2024. https://doi.org/10.1093/eurheartj/ehae176.
12. Schmidt B, Bordignon S, Neven K, et al. EUropean real-world outcomes with Pulsed field ablatiOn in patients with symptomatic atRIAl fibrillation: lessons from the multi-centre EU-PORIA registry. Europace 2023;25(7). https://doi.org/10.1093/europace/euad185.
13. Kueffer T, Bordignon S, Neven K, et al. Durability of pulmonary vein isolation using pulsed-field ablation. JACC Clin Electrophysiol 2024;10(4):698–708. https://doi.org/10.1016/j.jacep.2023.11.026.
14. Metzner A, Fiala M, Vijgen J, et al. Long-term outcomes of the pentaspline pulsed field ablation catheter for the treatment of paroxysmal atrial fibrillation: results of the prospective, multicenter FARA-Freedom Study. Europace 2024. https://doi.org/10.1093/europace/euae053.
15. Ruwald MH, Haugdal M, Worck R, et al. Characterization of durability and reconnection patterns at time of repeat ablation after single-shot pulsed field pulmonary vein isolation. J Intervent Card Electrophysiol 2023. https://doi.org/10.1007/s10840-023-01655-0.
16. Tohoku S, Chun KRJ, Bordignon S, et al. Findings from repeat ablation using high-density mapping after pulmonary vein isolation with pulsed field ablation. EP Europace 2022. https://doi.org/10.1093/europace/euac211.
17. Reddy VY, Anic A, Koruth J, et al. Pulsed field ablation in patients with persistent atrial fibrillation. J Am Coll Cardiol 2020;76(9):1068–80.
18. Rocca D, Marcon L, Magnocavallo M, et al. Pulsed electric field, cryoballoon, and radiofrequency for paroxysmal atrial fibrillation ablation: a propensity score-matched comparison. Europace 2023;26(1). https://doi.org/10.1093/europace/euae016.
19. Galuszka O, Baldinger S, Kueffer T, et al. Durability of pulmonary vein isolation with pulsed field ablation compared to radiofrequency ablation in patients with persistent atrial fibrillation: results from a prospective remapping study. Europace 2024;26(Supplement_1). https://doi.org/10.1093/europace/euae102.094.
20. Duytschaever M, De Potter T, Grimaldi M, et al. Paroxysmal AF ablation using a novel variable-loop biphasic pulsed field ablation catheter integrated with a 3D mapping system: 1-year outcomes of the multicenter

inspIRE study. Circ Arrhythm Electrophysiol 2023. https://doi.org/10.1161/circep.122.011780.

21. Turagam M, Neuzil P, Petru J, et al. AF ablation using a novel "single-shot" map-and-ablate spherical array pulsed field ablation catheter: 1-Year outcomes of the first-in-human PULSE-EU trial. Heart Rhythm 2024;21(8):1218–26.

22. Reddy VY, Peichl P, Anter E, et al. A focal ablation catheter toggling between radiofrequency and pulsed field energy to treat atrial fibrillation. JACC Clin Electrophysiol 2023. https://doi.org/10.1016/j.jacep.2023.04.002.

23. Reddy VY, Anter E, Peichl P, et al. First-in-Human clinical series of a novel conformable large-lattice pulsed field ablation catheter for pulmonary vein isolation. Europace 2024. https://doi.org/10.1093/europace/euae090.

24. Turagam MK, Neuzil P, Schmidt B, et al. Safety and effectiveness of pulsed field ablation to treat atrial fibrillation: one-year outcomes from the MANIFEST-PF registry. Circulation 2023;148(1):35–46.

25. Urbanek L, Stefano B, Schaack D, et al. Pulsed field versus cryoballoon pulmonary vein isolation for atrial fibrillation: efficacy, safety, and long-term follow-up in a 400-patient cohort. Circ Arrhythm Electrophysiol 2023;16(7):389–98.

26. Andrade JG, Deyell MW, Laurent M, et al. Healthcare utilization and quality of life for atrial fibrillation burden: the CIRCA-DOSE study. Eur Heart J 2022. https://doi.org/10.1093/eurheartj/ehac692.

27. Reddy VY, Mansour M, Calkins H, et al. Pulsed field vs conventional thermal ablation for paroxysmal atrial fibrillation: recurrent atrial arrhythmia burden. J Am Coll Cardiol 2024;84(1):61–74.

28. Hoffmann E, Straube F, Wegscheider K, et al. Outcomes of cryoballoon or radiofrequency ablation in symptomatic paroxysmal or persistent atrial fibrillation. Europace 2019;21(9):1313–24.

29. Badertscher P, Weidlich S, Knecht S, et al. Efficacy and safety of pulmonary vein isolation with pulsed field ablation vs. novel cryoballoon ablation system for atrial fibrillation. Europace 2023;25(12). https://doi.org/10.1093/europace/euad329.

30. Anter E, Mansour M, Nair DG, et al. Dual-energy lattice-tip ablation system for persistent atrial fibrillation: a randomized trial. Nat Med 2024;30:2303–10.

31. Kuck KH, Brugada J, Fürnkranz A, et al. Cryoballoon or radiofrequency ablation for paroxysmal atrial fibrillation. N Engl J Med 2016;374(23):2235–45.

32. Alessio FZ, Olson J, Scheel S, et al. Procedural efficiency is enhanced combining the pentaspline pulsed field ablation catheter with three-dimensional electroanatomical mapping system for pulmonary vein isolation. J Intervent Card Electrophysiol 2024. https://doi.org/10.1007/s10840-024-01846-3.

33. Iacopino S, Colella J, Dini D, et al. Sedation strategies for pulsed-field ablation of atrial fibrillation: focus on deep sedation with intravenous ketamine in spontaneous respiration. Europace 2023. https://doi.org/10.1093/europace/euad230.

34. Natale A, Mohanty S, Liu PY, et al. Venous vascular closure system versus manual compression following multiple access Electrophysiology procedures: the AMBULATE trial. JACC Clin Electrophysiol 2020;6(1):111–24.

Role of Catheter-Tissue Contact in Pulsed Field Ablation

Jacopo Marazzato, MD, PhD[a,b], Fengwei Zou, MD[a],
Xiaodong Zhang, MD, PhD[a], Luigi Di Biase, MD, PhD[a,*]

KEYWORDS

• Pulsed field ablation • Irreversible electroporation • Pulsed electrical field energy • Contact force

KEY POINTS

• Contact force is pivotal during radiofrequency ablation but the role of catheter-tissue contact is less clear for pulsed field ablation.
• Pre-clinical "in vivo" studies on ventricular swine models generally suggest that the higher the force, the deeper the lesions and the interplay between catheter-tissue contact and PFA dose synergistically impact on lesion formation.
• Likewise, clinical studies on patients undergoing pulmonary vein isolation with pulsed field ablation underscore the feasibility of the procedure provided that adequate catheter-tissue contact is warranted.
• Nevertheless, further clinical studies are required to investigate the long-term clinical impact of contact-force-guided pulsed field ablation in a variety of arrhythmogenic substrates.

INTRODUCTION

Radiofrequency (RF) energy requires a resistive load between the catheter tip and the myocardial tissue, which allows for electro-mechanical coupling that is known to be critical for lesion formation. Therefore, the higher the catheter-tissue contact during RF ablation, the deeper the lesion created.[1,2] Moreover from a safety perspective, monitoring contact force (CF) during RF ablation is proved to prevent steam pop, collateral damage, and risk of cardiac tamponade.[3]

Based on the biophysics of irreversible electroporation, pulsed electrical field (PEF) energy is a novel and minimally thermal energy source that proved to be highly selective for the myocardial tissue and capable of avoiding collateral damage to the neighboring organs.[4] Even though tissue compression provided by improved catheter tip stability should theoretically lead to deeper lesion formation due to greater PEF energy deployed to the myocardial tissue during high CF applications, the role of CF during pulsed field ablation (PFA) is controversial. In fact, PEF energy greatly differs from other thermal energy sources since it is highly customizable per se thanks to several ablation parameters (**Box 1**) that can be modulated during ablation, thus potentially limiting the role of catheter-tissue contact in this setting.[5–7] In contrast, other pre-clinical and clinical studies suggest the positive impact of CF-guided PFA.[8–15]

The purpose of this review is, therefore, to clarify the role of catheter-tissue contact during PFA

a Department of Cardiology, Montefiore Medical Center, 111 East 210th Street, Bronx, NY 10467, USA;
b Electrophysiology and Cardiac Pacing Unit, Humanitas Mater Domini, Via Gerenzano 2, Castellanza, Varese 21053, Italy
* Corresponding author. Electrophysiology and Cardiac Pacing Unit, Humanitas Mater Domini, Via Gerenzano 2, Castellanza, Varese 21053, Italy.
E-mail address: dibbia@gmail.com

Card Electrophysiol Clin 17 (2025) 191–203
https://doi.org/10.1016/j.ccep.2025.02.007

Abbreviations	
3D	3 dimensional
A	Ampere
CF	contact force
CTI	cavotricuspid isthmus
LA	left atrial
LI	local impedance
LTD	lesion tag distance
LV	left ventricle
MVA	mitral valvular area
pAF	paroxysmal atrial fibrillation
peAF	persistent atrial fibrillation
PEF	pulse electrical field
PFA	pulsed field ablation
PFI	pulsed field ablation index
PVI	pulmonary vein isolation
R	randomized
RF	radiofrequency
RIPV	right inferior pulmonary vein
RSPV	right superior pulmonary vein
RV	right ventricle
SAE	side adverse events
SVC-IVC	line connecting the superior to the inferior vena cava
TC	tissue contact
V	volts

through research of the available literature in the field.

METHODS

We performed bibliographic research on Medline considering articles published up to September

Box 1 Pulsed field ablation parameters
Biophysical properties:
• Amplitude voltage
• Duration width of pulses
• Number of pulses
• Packets of pulses
• Pause between packets
• Number of trains
• Time between trains
Catheter shape:
• Linear, solid tip
• Circular
• Basket
Modality of pulsed electrical field delivery:
• Unipolar biphasic
• Bipolar biphasic

2024. The following research terms were used: "Pulsed Field Ablation," "Irreversible Electroporation," and "Contact Force." Only original articles in English language were included. Abstracts, editorials, and research letters were excluded. The literature research was independently conducted by 2 authors (JM and LDB) and then revised by the other authors who reached a shared decision by consensus in case of discordance. Through nonsystematic research of the literature in the field, 11 studies[5–15] published from 2022[5] to 2024[6–15] were collected. Three studies were conducted on isolated porcine heart or vegetal models ("ex vivo" set-up),[5,6,8] 6 on "in vivo" animal models,[7–12] and, finally, 2 on human beings.[14,15] The features of all these studies are reported in **Tables 1** and **2**. For each study, data on the experimental setting, study population, PFA catheter and settings, CF evaluation, study endpoints, and results were all collected. In the preclinical animal studies, the attention was more focused on the impact of catheter-tissue contact, PFA dose, and their interplay on lesion formation (ie, lesion depth). On the other hand, in human studies, we investigated the adjunct role of CF on the clinical outcome of patients undergoing pulmonary vein isolation (PVI) with PFA.

PRECLINICAL STUDIES

The features of these studies[5–13] are reported in **Table 1**. With the only exception of one article,[6] the "ex vivo" preclinical studies[5,8] showed that even a small amount of catheter-tissue contact is required to achieve lesion formation during PFA. However, these results were not consistent between studies. Di Biase and colleagues[8] proved that both the interplay between adequate catheter-tissue contact (15–30 g) and PFA repetition led to deeper ventricular lesion formation, while Howard and colleagues showed that lesions can be created even with no direct contact with the myocardial tissue.[5] Likewise, Mattison and colleagues[6] demonstrated that CF had no impact on lesion depth when the force applied was less than 30 g.

The differences between study design can well explain these inconsistences (see **Table 1**). First, the experimental setup differed. While Di Biase and colleagues[8] utilized a benchtop vegetal potato model in which biphasic bipolar PFA was delivered upon each potato with different CF cutoffs to better estimate the interplay between CF and lesion depth,[16] in the other "ex vivo" experimental settings,[5,6] PFA applications were delivered to the epicardial surface of isolated swine hearts. Second, the evaluation of CF was not homogeneous. For instance, Mattison and

Table 1
Preclinical studies assessing the role of contact force during pulsed field ablation

Author, Year	Study Design	Experimental Setting	Ablation Catheter	PFA Settings	Methods and Contact Force Evaluation	Study Results	Overall Results on CF
Ex Vivo Studies							
Howard et al,[5] 2022	Non-R	Isolated porcine heart	4 array electrodes multipolar catheter (prototype)	4 trains of 1500 V biphasic bipolar energy	An offset toll allowed the catheter to be placed 0, 2, and 4 mm away from the epicardium. Histology followed to measure lesion depth. No further CF evaluation	*Lesion depth:* Zero CF: 4.3 ± 0.4 mm 2 mm off: 2.7 ± 0.4 mm 4 mm off: 1.3 ± 0.4 mm	Lesion formation can be achieved even without catheter-tissue contact
Mattison et al,[6] 2023	R	Modified Langerdoff experimental setup with porcine heart	Linear catheter (prototype)	Customized number of trains of 1500 V biphasic bipolar energy	The catheter was attached to a force gauge perpendicular to the epicardium. Contact was recorded and histology followed to appraise lesion size. The range of CF values was 0–50 g	For each gram of CF, linear regression analysis showed an increase of 0.01 mm in depth, 0.03 mm in width and 2.20 mm^3 in volume	Weak effect of CF on lesion depth, width and volume
Di Biase et al,[8] 2024	Non-R	Benchtop vegetal potato model	VARIPULSE (Biosense Webster) circular catheter	$\times 1$, $\times 2$, $\times 3$, and $\times 6$ ablations (1 ablation = 3 applications) of 1800 V biphasic bipolar energy	Ablations were delivered with different CF cutoffs (ie, 2 mm distance from the surface, 0, 15, and 30 g). Potatoes were then sliced to expose lesion depth	*Lesion depth:* 2 mm off: 0.6 ± 0.5 mm 0 g CF: 2.3 ± 0.6 mm 15–30 g: 4.3 ± 0.4 mm No increase in lesion depth above 15–30 g (plateau effect)	CF is required to achieve deeper lesion depth. Moreover, CF and application repetition have a synergistic effect

(continued on next page)

Table 1
(continued)

Author, Year	Study Design	Experimental Setting	Ablation Catheter	PFA Settings	Methods and Contact Force Evaluation	Study Results	Overall Results on CF
In Vivo Studies							
Di Biase et al,[12] 2023	R	18 pigs	CF-sensing commercial Thermocool SmartTouch SF catheter (Biosense Webster)	×12 and ×24 pulses of unipolar biphasic energy	Both PFA and RF energy sources were evaluated during ablation of atrial sites (RSPV, LA roof, MVA, SVC-IVC, and CTI). During ablation CF was maintained in the 5–30g range. Histology followed at 30 d invasive re-evaluation	After 30 d re-evaluation, lesion transmurality was achieved in 95% of sites and 100% of pulmonary veins achieving similar results for both PFA and RF	Similarly to RF, CF is important to achieve lesion transmurality even during PFA. However, higher PFA dose does not prove better for PVI
Doshi et al,[7] 2024	Non-R	10 pigs	Large area focal catheter (prototype)	Unipolar biphasic PFA (25 A, 1.6 ms)	As a surrogate of direct CF evaluation, TC was assessed as LI (ohm) between splines and the central ring electrode. Three TC cutoffs were established: No TC (<10 Ω), Low TC (11–29 Ω), and High TC (>30 Ω). Lesion depth was histologically assessed on RV endocardial lesions (acutely) and atrial lesions (30 d re-evaluation)	*RV lesions:* No TC: • Depth 1.7 ± 1.2 mm • Width 6.0 ± 4.5 mm Low TC: • Depth 5.7 ± 2.0 mm • Width 16 ± 5.2 mm High TC: • Depth 5.7 ± 2.0 mm • Width 17 ± 4.4 mm No lesion gaps for atrial lesion set except for no TC	Contact *per se* is more important than the degree of CF

Study	Rand.	Animals	Catheter	Ablation Parameters	Methods	Results	Conclusions
Nakagawa et al,[9] 2024	Non-R	5 pigs	CF-sensing commercial Tacticath Ablation catheter	Unipolar biphasic PFE (28 mA and 35 mA for RV and LV, respectively)	PFA delivered to endocardial RV and LV with 4 CF level: Group (1) Low CF (4–14 g) Group (2) Moderate CF (15–29 g) Group (3) High CF (30–55 g) Group (4) No contact (2 mm away) Acute histologic evaluation followed to assess lesion depth	*RV lesion depth:* Group (1) 3.9 ± 0.7 mm Group (2) 4.9 ± 0.6 mm Group (3) 5.7 ± 0.6 mm *LV lesion depth:* Group (1) 4.0 ± 1.0 mm Group (2) 5.6 ± 1.5 mm Group (3) 6.8 ± 1.0 mm Greater lesion depth for higher PFA dose in LV. No detectable lesions for Group (4)	CF paramount for adequate lesion formation Synergistic effect between PFA dose and CF in achieving deeper lesions in the LV
Hua et al,[10] 2024	Non-R	8 pigs	Linear CF-sensing catheter (prototype)	*High-dose:* 1800 V/10trains *Mid-dose:* 1800 V/5 trains *Low-dose:* 800 V/5 trains Ablation dose was chosen based on the thickness of each site	1. RV and LV ablation targeting 5, 15, 25, 35 g of CF followed by 30 d histologic evaluation 2. Atrial ablation targeting SVC, CTI, RSPV and RIPV followed by acute remapping and 30 d histologic evaluation	1. *RV/LV lesion depth:* For 5 g: 4.0 ± 1.0 mm For 15 g: 6.8 ± 1.2 mm For 25 g: 7.2 ± 1.2 mm For 35 g: 7.4 ± 0.3 mm 2. *Atrial lesions:* CF ranged from 9.4 ± 1.5 and 17.2 ± 2.6 g. 100% acute conduction block and lesion transmurality at 30 d	The higher the CF value, the deeper the lesion plateauing for CF >15 g Regardless of CF, lesion depth is generally greater for higher PFA dose

(continued on next page)

Table 1
(continued)

Author, Year	Study Design	Experimental Setting	Ablation Catheter	PFA Settings	Methods and Contact Force Evaluation	Study Results	Overall Results on CF
Younis et al,[11] 2024	R	8 pigs	Linear, dual energy, CF-sensing catheter	2.0 kV Unipolar biphasic PFA with 10 packets of applications	1. Atrial ablation. Pigs were randomized to PFA and RF ablation and applications were delivered to the inter-caval line 2. PFA ablation at RV and LV maintain 3 different CF cutoffs: 5–15 g (CF1), 20–30g (CF2), and 35–45 g (CF3). Histology evaluation followed at 7 d evaluation	1. *Atrial ablation:* Mean CF was 14 ± 6 g. PFA was associated with wider and longer transmural lesions compared to RF 2. *RV/LV lesion depth:* CF1: 4.4 ± 0.9 mm CF2: 6.6 ± 1.2 mm CF3: 9.2 ± 1.0 mm	CF is paramount to achieve adequate lesion depth during PFA and allows for improved catheter stability during ablation
Di Biase et al,[13] 2024	Non-R	17 pigs	Multipolar Basket Catheter OMNYPULSE (Biosense Webster Inc, Irvine, CA)	N/A	Impact on acute ventricular lesion depth was appraised for 1) ×3, ×6, ×9, ×12 PFA packets and 2) CF (CF 1: 5–26g, CF2: 26–50g, and CF3: 51–80g) and their integration in the PFI (300, 450, and 600)	Lesion depth was 4.4 ± 0.9 (CF1), 6.6 ± 1.2 (CF2), and 9.2 ± 1.0 mm (CF3) with depth ranging from 2.9 ± 0.7 mm to 4.4 ± 0.9 mm for low to high-dose PFA, respectively. PFI/100 predicts lesion depth.	CF and PFA dose predict lesion depth. Their interplay in the PFI synergistically impact on lesion size. Plateau effect on lesion depth >50g

Abbreviations: A, ampere; CF, contact force; CTI, cavotricuspid isthmus; LA, left atrial; LI, local impedance; LTD, lesion tag distance; LV, left ventricle; MVA, mitral valvular area; pAF, paroxysmal atrial fibrillation; peAF, persistent atrial fibrillation; PFA, pulsed field ablation; PFI, pulsed field ablation index; PVI, pulmonary vein isolation; R, randomized; RF, radio-frequency; RIPV, right inferior pulmonary vein; RSPV, right superior pulmonary vein; RV, right ventricle; SAE, side adverse events; SVC-IVC, line connecting the superior to the inferior vena cava; TC, tissue contact; V, volts.

Table 2
Clinical studies assessing the role of contact force during pulsed field ablation

Author, Year	Study Design	Patients (Age)	AF Type	Ablation Catheter	PFA Generator	Energy Settings	Study Endpoints	CF Evaluation	Results
Anic et al,[14] 2023	Non-R Prospective Multicenter study	82 (61 ± 9 y)	pAF (51%) peAF (49%)	CF-sensing TactiCath (Abbott) Intellanav Stablepoint (Boston Sc.) and Thermocool SmartTouch (Biosense Webster)	Centaury System	1. *Initial workflow development* Anterior: 22 A, 2.4 ms, 5 mm of LTD Posterior: 19–22 A, 1.4–2.4 ms, 3–5 mm of LTD 2. *Optimized PFA workflow* Anterior: 25 A, 2.4 ms, 4–6 mm LTD Posterior: 22 A, 2.4 ms, 4–6 mm LTD	1. Safety 2. Acute Efficacy 3. 90 d efficacy at invasive remapping	Ablation was carried out maintaining CF ≥5 g	1. Safety: 4.9% SAEs (3 hemorrhagic events and 1 cardiac tamponade) 2. Acute PVI in 100% and first pass isolation in 92.2% per vein 3. 90 d efficacy: (1) initial workflow cohort: 52% per vein (2) optimized PFA cohort: 89% per vein
Duytschaever et al,[15] 2024	Non-R Prospective multicenter single-arm study	137 (62 ± 8 y)	pAF (100%)	Dual-energy Thermocool SmartTouch (Biosense Webster)	TRUPULSE Generator toggling between PFA and RF	PFA was delivered to the postero-inferior region of the pulmonary veins RF was delivered to the anterior region, the Coumadin ridge and the carina between veins	1. Safety 2. Acute efficacy 3. 90 d durability in a subset of 30 patients	Ablation following a target index (VISITAG SURPOINT/PFI): • 550 (anterior, roof, ridge, carina) • 400 (posterior and inferior region) Tag size 3 mm and intertag ≤6	1. Safety: 4.4% SAEs (2 PV stenosis, 2 cardiac tamponade, 1 stroke and 1 pericarditis) 2. Acute PVI in 100% and first pass isolation in 96.8% per vein 3. 90 d efficacy 87% per vein

Abbreviations: A, ampere; CF, contact force; LTD, lesion tag distance; pAF, paroxysmal atrial fibrillation; peAF, persistent atrial fibrillation; PFA, pulsed field ablation; PFI, pulsed field ablation index; PVI, pulmonary vein isolation; R, randomized; RF, radiofrequency; SAE, side adverse events.

colleagues[6] used a wide range of CF values (0–50 g) applied in a randomized manner to allow for an even distribution of forces on the ventricular epicardium. On the other hand, in another experimental setting, a dedicated offset tool was used to precisely control catheter-tissue contact or the distance of the PFA electrodes from the epicardial surface of the heart.[5] Third, different ablation catheters and PFA settings were implemented. In fact, multipolar,[5] linear,[6] or circular[8] ablation catheters were utilized in different experimental settings, and the PEF energy dose was applied with variable voltage amplitudes, pulse widths, and number of delivered packets of pulses.[4]

More consistent results on the role of CF during PFA were provided by 6 "in vivo" preclinical studies conducted on animals[7,9–13] (randomized[11,12] vs nonrandomized[7,9,10,13]), and their characteristics are illustrated in **Table 1**.

All these studies were conducted on pigs including up to 18 animals.[12] Three-dimensional (3D) mapping of the atrial[7,10–12] and ventricular chambers[7,9–11,13] was carried out before ablation using RHYTHMIA,[7,11] EnSite,[9] CARTO,[12,13] or other mapping systems.[10] Only 2 studies implemented commonly used CF-sensing solid-tip ablation catheters such as the Thermocool SmartTouch (Biosense Webster Inc, Irvine, CA)[12] and TactiCath (Abbott, Abbott Park, North Chicago, IL)[9] while either linear[10,11] or basket-like[7,13] prototype catheters were utilized in other experimental settings. Unipolar biphasic PFA ablation was implemented in all studies through a variety of amplitude voltage, pulse width, packets and trains of pulses (see **Box 1, Table 1**). As for CF evaluation, one study investigated the variation of local impedance as a surrogate of CF,[7] and all others provided direct appraisal of CF measured in grams.[9–13] One study only explored the effect of 5 to 30 g CF on atrial lesion transmurality,[12] while in all the other experiences,[7,9–13] predefined CF cutoffs were identified to explore the impact of different levels of force on ventricular lesion size. Histologic evaluation occurred immediately,[7,9,13] 7 days[11] or 30 days after ablation.[10]

When ablating atrial targets, regardless of the implemented PFA dose, CF generally led to atrial lesion transmurality in 100% of the ablated pulmonary veins.[7,10,12] In other atrial sites, especially mitral isthmus region, lesion transmurality was often not fully achieved. Regarding the ventricular substrates, the correlation between the CF applied during ablation and the ventricular lesion size was evaluated in 5 "in vivo" studies.[7,9–13] Doshi and colleagues[7] showed that comparable lesion depths were obtained regardless of the PFA

dose, and all other studies demonstrated that the higher the CF value, the deeper the lesion formation even though a plateaux effect could be expected beyond 15 g[10] or 50 g[13] depending on catheter size and shape.

Last but not least, the interaction between the PEF dose and the CF applied during ablation was investigated in only one study[13] where the authors explored the impact of PEF energy dose (ie, ×3, ×6, ×9, and ×12 packets of pulses) and CF (ie, 5–26 g; 26–50 g; 51–80 g) on ventricular lesion depth.[13] The authors showed that increasing values of PFA ablation dose and catheter-tissue contact led to progressively deeper lesions. However, it was in fact the combination in the pulsed field ablation index (PFI) formula that synergistically and significantly had an impact ventricular lesion depth.[13] Moreover, PFI well correlated with lesion size and could also predict lesion depth as evaluated on histology, thus making PFI a good index of lesion quality for PFA (**Fig. 1**).[13]

CLINICAL STUDIES

To date, only 2 nonrandomized, prospective, multicenter clinical studies investigated how catheter-tissue contact impacted the outcome of patients undergoing PVI with PFA: The (Safety & Clinical Performance Study of Catheter Ablation With the Centauri System for Patients With Atrial Fibrillation [ECLIPSE AF][14] and the SmartfIRE Trials.[15] The features of these 2 studies are reported in **Table 2**.

In the ECLIPSE AF trial, Anic and colleagues[14] systematically evaluated the acute feasibility and chronic efficacy of focal PFA using the CENTAURI System (Galvanize Therapeutics, Redwood City, CA) using 3 commercial CF-sensing, sold-tip ablation catheters (ie, TactiCath SE, INTELLANAV STABLEPOINT, [Boston Scientific Corporation, Natick, MA], and Thermocool SmartTouch, [Biosense Webster Inc, Irvine, CA]) and related mapping systems (EnSite NavX Precision [Abbott, Abbott Park, North Chicago, IL], RHYTHMIA HDx [Boston Scientific Corporation, Natick, IL], and CARTO system, [Biosense Webster Inc, Irvine, CA]) for PVI in 82 patients with paroxysmal (51%) and persistent (49%) AF. The authors split the study population into 5 different study groups. Two were allotted into an initial workflow development strategy with prespecified PFA settings (see **Table 2**) using the TactiCath catheter only. In these patients, chronic durability was assessed at 90 days via invasive pulmonary vein remapping to optimize and validate the acute PFA parameters. The subsequent 3 cohorts were appraised each with the 3 commercial CF-sensing catheters with optimized PFA settings. During ablation, CF was maintained above 5 g.[17]

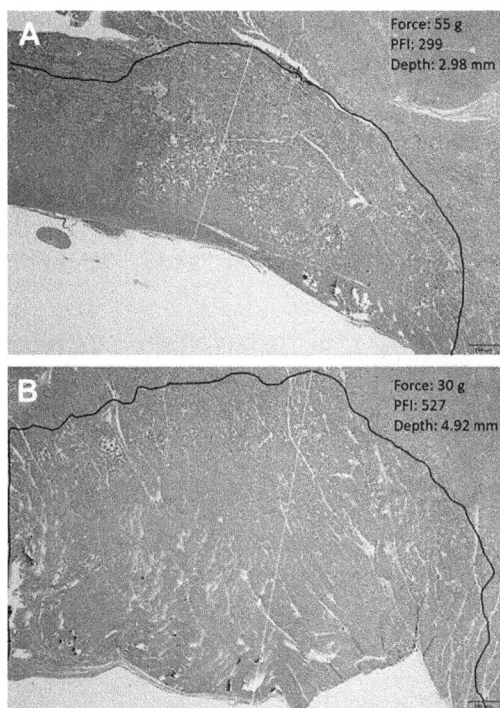

Fig. 1. *The histologic correlation among pulsed field electrical dose, contact force, and ventricular lesion depth during pulsed field ablation in the ventricular swine heart.* In the study by Di Biase and colleagues,[13] the authors proved that both contact force values and pulsed electrical field energy well correlated with the endocardial ventricular lesion depth on histologic examination through an asymptotically relationship. However, when contact force and pulsed field electrical dose were combined in a single formula—the pulsed field ablation index or PFI—it was proven that their interaction synergistically led to way deeper ventricular lesions. Furthermore, the pulsed field ablation index values divided by a factor of 100 (ie, PFI/100) could predict the actual lesion depth in millimeters. As reported in 2 different histologic specimens drawn from the study,[13] the PFI was clearly correlated with the average ventricular lesion depth. For instance, a PFI of 298 (A) and 527 (B) were associated with a mean ventricular lesion depth of 2.98 mm (A) and 4.92 mm (B), respectively, thus providing insights in the prediction of the lesion depth during pulsed field ablation.

Chronic invasive remapping followed. As shown in **Table 2**, the procedure proved safe with 4.9% incidence of adverse events and mostly composed of bleedings event. Acute PVI was achieved in 100% of cases with first pass isolation in roughly 92% per vein. Chronic efficacy tested at 90 day remapping showed durable isolation in 89% of the pulmonary veins ablated with optimized parameters compared with 52% chronic lesions in those ablated according to the initial workflow PFA settings.

In the SmartflRE trial,[15] Duytschaever and colleagues investigated the Dual-Energy CF-sensing, solid-tip Thermocool SmartTouch SF ablation catheter toggling from RF to PEF energy through the dual TRUPULSE generator (Biosense Webster Inc, Irvine, CA). Point-by-point PFA was delivered to the posterior and inferior region of the ablation line encircling the pulmonary veins while RF was applied to the thicker anterior region, ridge, and carina of these anatomic structures. Regarding CF evaluation, as shown in **Table 2**, specific target indexes for PEF and RF energy sources were utilized during ablation, PFI and VISITAG SUR-POINT module, respectively.[15] Different from the ECLIPSE AF trial, the SmartflRE study explored the acute feasibility and the chronic efficacy of patients with paroxysmal atrial fibrillation undergoing PVI using a combination of energy sources and not PEF energy only. Despite these inherent differences, the overall acute safety, efficacy, and chronic durable lesions were overlapping between studies.

DISCUSSION

When the impact of CF on lesion size is appraised during PFA, multiple preclinical and clinical studies suggest that catheter-tissue contact is paramount in achieving adequate lesion formation and that no contact provide absent or remarkably shallow lesions. Moreover, the higher the catheter-tissue contact, the deeper the lesions, which can be explained by the greater amount of PEF energy delivered to the myocardial tissue due to better catheter stability during high-contact applications.[11]

Different from RF energy, PEF is highly customizable via on a myriad of ablation parameters (see **Box 1**) that can theoretically lead to many combinations of PFA settings. Leveraging this combination of ablation parameters, the operator can select the actual amount of energy or PEF dose conveyed to the myocardium according to specific tissue requirements.[4] Even if low-dose PFA may be sufficient to achieve lesion transmurality at the pulmonary vein location,[12] increasing voltage amplitude and the number of applications seem necessary to achieve full lesion depth in thicker anatomic structures, such as the mitral isthmus region.[12] In addition, some studies also recorded "a plateau effect" for values of CF as low as 15 g[10] meaning that lesion size seems not to be affected by values of CF exceeding a contact threshold.

Therefore, it is the interplay between catheter-tissue contact and the amount of PEF energy dose delivered to the myocardial tissue in synergy that plays the most important role in achieving durable and transmural lesions.[13] Furthermore, as proven in vegetal models, specific ablation modalities related to PFA catheters, such as ablation stacking and catheter rotation, may further increase the chance to create bigger myocardial lesions[8] (**Fig. 2**). Whether these aspects translate into better clinical outcomes is yet to be established.

Currently, only 2 studies, the ECLIPSE AF and SmartfIRE trials,[14,15] were conducted on patients undergoing PVI using commercial CF-sensing, solid-tip catheters implementing either PFA or a combination of PEF and RF energy sources. Both studies proved the feasibility of the procedure in keeping with previous studies using the same ablation catheters delivering RF or PEF energy. Regarding safety, the incidence of side adverse

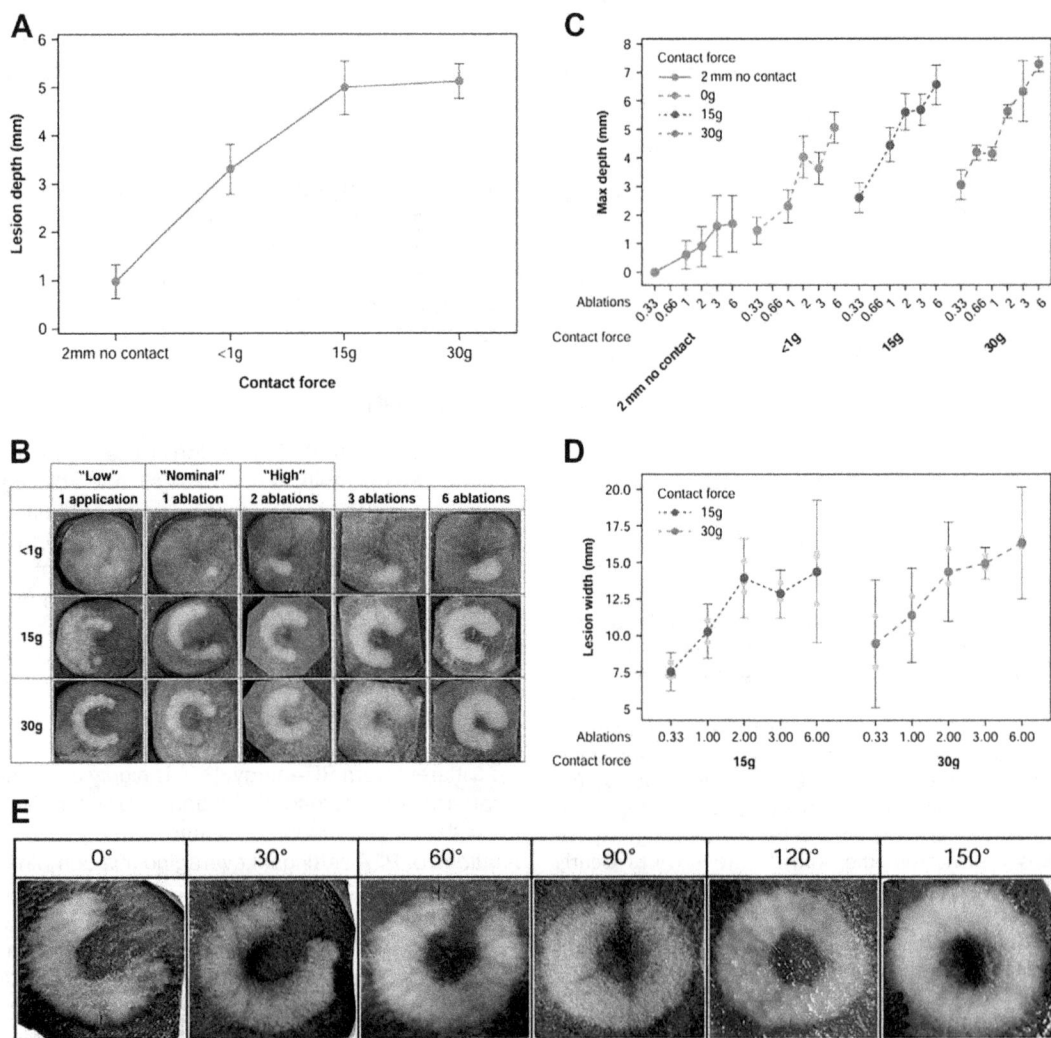

Fig. 2. *Impact of contact force and catheter rotation in lesion depth.* (*A*) An interval plot of lesion depth versus catheter contact in a vegetal model (*P*<.001). (*B*) Images of potato lesions corresponding to one application up to 6 ablations with 0, 15, and 30 g of contact force. The terms "low," "nominal," and "high" refer to the number of energy applications delivered before moving or rotating the catheter. Low dose entails 1 application, nominal dose entails 3 applications/1 ablation, and high dose entails 6 applications/2 ablations without moving the catheter. (*C*) An interval plot of lesion depth versus contact force (*P*<.001) and ablation dosage (*P*<.001). (*D*) An interval plot of lesion width versus contact force (*P* = .228) and ablation dosage (*P*<.001). (*E*) The degree measures indicate the angle to which the tip of the variable loop circular catheter is rotated (0°–180°) around the center point of the loop from the position of the first ablation to the position of the second stacked ablation. (*Data from* Di Biase L, Marazzato J, Gomez T, et al. Application repetition and electrode-tissue contact result in deeper lesions using a pulsed-field ablation circular variable loop catheter. Europace 2024;26(9):euae220. https://doi.org/10.1093/europace/euae220.)

events recorded in the ECLIPSE AF and SmartflRE trials was similar to past experiences using RF, CF-sensing catheters.[18] As for acute efficacy, the rate of first pass PVI was even higher when compared to RF ablation delivered with the same CF-sensing ablation catheters (92.2%[14]–96.8%[15] vs 73%–83%[19–21]). Chronic assessment was carried out in the ECLIPSE AF and SmartflRE trials through invasive remapping 90 days postprocedure. The overall chronic PVI rate was 87% to 89% (60% per patient) on average. This figure is in keeping with studies conducted with RF[22] or PEF field energy systems implementing non-CF-sensing catheters—such as the AFFERA (Medtronic, Minneapolis, MN)[23] and the FARAPULSE (Boston Scientific Corporation, Natick, MA) system[24]—where chronic remapping was mandatory after the index procedure. However, the rate of pulmonary vein reconnections is known to be higher in patients undergoing redo procedures for symptomatic arrhythmia recurrence after an initially successful PVI performed with thermal energy sources, such as RF, cryoablation, or laser ablation.[25] Likewise, similar findings were also observed in patients undergoing 3D remapping for symptomatic atrial fibrillation after PVI with the FARAPULSE systems[26,27] in which the rate of durable PVI was as low as 63%[26] to 69%[27] of the veins and 21%[26] to 42%[27] of the appraised patients.

In terms of reconnection sites, electrical gaps were more frequently found at the right-sided anterior carina region. Although the bulky FARAPULSE system and trans-septal sheath apparatus might make energy delivery difficult at the right inferior pulmonary vein and the thickness of the muscular sleeves of this anatomic structure may prevent deep and transmural lesions,[28] inadequate catheter-tissue contact, including risk of capturing the right phrenic nerve leading to chest movement during ablation, may in fact explain the remarkably high rate of reconnection observed at this site.[26,27] In fact, despite using different technologies, the ECLIPSE AF and SmartflRE trials found similar sites of reconnections at 90 day evaluation. When a review of the ablation set in the index PVI was performed to compare it with the location of the reconnection sites observed during redo procedure in the SmartflRE trial, it was found that reconnection was mostly due to lesion discontinuity or nontransmurality from low PFI parameters.[15] These findings would further suggest that both adequate catheter-tissue contact and the amount of PEF dose delivered to the myocardial tissue are paramount to achieve adequate lesion formation.

While ECLIPSE AF and SmartflRE provide the first systematic evaluation of an ablation strategy based on commercial CF-sensing catheters using PEF energy for PVI, several study limitations should be acknowledged. First, both trials have no control arms, thereby no comparison between RF (standard of care) versus PEF energy was appraised. Furthermore, the study methodology greatly differed. Not only were the PFA generators different, but the study protocol also was nonhomogeneous. In fact, while the ECLIPSE AF trial analyzed PEF energy only,[14] the SmartflRE study evaluated a combination of PEF and RF energy to achieve PVI.[15] Second, a clinical follow-up was not appraised, and whether 90 day evaluation translates into good long-term outcome is not clear. To further complicate things, durability assessment was not mandatory in the SmartflRE trial and was assessed in 30 patients only. Third, no evaluation of catheter stability was carried out with PFA and ablation tags were applied without respiratory gating.[14,15] Finally, as for PEF dose, although in the ECLIPSE trial the authors optimized the PFA parameters on the basis of an initial workflow, the variability of tissue thickness may require higher PEF dose to achieve better results.

SUMMARY

PEF energy is a highly customizable minimally thermal energy source that relies on specific ablation parameters and can be chosen by operators, potentially leading to a myriad of different PFA recipes. What is the best PEF energy dose to be delivered in accordance with the myocardial tissue thickness of the selected ablation target is yet to be ascertained. These observations notwithstanding, recent preclinical and clinical studies clearly suggest that regardless of the selected PEF energy dose, catheter-tissue contact is pivotal in achieving deeper lesion formation, and the higher the amount of CF, the deeper the lesion. Data on PFA of atrial targets beyond pulmonary veins are lacking and clinical data are scarce, and there is an urgent need to appraise the clinical role of CF during PFA for atrial and ventricular arrhythmias to unveil the black box on one of the most intriguing technologies in cardiac electrophysiology of the last decades.

CLINICS CARE POINTS

- While the importance of CF is well acknowledged during RF ablation, the role of catheter-tissue contact is far less clear for PFA.
- Although better catheter tip stability, tissue compression and envelopment provided by high catheter-tissue contact would

potentially lead to deeper lesion from greater electrical field conveyed to the myocardial tissue, recent literature on the role of CF is controversial.

- With only few exceptions, preclinical "in vivo" studies on ventricular swine models suggest that the higher the force, the deeper the lesions. More specifically, it is the interplay between CF and the amount of PEF energy delivered to the myocardium that synergistically impact lesion formation.

- Clinical studies conducted on patients undergoing PVI with PFA underscore the high safety and efficacy this novel energy source provided that adequate catheter-tissue contact is warranted.

- Further clinical studies are required to investigate the long-term clinical impact of contact-force-guided PFA in a variety of arrhythmogenic substrates.

DISCLOSURE

Dr L. Di Biase is a consultant for Stereotaxis, Biosense Webster, Boston Scientific, Abbott Medical, I-Rhythm, Siemens Medtronic, AtriCure, Biotronik, and Zoll. None for the other authors. No funding sources to be acknowledged.

REFERENCES

1. Thiagalingam A, D'Avila A, Foley L, et al. Importance of catheter contact force during irrigated radiofrequency ablation: evaluation in a porcine ex vivo model using a force-sensing catheter. J Cardiovasc Electrophysiol 2010;21(7):806–11.

2. Shah DC, Lambert H, Nakagawa H, et al. Area under the real-time contact force curve (force-time integral) predicts radiofrequency lesion size in an in vitro contractile model. J Cardiovasc Electrophysiol 2010; 21(9):1038–43.

3. Yokoyama K, Nakagawa H, Shah DC, et al. Novel contact force sensor incorporated in irrigated radiofrequency ablation catheter predicts lesion size and incidence of steam pop and thrombus. Circ Arrhythmia Electrophysiol 2008;1(5):354–62.

4. Julian Chun KR, Miklavčič D, Vlachos K, et al. State-of-the-art pulsed field ablation for cardiac arrhythmias: ongoing evolution and future perspective. Europace 2024;26(6):1–14.

5. Howard B, Verma A, Tzou WS, et al. Effects of electrode-tissue proximity on cardiac lesion formation using pulsed field ablation. Circ Arrhythmia Electrophysiol 2022;15(10):706–13.

6. Mattison L, Verma A, Tarakji KG, et al. Effect of contact force on pulsed field ablation lesions in porcine cardiac tissue. J Cardiovasc Electrophysiol 2023; 34(3):693–9.

7. Doshi SK, Flaherty MC, Laughner J, et al. Catheter–tissue contact optimizes pulsed electric field ablation with a large area focal catheter. J Cardiovasc Electrophysiol 2024;35(4):765–74.

8. Di Biase L, Marazzato J, Gomez T, et al. Application repetition and electrode-tissue-contact results in deeper lesions using a pulsed-field ablation circular variable loop catheter. Europace 2024;26:1–18.

9. Nakagawa H, Castellvi Q, Neal R, et al. Effects of contact force on lesion size during pulsed field catheter ablation: histochemical characterization of ventricular lesion boundaries. Circ Arrhythmia Electrophysiol 2024;17(1):11–23.

10. Hua J, Xiong Q, Kong Q, et al. A novel contact force sensing pulsed field ablation catheter in a porcine model. Clin Cardiol 2024;47(2):1–8.

11. Younis A, Santangeli P, Garrott K, et al. Impact of contact force on pulsed field ablation outcomes using focal point catheter. Circ Arrhythm Electrophysiol 2024;17(6):e012723.

12. Di Biase L, Marazzato J, Zou F, et al. Point-by-Point pulsed field ablation using a multimodality generator and a contact force-sensing ablation catheter: comparison with radiofrequency ablation in a remapped chronic swine heart. Circ Arrhythmia Electrophysiol 2023;16(12):663–71.

13. Di Biase L, Marazzato J, Govari A, et al. Pulsed field ablation index-guided ablation for lesion formation: impact of contact force and number of applications in the ventricular model. Circ Arrhythmia Electrophysiol 2024;17(4):E012717.

14. Anić A, Phlips T, Brešković T, et al. Pulsed field ablation using focal contact force-sensing catheters for treatment of atrial fibrillation : acute and 90-day invasive remapping results. Europace 2023;25(6):1–11.

15. Duytschaever M, Račkauskas G, Potter T De, et al. Dual energy for pulmonary vein isolation using dual-energy focal ablation technology integrated with a three-dimensional mapping system : SmartfIRE 3-month results. Europace 2024;26(5):1–10.

16. Gasperetti A, Assis F, Tripathi H, et al. Determinants of acute irreversible electroporation lesion characteristics after pulsed field ablation: the role of voltage, contact, and adipose interference. Europace 2023;25(9):1–9.

17. Phlips T, Taghji P, El Haddad M, et al. Improving procedural and one-year outcome after contact force-guided pulmonary vein isolation: the role of interlesion distance, ablation index, and contact force variability in the 'CLOSE'-protocol. Europace 2018; 20(FI3):f419–27.

18. Mansour M, Calkins H, Osorio J, et al. Persistent atrial fibrillation ablation with contact force–sensing catheter: the prospective multicenter PRECEPT trial. JACC Clin Electrophysiol 2020;6(8):958–69.

19. Duytschaever M, Vijgen J, De Potter T, et al. Standardized pulmonary vein isolation workflow to enclose veins with contiguous lesions: the multicentre VISTAX trial. Europace 2020;22(11):1645–52.

20. Di Biase L, Monir G, Melby D, et al. Composite index tagging for PVI in paroxysmal AF: a prospective, multicenter postapproval study. JACC Clin Electrophysiol 2022;8(9):1077–89.

21. Okumura K, Inoue K, Goya M, et al. Acute and mid-Term outcomes of ablation for atrial fibrillation with VISITAG SURPOINT: the Japan MIYABI registry. Europace 2023;25(9):1–10.

22. Galuszka OM, Baldinger SH, Servatius H, et al. Durability of CLOSE-guided pulmonary vein isolation in persistent atrial fibrillation. JACC Clin Electrophysiol 2024;10(6):1090–100.

23. Turagam MK, Neuzil P, Petru J, et al. PV isolation using a spherical array PFA catheter: application repetition and lesion durability (PULSE-EU study). JACC Clin Electrophysiol 2023;9(5):638–48.

24. Reddy VY, Dukkipati SR, Neuzil P, et al. Pulsed field ablation of paroxysmal atrial fibrillation: 1-year outcomes of IMPULSE, PEFCAT, and PEFCAT II. JACC Clin Electrophysiol 2021;7(5):614–27.

25. Nery PB, Belliveau D, Nair GM, et al. Relationship between pulmonary vein reconnection and atrial fibrillation recurrence: a systematic review and meta-analysis. JACC Clin Electrophysiol 2016;2(4):474–83.

26. Kueffer T, Stefanova A, Madaffari A, et al. Pulmonary vein isolation durability and lesion regression in patients with recurrent arrhythmia after pulsed-field ablation. J Interv Card Electrophysiol 2024;67(3):503–11.

27. Ruwald MH, Haugdal M, Worck R, et al. Characterization of durability and reconnection patterns at time of repeat ablation after single-shot pulsed field pulmonary vein isolation. J Interv Card Electrophysiol 2024;67(2):379–87.

28. Ho SY, Cabrera JA, Sanchez-Quintana D. Left atrial anatomy revisited. Circ Arrhythmia Electrophysiol 2012;5(1):220–8.

Pulsed Field Ablation in Ventricular Arrhythmias

Josef Kautzner, MD, PhD*, Petr Peichl, MD, PhD

KEYWORDS

- Ventricular arrhythmias • Ventricular premature beats • Ventricular tachycardia • Catheter ablation
- Pulsed field energy

KEY POINTS

- Pulsed field ablation (PFA) is potentially useful for ablation of ventricular arrhythmias, being safer with better penetration through scar tissue compared to thermal energies.
- Solid-tip PFA within the great cardiac vein appears to be useful for arrhythmias originating in the left ventricular summit.
- Large-footprint catheter that toggles between radiofrequency current and PFA allows creation of larger lesions and better penetration through the scar tissue.

INTRODUCTION

In the last 2 decades, catheter ablation (CA) has become a well-established strategy for management of a broad spectrum of ventricular arrhythmias (VA).[1] Until now, radiofrequency current was the main energy source for these kinds of procedures. In idiopathic focal ventricular premature beats (VPBs) or ventricular tachycardias (VTs), radiofrequency CA has demonstrated very high efficacy and an excellent safety profile. In subjects with arrhythmia-induced cardiomyopathy, CA improves left ventricular function. Therefore, it is considered in the guidelines of the European Society of Cardiology (ESC). However, there are some locations of the focus, which may be difficult to reach. Typical examples are the left ventricular summit or papillary muscles.

In patients with structural heart disease and recurrent VTs, CA of the arrhythmogenic substrate is an important strategy for the prevention of these arrhythmias. Based on the current evidence, it decreases VT burden and number of hospitalizations. Some recent studies have shown improvement of prognosis.[2,3] The problem with this kind of ablation is that the substrate is often extensive and its modification requires many lesions. In addition, some parts of the substrate may not be accessible to CA. Examples include midmyocardial location, the presence of old thrombus or inability to obtain pericardial access because of severe adhesions after previous surgery or pericarditis.[4] Another problem could be the inadequate endpoint of CA due to the noninducibility of VT. Finally, genetic studies suggest that the substrate could be diffuse in some genetic variants and CA has poor results.[5] These patients often rapidly progress with heart failure, and implantation of left ventricular assist device or heart transplant are better options.

In recent years, a new energy source has been introduced into the clinical arena, called pulsed field ablation (PFA).[6–9] In addition, novel catheter designs are being developed with large-footprint electrodes that can both map and ablate.[10] Some may even toggle between pulsed field energy and high-energy radiofrequency current.[11] The aim of this review is to summarize current evidence on the use of PFA for ablation of VA.

Department of Cardiology, Institute for Clinical and Experimental Medicine (IKEM), Videnska 1958/9, 14021 Prague, Czech Republic
* Corresponding author.
E-mail address: josef.kautzner@ikem.cz

Card Electrophysiol Clin 17 (2025) 205–212
https://doi.org/10.1016/j.ccep.2025.02.008
1877-9182/25/© 2025 Elsevier Inc. All rights reserved, including those for text and data mining, AI training, and similar technologies.

Abbreviations	
CA	catheter ablation
PFA	pulsed field ablation
VA	ventricular arrhythmias
VPB	ventricular premature beats
VT	ventricular tachycardias

POTENTIAL ADVANTAGES AND DISADVANTAGES OF PULSED FIELD ABLATION IN THE VENTRICLES

Based on preclinical studies, PFA is a highly selective and nonthermal ablation energy, which induces cell apoptosis, resulting in cellular death. Importantly, cardiomyocytes require a lower electric field intensity for inducing irreversible electroporation than the extracellular matrix, blood vessels, or nerves.[12,13] Therefore, PFA mitigates the risk of collateral damage to adjacent tissues. For this reason, it may be advantageous for the treatment of VA, particularly those that involve ablation close to coronary vessels or nerves.

The other potential advantage may be better penetration through the scar tissue as compared to radiofrequency current. One study in postmyocardial infarction swine documented that the monopolar PFA produced uniform and well-demarcated lesions exhibiting irreversible injury characterized by cardiomyocyte death, contraction bands, and lymphocytic infiltration, and that the width and depth of the ablation lesions surpassed radiofrequency lesions, with a greater transmurality rate (73% vs 30%).[14] Importantly, PFA extended from the subendocardium through collagen and fat to the epicardial layers, which was not the case in radiofrequency lesions. Radiofrequency lesions were less uniform and largely limited to the subendocardium with minimal effect on viable myocardium deeper to separating layers of collagen and fat. Another preclinical study demonstrated that the depth of lesions created by monopolar PFA in scared ventricular myocardium was smaller than in healthy myocardium, while their widths were similar.[15]

Similar data were published for bipolar PFA in swine model of myocardial infarction using linear and basket catheter designs.[16] In scar tissue, the lesion depth was greater for PFA as compared to radiofrequency lesions (PFA vs radiofrequency ablation depth, 5.7 ± 0.8 mm vs 4.8 ± 1.4 mm; $P = .012$). There was no difference in lesion depth between the 2 catheter designs, only basket catheter lesions were broader. Another study with bipolar, biphasic PFA in swine scarred myocardium showed better penetration in infarct or iatrogenic scar with deeper lesions.[17]

Repetition dependency is another potentially useful feature of PFA. In an animal study with monopolar PFA and large-footprint catheter, the average lesion depth increased with repetitive applications significantly, both acutely and chronically.[18] The underlying mechanism of repetition dependency may include the gradual destruction of a larger section of the sarcolemmal membrane. The lesion depth in chronic phase was between 7 to 8 mm. Another in vivo experimental study showed that repeated PFA deliveries on papillary muscles or moderator band achieve lesion depth of around 6 mm.[19] Repeated epicardial deliveries resulted in lesion as deep as 9 mm. The authors tested also a possibility to create bipolar lesions between 2 lattice-tip catheters across the interventricular septum or left ventricular free wall. An 87% transmurality rate and a mean depth of 14.3 ± 4.7 mm were achieved without evidence of thermal injury or tissue disruption and with evidence of fibrotic healing.

However, compared to pulmonary vein isolation, where remapping at 3 months can show gaps and lead to tuning of the pulse field characteristics until practically 100% durability is reached,[20,21] there is no such clear end-point in clinical VT ablation. Currently, we lack optimally tuned pulsed field energy for VT ablation. The problem is that once one delivers PFA, local electrograms disappear and the only proof of lesion quality may be local noncapture. However, it does not necessarily mean that the lesion will be durable and deep enough to modify the substrate. Noninducibility of VT is also not a very reliable means to check for completeness of substrate modification. One theoretically useful option could be to employ a short, reversible pulse of PFA to terminate VT in the critical region of the substrate.[22,23] So far, this strategy of the so-called pulsed field mapping has been tested in human in atypical flutter and in atrioventricular nodal reentry tachycardia.[23]

Regarding safety, concerns for coronary artery vasospasm and/or stenosis[24,25] secondary to neointimal hyperplasia, as well as nerve damage,[26] have been raised. However, current experience suggests a lower risk of these complications compared to the thermal catheter-based ablation modalities used for comparable substrates. Data on the safety of PFA for atrial fibrillation are also reassuring that the risk of collateral damage is low.[27]

AVAILABLE PULSED FIELD ABLATION TECHNOLOGIES

As for now, several technologies of PFA have been approved for the clinical use, mainly for ablation of atrial fibrillation.

Farapulse System

The key parts of this system are a pentaspline catheter Farawave and the generator Farapulse (Boston Scientific). During early clinical studies, the characteristics of the pulse were optimized based on remapping data.[20] The optimized pulse resulted in excellent durability of lesions. This platform is currently the most widespread PFA tool and the total number of procedures for atrial fibrillation already exceeded 100,000. It has demonstrated a favorable safety profile by avoiding much of the collateral damage seen with conventional thermal ablation.[27]

Several case reports in Europe have demonstrated the potential safety and efficacy of pentaspline catheter and PFA for scar-related VT.[28–31] In the case series, PFA applications changed both the morphology and amplitude of ventricular electrograms (decreasing the mean amplitude by 30% after a first application and 56% after a complete set).

Although this is an off-label indication, reports considered potential advantages for modification of the scar-related substrate. These included wider area ablation for substrate modification, efficiency, and lack of significant irrigation requirement. No complications have been reported. These pioneering attempts suggest a great promise of PFA for VT ablation.

Centauri System

The Centauri system (CardioFocus) is a novel pulsed field generator that enables PFA using different commercially available catheters. Its safety and efficacy were evaluated for ablation of atrial fibrillation.[32] Anecdotally, this generator has been used for VA ablation, but so far, data on efficacy and safety are limited to case reports[33] and small case series.[34] In a cohort of 20 patients from 2 centers, the Centautri system was used together with a contact-force-sensing catheter and 3D mapping system for ablation of VPBs. Altogether 55% of procedures were performed under general anesthesia. Median procedural and fluoroscopy times reached 95.5 and 6.55 min, respectively. The median number of PFA applications reached 8 with a median contact force of 10 g. A significant reduction of electrogram voltage was observed and acute success reached 85%. Interestingly, 2 patients with procedural failure showed late success in reduction of ectopic activity greater than 80%. The median follow-up was 120 days and 85% success in suppression of VPBs. Transient ST segment depression occurred in 1 patient and permanent right bundle block in another patient.

Affera System

The third approved technology for the clinical use of PFA in atrial fibrillation ablation is the Affera system (Medtronic) with a large-footprint catheter called Sphere 9.[20,21] This system was optimized for use in atria for atrial fibrillation or atrial tachycardia with very promising results. Few ablations with radiofrequency current were done for ventricular substrate during the development phase of the system. Later, the clinical use of a lattice tip for VT ablation has been reported in a case report and small case series.[35,36] The latter study reported on experience with the use of lattice-tip catheter in 4 patients with structural heart disease, 3 had previous ablation procedure. The diagnoses were Brugada syndrome, arrhythmogenic right ventricular cardiomyopathy, and ischemic or non-ischemic cardiomyopathy. In 2 patients with right ventricular substrates, PFA was used first. In others, radiofrequency ablation from the lattice-tip electrode was initially employed. There was a significant increase of low-voltage area after ablation. No procedural complications were noted. At a median follow-up of 5 months, no recurrences of VT were observed.

OUR EXPERIENCE WITH FOCAL PULSED FIELD ABLATION IN VENTRICULAR ARRHYTHMIAS

Our 2-center study aimed to analyze the safety and efficacy of focal PFA delivered by the Centauri generator through a contact-force-sensing ablation catheter (Smart Touch, Biosense Webster) and a 3-dimensional electroanatomical mapping system.[37] Both patients with frequent VPBs and scar-related VT were recruited. The procedures were performed under conscious sedation with fentanyl and midazolam, or on propofol. Applications (25A) were delivered using the Centauri generator and repeated at each target site up to 3 times to maximize the lesion size. Whenever PF was applied within the great cardiac vein, coronary angiography was performed before and after the PFA to exclude coronary artery spasm. No nitrates were applied prophylactically before PFA. Following CA, patients were evaluated in the departmental outpatient clinic in 3-month intervals.

The population consisted of 44 patients from the 2 centers. Twenty-one (48%) patients had frequent VPBs with a mean burden of $27 \pm 12\%$ on a 24-h Holter monitoring and the rest had scar-related VT. A total of 57% of patients had previously failed RF ablation procedure(s) for VA. The mean procedural duration was 113 ± 46 minutes, and the fluoroscopy time reached 6.9 ± 4.3 minutes. On average, 16 ± 15 PF applications were delivered per patient. Importantly, PF deliveries did not induce sustained VT or ventricular fibrillation in any of the patients. In 9 patients (20%), additional lesions with RF energy were delivered (2 ± 7 applications per patient).

We have made several important observations: (1) compared to radiofrequency energy, focal PFA within the great cardiac vein was not limited by a high impedance or poor catheter-tip cooling, (2) PFA inside the great cardiac vein was not associated with coronary artery spasm (**Fig. 1**), (3) in scar-related VT, abolition of local electrograms cannot be considered an endpoint of CA (in contrast to radiofrequency ablation), (4) since PFA lesions have larger zone of a reversible injury, also noninducibility of VT may not be an adequate endpoint, (5) unexpected conduction system block was observed during retrograde CA in the left ventricle due to current leakage from the proximal, shaft-visualizing electrodes of the ablation catheter (this adverse event was never observed when the transseptal approach to the left ventricle was chosen); (6) focal PFA was not associated with excessive myocardial damage as assessed by troponin levels postablation.

More recently, we observed another interesting phenomenon while performing focal PFA in VA. Delivery of PF energy in specific regions of a substrate captured locally the myocardium and led to intermittent stimulation. Disappearance of such capture might indicate creation of a good ablation lesion (**Fig. 2**).

OUR EXPERIENCE WITH LARGE-FOOTPRINT PULSED FIELD ABLATION IN VENTRICULAR ARRHYTHMIAS

Our recent analysis of 18 patients (aged 55 ± 15 years, 1 woman) with recurrent sustained VT is currently submitted for publication.[38] A total of 66% of patients had failed previous endocardial radiofrequency CA with conventional irrigated-tip catheter. Mapping/ablation was performed using the novel electroanatomical mapping system Affera. Just to recap briefly the technology, the nitinol lattice-tip electrode has 9 microelectrodes distributed around an equator and on the top. These microelectrodes collect close unipolar signals against indifferent central electrode on the shaft. Such an arrangement allows fast high-density mapping of ventricular substrate and/or activation mapping during tolerated VT (**Fig. 3**). The system provides an option to deliver high-energy radiofrequency or PF energy.

All procedures were performed under general anesthesia. Ablation using high-energy radiofrequency current was used as the primary ablation strategy. PFA applications were added to further consolidate the lesions if VT suppression or

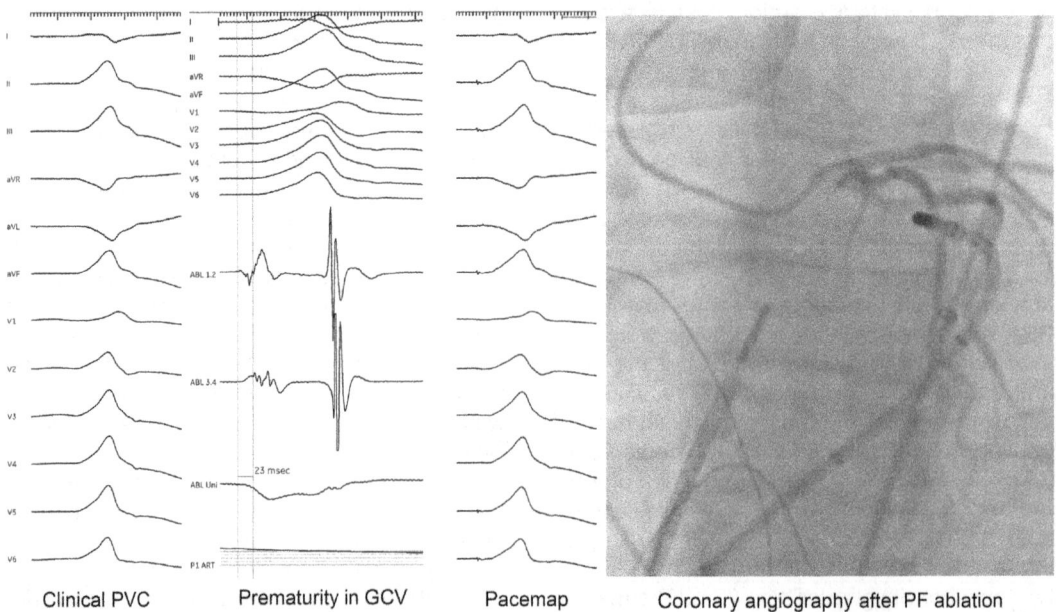

| Clinical PVC | Prematurity in GCV | Pacemap | Coronary angiography after PF ablation |

Fig. 1. An illustrative case of a patient with frequent VPBs originating from the great cardiac vein. The panels show from left to right the morphology of the clinical VPB, local electrogram at the site of the earliest activity, the pacemap with 12/12 match with clinical VPB, and the angiogram of the left main coronary artery. No spasm was noted after PFA, which successfully eliminated the clinical VPB.

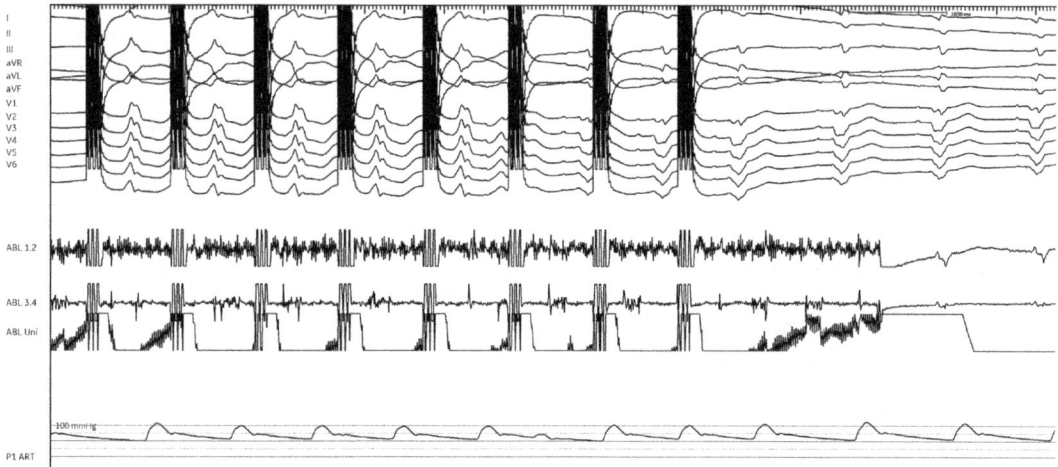

Fig. 2. Surface ECG and intracardiac electrograms during PFA using focal 4mm-tip catheter and Centauri generator. The initial pulses lead to local myocardial capture with long pulse-to-QRS interval. Note that the capture is lost for the last 3 pulses, which might indicate the creation of a good ablation lesion. Abl 1.2, distal bipole of the ablation catheter; Abl 3.4, proximal bipole of ablation catheter; ABl uni, unipolar signal from the distal electrode; P1 ART, arterial blood pressure.

adequate substrate modification could not be achieved by radiofrequency ablation only. PFA was not used in close vicinity to the proximal ventricular conduction system. On the other hand, in epicardial space, only PFA was used.

This more recent experience with a large-footprint catheter and the use of both radiofrequency current and PFA has provided another interesting observation: (1) high-density mapping with the large-footprint catheter was efficient; however, entrainment mapping was limited due to frequently observed noncapture from microelectrodes, (2) a combination of high-energy radiofrequency current and PF allowed fast and effective modification of the endocardial substrate, (3) epicardial use of PFA was safe and there

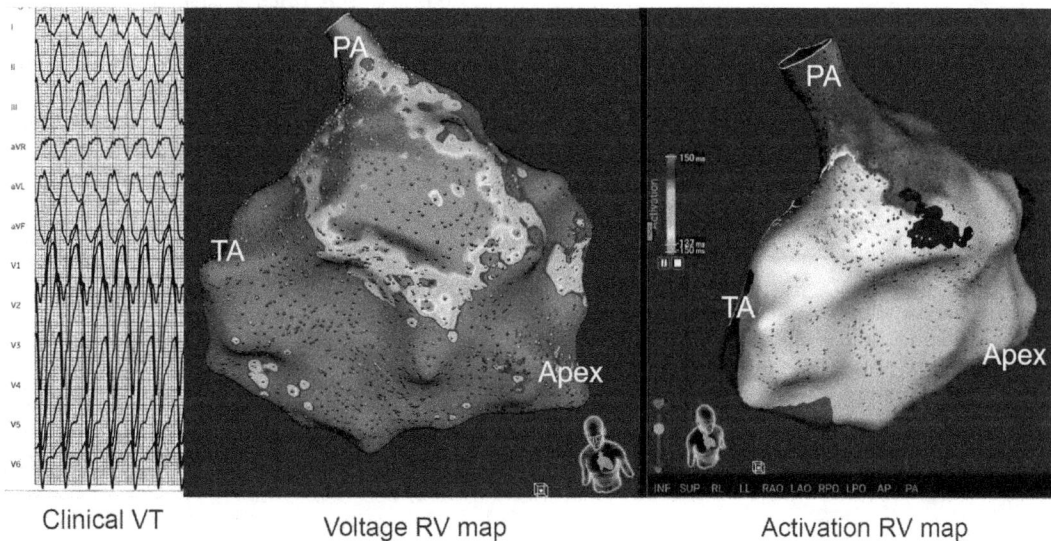

Clinical VT   Voltage RV map   Activation RV map

Fig. 3. An illustrative case of a patient with grown-up congenital heart disease after surgical correction (double outlet right ventricle). The panels show from left to right the ECG morphology of clinical VT, voltage map of the right ventricular with a large scar in the outflow tract that corresponds to a patch, and an activation map during VT that depicts reentry encircling the low-voltage area in the outflow tract. Ablation from the scar toward the tricuspid annulus successfully terminated VT. Apex, apical region of the right ventricle; PA, pulmonary artery; TA, tricuspid annulus.

was no risk of phrenic nerve palsy, (4) PF energy allowed ablation close to coronary arteries, only with a risk of spasm that resolved after administration of nitrates, (5) some regions of the heart are difficult to reach with 9 mm electrode (eg, below the tricuspid or mitral valve or some trabeculated areas).

Precise positioning of the large-footprint electrode within the heart underscores the role of intracardiac echocardiography that enables detailed visualization of the lattice tip and its tailored placement. This is much easier in ischemic cardiomyopathy since scarring and remodeling after myocardial infarction results in thinning and smoothing of the myocardial wall. Such conditions facilitate mapping and CA with the lattice-tip electrode. It differs from patients with nonischemic cardiomyopathy since they often have prominent trabeculations and variable wall thickness. The critical components of the substrate may be localized more frequently intramurally and more difficult to be described and successfully ablated.

SUMMARY

Early experience with PFA in VA is promising. PFA allows safe energy delivery in the great cardiac vein or epicardially close to coronary arteries or phrenic nerve. Also, PFA within the scar tissue seems to be more efficacious than using radiofrequency current. However, we still do not know which pulse characteristics are optimal for VA ablation. It is therefore much more difficult to tune up the characteristics of the pulse than in ablation of atrial fibrillation. Remapping after 3 months showed clearly gaps in the ablation lines around the pulmonary vein ostia. This strategy has been used when developing Farapulse or Affera system for ablation of atrial fibrillation. In structural heart disease VT, we lack similar studies on the efficacy of PFA. The best proof would be remapping of the core isolated region of the scar. A surrogate endpoint could be the noninducibility of arrhythmia, which may not reflect the true durability of the PFA lesions. The other option is to wait for long-term effects using VT burden assessment from implanted ICD.

Despite all the above difficulties we feel that PFA of VA is a new avenue that has to be explored.

CLINICS CARE POINTS

- Pulsed field ablation (PFA) is a novel non-thermal energy source for catheter ablation, which is potentially useful also for ablation of ventricular arrhythmias (VA).

- The main advantages are minimal risk for a collateral damage and better penetration through the scar tissue compared to thermal energies.

- So far, few technologies have been employed successfully in VA ablation.

- Solid-tip PFA appears to be particularly useful within the great cardiac vein or other cardiac veins adjacent to arrhythmogenic focus or substrate, and for ablation on the papillary muscles or in the periannular region.

- A large-footprint catheter that toggles between PFA and radiofrequency ablation allows the creation of large lesions to modify the myocardial substrate and better penetrate through the scar tissue.

- Side effects of PFA are minimal and include the risk of coronary spasm, transient phrenic nerve palsy, or hemolysis.

DISCLOSURES

J. Kautzner reports personal fees from Biosense Webster, Boston Scientific, GE Healthcare, Medtronic, and St. Jude Medical (Abbott) for participation in scientific advisory boards and has received speaker honoraria from Biosense Webster, Biotronik, Boston Scientific, Medtronic, ProMed CS, St. Jude Medical (Abbott), and Viatris. P. Peichl has received speaker honoraria from St Jude Medical (Abbott) and has served as a consultant for Biotronik and Boston Scientific. This study was supported by the project National Institute for Research of Metabolic and Cardiovascular Diseases (Programme EXCELES, Project No. LX22NPO5104)—Funded by the European Union-Next Generation EU. This work was also funded by the project (Ministry of Health of the Czech Republic) for development of research organization 00,023,001 (IKEM, Prague, Czech Republic)—Institutional support.

REFERENCES

1. Zeppenfeld K, Tfelt-Hansen J, de Riva M, et al. 2022 ESC Guidelines for the management of patients with ventricular arrhythmias and the prevention of sudden cardiac death. Eur Heart J 2022; 43(40):3997–4126.

2. Della Bella P, Baratto F, Vergara P, et al. Does timing of ventricular tachycardia ablation affect prognosis in patients with an implantable cardioverter defibrillator? Results from the multicenter randomized PARTITA trial. Circulation 2022;145:1829–38.

3. Ravi V, Poudyal A, Khanal S, et al. A systematic review and meta-analysis comparing radiofrequency

catheter ablation with medical therapy for ventricular tachycardia in patients with ischemic and non-ischemic cardiomyopathies. J Interv Card Electrophysiol 2023;66:161–75.

4. Tokuda M, Kojodjojo P, Tung S, et al. Acute failure of catheter ablation for ventricular tachycardia due to structural heart disease: causes and significance. J Am Heart Assoc 2013;2(3):e000072.

5. Ebert M, Wijnmaalen AP, de Riva M, et al. Prevalence and prognostic impact of pathogenic variants in patients with dilated cardiomyopathy referred for ventricular tachycardia ablation. JACC Clin Electrophysiol 2020;6(9):1103–14.

6. Moshkovits Y, Grynberg D, Heller E, et al. Differential effect of high-frequency electroporation on myocardium vs. non-myocardial tissues. Europace 2023;25(2):748–55.

7. Chen C. Pulsed-field ablation opening a new era in cardiac arrhythmia therapy. Int J Cardiol 2024;19:132588.

8. Repp ML, Chinyere IR. Opportunities and challenges in catheter-based irreversible electroporation for ventricular tachycardia. Pathophysiology 2024;31:32–43.

9. Ezzeddine FM, Asirvatham SJ, Nguyen DT. Pulsed field ablation: a comprehensive update. J Clin Med 2024;13(17):5191.

10. Kawamura I, Reddy VY, Wang BJ, et al. Pulsed field ablation of the porcine ventricle using a focal lattice-tip catheter. Circ Arrhythm Electrophysiol 2022;15(9):e011120.

11. Reddy VY, Peichl P, Anter E, et al. A focal ablation catheter toggling between radiofrequency and pulsed field energy to treat atrial fibrillation. JACC Clin Electrophysiol 2023;9(8 Pt 3):1786–801.

12. Aycock KN, Campelo SN, Davalos RV. A comparative modeling study of thermal mitigation strategies in irreversible electroporation treatments. J Heat Transfer 2022;144:031206.

13. Teng P, Wu Y, Chen R, et al. Pulsed field ablation as a precise approach for cardiac arrhythmia treatment via cardiac microenvironment remodeling. Bioelectrochemistry 2023;154:108502.

14. Younis A, Zilberman I, Krywanczyk A, et al. Effect of pulsed-field and radiofrequency ablation on heterogeneous ventricular scar in a swine model of healed myocardial infarction. Circ Arrhythm Electrophysiol 2022;15(10):e011209.

15. Sandhu U, Alkukhun L, Kheiri B, et al. In vivo pulsed-field ablation in healthy vs. chronically infarcted ventricular myocardium: biophysical and histologic characterization. Europace 2023;25:1503–9.

16. Im SI, Higuchi S, Lee A, et al. Pulsed field ablation of left ventricular myocardium in a swine infarct model. JACC Clin Electrophysiol 2022;8:722–31.

17. Kawamura I, Reddy VY, Santos-Gallego CG, et al. Electrophysiology, pathology, and imaging of pulsed field ablation of scarred and healthy ventricles in swine. Circ Arrhythm Electrophysiol 2023;16(1):e011369.

18. Yavin HD, Higuchi K, Sroubek J, et al. Pulsed-field ablation in ventricular myocardium using a focal catheter: the impact of application repetition on lesion dimensions. Circ Arrhythm Electrophysiol 2021;14:e010375.

19. Nies M, Watanabe K, Kawamura I, et al. Preclinical study of pulsed field ablation of difficult ventricular targets: intracavitary mobile structures, interventricular septum, and left ventricular free wall. Circ Arrhythm Electrophysiol 2024;17(6):e012734.

20. Reddy VY, Neuzil P, Koruth JS, et al. Pulsed field ablation for pulmonary vein isolation in atrial fibrillation. J Am Coll Cardiol 2019;74(3):315–26.

21. Reddy VY, Peichl P, Anter E, et al. A focal ablation catheter toggling between radiofrequency and pulsed field energy to treat atrial fibrillation. JACC Clin Electrophysiol 2023;9(8 Pt 3):1786–801.

22. van Zyl M, Ladejobi AO, Tri JA, et al. Reversible atrioventricular conduction impairment following bipolar nanosecond electroporation of the inter- ventricular septum. J Am Coll Cardiol EP 2021;7(2):255–7.

23. Koruth JS, Neuzil P, Kawamura I, et al. Reversible pulsed electrical fields as an in vivo tool to study cardiac electrophysiology: the advent of pulsed field mapping. Circ Arrhythm Electrophysiol 2023;16(10):e012018.

24. Ladejobi A, Christopoulos G, Tan N, et al. Effects of pulsed electric fields on the coronary arteries in swine. Circ Arrhythm Electrophysiol 2022;15:e010668.

25. Higuchi S, Im SI, Stillson C, et al. Effect of epicardial pulsed field ablation directly on coronary arteries. JACC Clin. Electrophysiol 2022;8:1486–96.

26. Pansera F, Bordignon S, Bologna F, et al. Catheter ablation induced phrenic nerve palsy by pulsed field ablation-completely impossible? A case series. Eur Heart J Case Rep 2022;6:ytac361.

27. Ekanem E, Neuzil P, Reichlin T, et al. Safety of pulsed field ablation in more than 17,000 patients with atrial fibrillation in the MANIFEST-17K study. Nat Med 2024;30(7):2020–9.

28. Ouss A, van Stratum L, van der Voort P, et al. First in human pulsed field ablation to treat scar-related ventricular tachycardia in ischemic heart disease: a case report. J Interv Card Electrophysiol 2023;66(3):509–10.

29. Adragao P, Matos D, Carmo P, et al. Pulsed-field ablation vs radiofrequency ablation for ventricular tachycardia: first in-human case of histologic lesion analysis. Heart Rhythm 2023;20(10):1395–8.

30. Lozano-Granero C, Hirokami J, Franco E, et al. Case series of ventricular tachycardia ablation with pulsed-field ablation: pushing technology further (into the ventricle), JACC Clin. Electrophysiol 2023;9(9):1990–4.

31. Martin CA, Zaw MT, Jackson N, et al. First worldwide use of pulsed-field ablation for ventricular tachycardia ablation via a retrograde approach. J Cardiovasc Electrophysiol 2023;34(8):1772–5.

32. Anić A, Phlips T, Brešković T, et al. Pulsed field ablation using focal contact force-sensing catheters for treatment of atrial fibrillation: acute and 90-day invasive remapping results. Europace 2023;25(6): euad147.

33. Compagnucci P, Valeri Y, Conti S, et al. Technological advances in ventricular tachycardia catheter ablation: the relentless quest for novel solutions to old problems. J Interv Card Electrophysiol 2024; 67(4):855–64.

34. Della Rocca DG, Cespón-Fernandez M, Keelani A, et al. Focal pulsed field ablation for premature ventricular contractions: a multicenter experience. Circ Arrhythm Electrophysiol 2024;17(9):e012826.

35. Yokoyama M, Vlachos K, Duchateau J, et al. Pulsed field epicardial ablation for VT storm: a case report of bail-out therapy. Heart Rhythm 2024. S1547-5271(24)03140-0.

36. Pannone L, Doundoulakis I, Cespón-Fernández M, et al. A large footprint focal catheter toggling between pulsed field and radiofrequency energy: first clinical experience for ventricular tachycardia ablation. Europace 2024;26(7):euae193.

37. Peichl P, Bulava A, Wichterle D, et al. Efficacy and safety of focal pulsed-field ablation for ventricular arrhythmias: two-centre experience. Europace 2024; 26:euae192.

38. Peichl P, Wichterle D, Schlosser F, et al. Ablation of ventricular tachycardia using dual-energy, lattice-tip, mapping and ablation system: early feasibility and safety study. Europace 2024;26(11):euae275.

Current Safety Profile of Pulse Field Ablation
Not Everything that Shines Is Gold

Aashish Katapadi, MD[a], T. Jared Bunch, MD[b], Rajesh Kabra, MD[a],
Thomas F. Deering, MBA, MD[c], Dhanunjaya Lakkireddy, MBA, MD[a],*

KEYWORDS

• Atrial fibrillation • Complications • Electroporation • Pulse field ablation • Safety • Thermal ablation

KEY POINTS

- Pulse field ablation is a promising technology with a potentially improved clinical safety profile compared to traditional thermal energy sources.
- Complications related to pulse-field ablation can be separated into traditional complications of intracardiac procedure and thermal injury and complications unique to electroporation.
- The technology has inherent advantages and disadvantages, as well as additional considerations and controversies, that must be considered and require future study.

INTRODUCTION

Catheter ablation (CA) is an effective treatment option for atrial fibrillation (AF) and is recommended as a first-line therapy in select patients. Despite improvements in procedural outcomes and techniques, the primary energy source remains radiofrequency ablation (RFA) or cryoablation (CRA), with the potential for collateral damage to surrounding structures.

Pulse field ablation (PFA) is a novel, nonthermal energy source alternative that utilizes electroporation, in which brief applications of electric field gradient create reversible pores in the cell plasma membrane.[1] High voltages and long application durations result in cell apoptosis and necrosis, affecting particular tissues more than others. Cardiomyocytes are more susceptible to its effects due to a lower electric field threshold.[2] While each PFA system requires individual testing to optimize for cellular vulnerability and irreversible cellular damage, the goal is to create durable transmural lesions without collateral damage.

Several studies demonstrate that PFA results in similar efficacy, shorter procedure times, and acceptable complication rates compared to existing thermal ablation tools.[3–6] Complications measured in these studies included traditional and thermal injury risks and those unique to PFA. Since PFA causes injury to the cell without significant heat generated, evaluating it using thermal injury risks may underestimate its true safety. Additionally, symptoms and timing of PFA-specific risks may significantly differ from those of RFA or CRA.

As PFA use grows, the authors anticipate a better understanding of the technology and its unique complications. A solid grasp of current knowledge and electroporation-specific risks is essential. Consequently, this review covers the evolution and current safety profile of PFA.

a Department of Clinical Electrophysiology, Kansas City Heart Rhythm Institute, 5100 West 110th Street, Suite 200, Overland Park, KS 66210, USA; b Division of Cardiovascular Medicine, Department of Internal Medicine, University of Utah Health, 30 North 1900 East, Room 4A100, Salt Lake City, UT 84132, USA; c Department of Electrophysiology, Piedmont Heart of Buckhead Electrophysiology, Piedmont Heart Institute, 95 Collier Road Northwest, Suite 6000, Atlanta, GA 30309, USA
* Corresponding author.
E-mail address: dhanunjaya.lakkireddy@hcahealthcare.com

Card Electrophysiol Clin 17 (2025) 213–225
https://doi.org/10.1016/j.ccep.2025.02.009
1877-9182/25/© 2025 Elsevier Inc. All rights are reserved, including those for text and data mining, AI training, and similar technologies.

Abbreviations	
AF	atrial fibrillation
AKI	acute kidney injury
CA	catheter ablation
CAS	coronary artery vasospasm
CRA	cryoablation
PFA	pulse field ablation
PV	pulmonary vein
RFA	radiofrequency ablation
TIA	transient ischemic attack

EARLY SAFETY DATA

The current form of PFA evolved from early attempts at direct current ablation, which was effective for His bundle and ventricular tachycardia ablation.[7] However, it required general anesthesia, was pro-arrhythmic immediately post-procedure, and was associated with barotrauma and electrical arcing.[8,9] The development of low-energy direct current ablation addressed these issues, but the advent of RFA quickly replaced these techniques until recently.[10]

Preclinical and Animal Studies

Early animal studies on PFA showed promising safety (**Table 1**).[11] These studies revealed transmural lesions near the pulmonary vein (PV) without stenosis, which have been confirmed by many. They also demonstrated no esophageal injury, including luminal stenosis, erosion or ulcer, or fistula formation, up to 16 weeks post-ablation.[12] A meta-analysis of 16 early studies demonstrates PFA safety, with minimal complications that include ventricular arrhythmia, arcing, pericarditis, and unexplained hemodynamic instability; none were linked to direct electroporation.[13]

Early Clinical Trials

The safety of PFA was further confirmed in early human trials and clinical trials (**Table 2**).[14,15] Notable first-in-human studies are those by Reddy and colleagues[16] and Loh and colleagues[17], in which no major complications were reported; however, 9 out of 10 patients experienced reversible ST-segment elevation in the latter.

The first trials assessing PFA were the IMPULSE and PEFCAT trials, which reported one pericardial effusion 120 days after the procedure.[2] Their extension, PEFCAT II, reported a 2.5% incidence of early or late adverse events over 1 year. Later trials and registries, such as PULSED-AF, MANIFEST-PF, and EU-PORIA, demonstrate similar safety.[4,18,19] In ADVENT, prespecified device and procedure-related adverse events (2.1% vs 1.5%, 95% Bayesian CI -1.5–2.8) were non-inferior, but PV cross-sectional changes (−0.9% vs −12.0%) were superior with PFA than thermal ablation.[5] A meta-analysis of 24 studies with 5203 total patients further reveals fewer complications (2.05% vs 7.75%, $P = .001$) with PFA than thermal ablation.[20] Yet, awareness and understanding of these complications (**Fig. 1**) remain essential.

TRADITIONAL COMPLICATIONS OF CARDIAC ABLATION PROCEDURES

PFA uses cannulation, cardiac access, and catheter manipulation techniques like other CA tools. Thus, procedure-related complications, like vascular issues, pericardial effusion, and stroke—listed in order of decreasing frequency—still occur.[21] Periprocedural complications occurred in only 1.4% of CA procedures from 2005 to 2020 despite doubling procedures and declined in 2018 to 2022 from 2013 to 2017 (3.77% vs 5.31%, $P = .043$).[21,22] Monitoring for them, though, remains an integral part of any catheter-based procedure.

Pericardial Tamponade and Cardiac Perforation

Pericardial effusion, with or without tamponade, is a recognized complication of CA procedures, often caused by trauma or perforation (micro- or macro-).[23] Diagnosis necessitates intracardiac echocardiography and hemodynamic monitoring with a low index of suspicion.[24] The risk of effusion increases with anticoagulation status and transvenous puncture, but patients show no increase in mortality, stroke, or hospitalization (HR 1.22, 95% CI 0.79–1.88).[25,26] Patients should be treated with pericardiocentesis or surgery when indicated. Given that many PFA catheters are single-shot tools with larger sizes, the potential for trauma and effusion should be considered, as the incidence of tamponade is still 0.36% in PFA.[6]

Cerebral Embolic and Microembolic Events

Even though CA aims to reduce stroke, it is still a recognized periprocedural risk in ablation procedures, with an estimated incidence of 0.97%.[27] The risk remains unchanged with PFA compared to RFA and CRA (0.6% vs 0.3% vs 0%, $P = .61$) and persists 24 to 48 hours post-procedure.[28,29] It also increases with a CHA_2DS_2VASC score 2 or more (OR 7.1, $P = .02$) and a history of stroke (OR 9.5, $P<.01$).[29] In contrast, periprocedural anticoagulation decreases (OR 13, 95% CI 3.1–55.6, $P<.001$ when discontinuing Warfarin) but does not eliminate risk.[30,31]

Table 1
Initial complications seen in animal studies

Study, Year	Animal	Described Adverse Events
Lavee et al, 2007	Pig	No local temperature change; no peripheral damage
Hong et al, 2009	Sheep	Endothelial denudation of intralesional veins; mild esophageal injury; arcing
Wittkampf et al, 2012	Pig	None
Du Pre et al, 2013	Pig	No intimal hyperplasia of coronary arteries
Neven et al, 2014	Pig	Local epicardial hematoma
Van Driel et al, 2014	Pig	None
Zager et al, 2016	Rat	None. Increasing myocardial injury with greater voltage
Madhavan et al, 2016	Dog	Ventricular fibrillation
Hirano et al, 2018	Pig	Expected endomyocardial injury. No macroscopic injury
Koruth et al, 2019	Pig	Monophasic: brief episodes of tachycardia; insignificant ST elevation and T-wave peaking. Biphasic: involuntary muscle and diaphragmatic stimulation. Phrenic nerve was spared
Padmanabhan et al, 2019	Dog	One dog died due to procedural and pericardial puncture complication. Spillover ganglionic lesions; mild damage to posterior wall of pulmonary artery; minor damage to pulmonary vein myocardium
Sugrue et al, 2020	Dog	Minimal myocardial damage; ventricular tachycardia
Yavin et al,[73] 2020	Pig	Mild esophageal edema

Minimal complications are demonstrated even in pre-clinical animal studies, and few even reported no complications.
Abbreviations: CI, confidence interval; HR, hazard ratio; OR, odds ratio.
Di Monaco A et al., Pulsed Field Ablation to Treat Atrial Fibrillation: A Review of the Literature. Journal of Cardiovascular Development and Disease. 2022; 9(4):94. https://doi.org/10.3390/jcdd9040094.

Silent cerebral lesions (**Fig. 2**)[32] are another often overlooked complication without clear clinical implications. In one study of 54 patients undergoing CA for AF, 6 developed asymptomatic lesions on diffusion-weighted MRI.[33] Multi-phased RFA procedures showed a higher incidence than single phase or CRA (37.5% vs 7.4% vs 4.3%, $P = .003$).[34] The incidence of PFA is lower, with one study reporting risk in 1 out of 18 on post-CA imaging and another more recent study reporting no lesions in 30 patients.[3,35] Risks may be mitigated by minimizing dwell times, avoiding extensive left atrial ablation, intraprocedural, or post-procedural cardioversion for up to 4 weeks, and maintaining adequate anticoagulation times.[36] Catheter and sheath geometry may also influence risk, but further study is needed to understand it, its factors, and long-term implications.

TRADITIONAL COMPLICATIONS OF THERMAL INJURY

Adverse events related to thermal energy can be mitigated through thermodynamic principles, such as adjusted power settings and decreased dwell times. These strategies have helped lower but not eliminate this risk.[37] PFA generates modest heat, so similar complications may arise. In the MANIFEST-17K study—the most extensive analysis of PFA safety thus far—major and minor complications occurred in 0.98% and 3.21% of all cases, respectively; energy-related complications included esophageal injury, PV stenosis, phrenic nerve injury, coronary artery spasm (CAS), and hemolysis-related acute kidney injury (AKI), with only 0.23% attributed to PFA.[6] Compared to the original cohort, this study had fewer major (0.98% vs 1.65%) and minor (3.35% vs 3.86%) complications, suggesting improvement as operators gained experience. This coincides with a learning curve anticipated with all technologies influencing safety and efficacy. However, unlike RFA or CRA, which allows a more global approach to enhancing safety and efficacy, PFA requires individually optimized dosing and application across all available systems.

Esophageal Injury

Esophageal injury, particularly atrioesophageal fistula, is a serious concern in ablation, especially when ablating near the right-sided PVs. This injury can be prevented using esophageal monitoring, deviation, and active cooling. With PFA, the main

Table 2
Complications from first clinical trials and registries

Study, Year	Study Size[a]	Described Adverse Events
Reddy et al,[16] 2018	22	None.
Reddy et al,[2] 2019	81	Pericardial tamponade (1).
Loh et al,[17] 2020	10	Stroke (1); ST-segment elevation (9).
Reddy et al, 2021	121	Cardiac perforation or tamponade (2); vascular complications (1).
Nakatani et al, 2021	18	Groin hematoma (1).
Cochet et al,[59] 2021	18	No esophageal injury; aortic lesions (6).
Gunawardane et al, 2021	20	CAS (1).
Reddy et al,[54] 2022	50	Temporary ST-segment depression. However, Nitroglycerin was effective at prevention.
PULSED AF, 2022	300	Pericardial effusion (1).
MANIFEST-PF, 2022	1758	Pericardial tamponade (17); stroke (7); transient phrenic nerve paresis (8); CAS (1); vascular complications (43).
Blockhaus et al, 2022	23	Stroke (1); transient hypotension or bradycardia.
Futing et al, 2022	40	Pericardial tamponade (1).
Musikantow et al, 2023	121	Pericardial tamponade (1); TIA (1); hematoma (1).
ADVENT, 2023	305	Cardiac tamponade or perforation (2); pulmonary edema (1); TIA (1); vascular complication (1).
Maury et al, 2023	2	Pulmonary hemorrhage.
EU-PORIA, 2023	1233	Pericardial tamponade (14); stroke (5); TIA (2); vascular complication (12); phrenic nerve dysfunction (4); CAS (1); air ebolism (3).
MANIFEST-17K, 2024	17642	Stroke (22); pericardial tamponade (63); vascular complication (441); CAS (53); renal failure (6); TIA (21); transient phrenic nerve injury (11).

Although preclinical studies suggest a favorable safety profile, there are still described adverse events. Many of these are procedure related, though few continue to be energy related.

Abbreviations: CAS, coronary artery spasm; TIA, transient ischemic attack.

[a] Only number of subjects undergoing pulsed-field ablation.

Adapted from Iyengar SK, Iyengar S, Srivathsan K. The promise of pulsed field ablation and the challenges ahead. *Front Cardiovasc Med.* 2023;10:1235317. https://doi.org/10.3389/fcvm.2023.1235317; Amin AM, Nazir A, Abuelazm MT, et al. Efficacy and safety of pulsed-field versus conventional thermal ablation for atrial fibrillation: A systematic review and meta-analysis. Journal of Arrhythmia. 2024/07/18 2024;n/a(n/a)doi:https://doi.org/10.1002/joa3.13118.

advantage is its minimal, if any, impact on the esophagus. Animal and clinical studies support this, and one showed no esophageal injury with PFA compared to 43% with thermal ablation on post-ablation cardiac MRI despite similar contact rates.[38] Similar results have been observed using endoscopy and electrogastrography.[39] Rare incidences of injury seem to resolve within 21 days without long-term damage.[40] However, a slight increase in esophageal temperature ($0.8\pm0.6°$ C) during PFA suggests that heat generation is still relevant.[41]

Additionally, vigilance is necessary for potential complications from electrical injury to the nervous or vasculature systems of the esophagus, such as dysmotility, smooth muscle dysfunction, or macrovascular arterial injury. Although direct tissue injury may be absent, the short-term and long-term effects on the autonomic nerves and vasculature supplying the gut are poorly understood.

Pulmonary Vein Stenosis

PV stenosis is another complication that PFA effectively eliminates. This occurs due to fibrosis or scarring—which some individuals may have a higher propensity for as part of their bodies' healing process—that is detected with post-ablation imaging. In a study of 10,368 patients undergoing RFA, severe stenosis occurred in 0.5% of cases and was linked to significant morbidity, with symptoms like dyspnea, cough, and fatigue.[42] In contrast, studies show that PFA results in significantly less mild (30%–49% ostial decrease; 0% vs 9%, $P<.001$), moderate (50%–69% ostial decrease;

Complications With Ablation Procedures

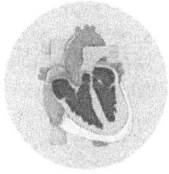

Cardiac
- Cardiac perforation
- Pericardial effusion or tamponade
- Malignant arrhythmias
- Sinus node dysfunction
- Aortic wall injury
- Coronary artery spasm
- Severe troponemia

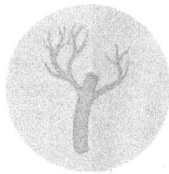

Vascular
- Hematoma
- Aneurysm or pseudoaneurysm
- Ischemic limb
- Retroperitoneal bleed

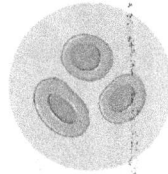

Hematologic
- Excessive hemolysis

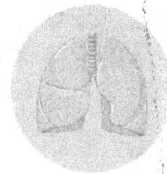

Pulmonary
- Pulmonary edema
- Phrenic nerve injury
- Pneumonia
- Pulmonary vein stenosis
- Air embolism

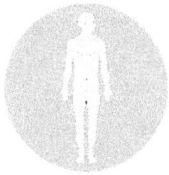

Systemic
- Death
- Gaseous microbubbles

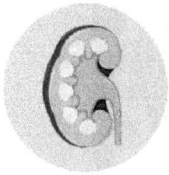

Renal
- Contrast-induced, dehydration, or hemolysis-induced renal injury

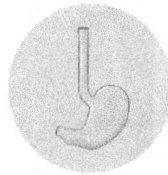

Esophagus
- Atrio-esophageal fistula
- Autonomic dysfunction with gastrointestinal dysmotility

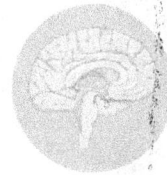

Neurologic
- Stroke or transient ischemic attack
- Silent cerebral events

Injury more commonly seen in pulsed-field energy source
Injury more commonly seen in thermal (radiofrequency or cryothermal) energy sources

Fig. 1. Procedural and energy-dependent complications. Complications can be divided into procedural and energy-dependent, highlighted in color. Energy-dependent can be further divided into commonly seen in all thermal sources (*red*) or PFA (*blue*), though this division is not exclusive.

0% vs 1.8%, $P<.001$), and severe (70%–100% ostial decrease; 0% vs 1.2%, $P<.001$) stenosis than RFA.[43] These findings have been consistently replicated, with no reported cases of PFA causing PV stenosis.[44] These encouraging results suggest that this complication may no longer be relevant with current PFA technologies. However, the long-term implications of this injury in susceptible individuals are largely unknown, and sequential cardiac computer tomography and studies for each specific PFA system are still necessary.

Phrenic Nerve Injury

Phrenic nerve injury, whether reversible or irreversible, is another recognized complication of existing ablation techniques. The Netherlands Heart Registry demonstrated an incidence of 0.7% in 9549 cases using thermal energy, with recovery in 70% of those affected.[45] The incidence of phrenic nerve

injury with PFA was anticipated to be rare, but transient and permanent damage has been consistently observed.[46] Phrenic nerve monitoring or sequential diaphragmatic compound motor action potentials—previously used in CRA systems—may be beneficial.[47] Like thermal energy, the risk of injury is influenced by the proximity of the PFA catheter to the phrenic nerve and dose levels, but unlike traditional tools, these factors differ among PFA systems.[48] The extensive catheter profile must also be considered, as it may increase the risk of injury. Nevertheless, this risk appears to decrease more than tenfold with PFA, though no study has compared it to thermal sources.[6]

COMPLICATIONS UNIQUE TO PULSED-FIELD ABLATION AND ELECTROPORATION

In addition to those discussed previously, PFA introduces unique complications that arise from

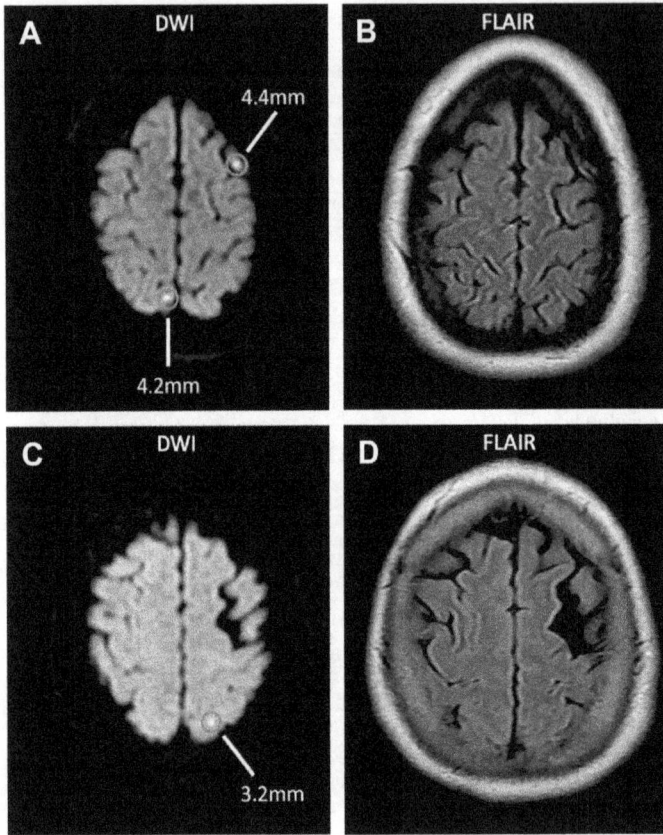

Fig. 2. MRI of cerebral silent ischemia. T2-weighted DWI (*A*) with lesions highlighted in red and FLAIR imaging (*B*) of a patient with silent cerebral ischemia. Another examples of DWI and FLAIR are provided in (*C*) and (*D*), respectively. *Abbreviations*: DWI, diffuse-weighted imaging; FLAIR, fluid-attenuated inversion recovery; mm, millimeters. (*From* Patel C, Gerstenfeld EP, Gupta SK, et al. Comparison of cerebral safety after atrial fibrillation using pulsed field and thermal ablation: Results of the neurological assessment subgroup in the ADVENT trial. Heart Rhythm. https://doi.org/10.1016/j.hrthm.2024.05.048.)

electroporation despite tissue selectivity. Many of these issues may still occur with thermal ablation but at much lower frequencies.

Gaseous Microbubbles

Microbubble formation is inherent to electroporation in PFA and caused by hydrolysis and nitrogen displacement.[49] Microbubbles were also seen in RFA due to tissue heating and linked to steam pops, perforation, myocardial ulceration, and thromboembolism.[50] The presence and severity of microbubble formation depend on power settings affecting the speed and extent of tissue heating. They are also associated with irrigated tip catheters designed to minimize tissue disruption and endothelial injury.[51] Similarly, each PFA system may carry unique microbubble risks, but mitigation opportunities may be limited since its genesis is inherent in the technology. Further study is needed to evaluate the significance of these microbubbles on end-organ function.

Coronary Artery Spasm

Again, CAS is a known complication of existing CA modalities (**Fig. 3**A-D), with a 0.19% incidence in a study of 22,232 patients.[52] It presents with ST-segment changes and, though more subclinical, may cause death. Coronary atherosclerosis, implantation of drug-eluting stents, and smoking may predispose some patients, and CAS can be triggered by medication infusion before, during, or after ablation.[52,53] With PFA, energy delivery near the coronary arteries—especially the right coronary adjacent to the cavotricuspid isthmus and left circumflex next to the mitral isthmus—is a major provoking factor.[54,55] There exist rare cases of CAS-related cardiac arrest resulting in patient death, but they are undergoing litigation before being made public.

CAS is often spontaneous or can be resolved with immediate intracoronary nitroglycerin. Prophylactic nitroglycerin administration or alternative energy sources when ablating near the coronary arteries may also prevent it. However, the long-term effects of CAS are unclear. While clinical data show no lasting coronary lesions, a porcine study suggested that intimal hyperplasia may occur even with nitroglycerin (see **Fig. 3**E-F).[56,57] There are also no data on disease progression or risk of injury in patients with known coronary artery disease.

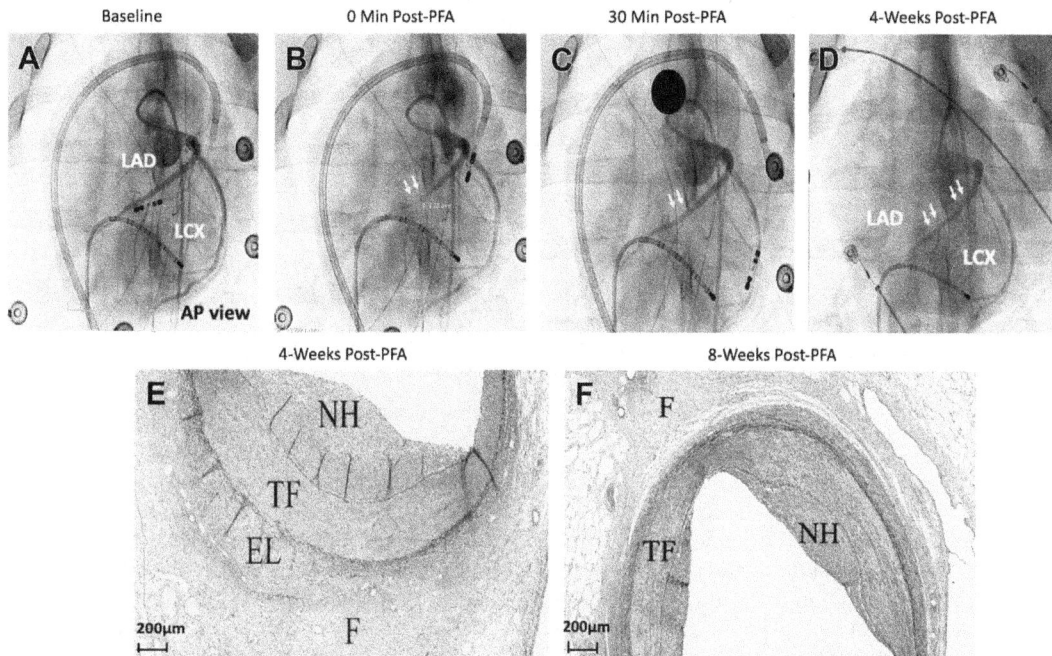

Fig. 3. Coronary artery spasm overtime. Coronary angiography of a patient demonstrates a distal site (*A*) that exhibits significant narrowing immediately after PFA application (*B*) and 30 minutes after (*C*). By 4 weeks, evidence of stenosis has resolved (*D*). Histologic changes at 4 (*E*) and 8 (*F*) weeks demonstrate improving neointimal hyperplasia and tunica media fibrosis. *Abbreviations*: AP, anterior–posterior; EL, (adventitial) elastic fiber; F, (adipose tissue) fibrosis; NH, neointimal hyperplasia; LAD, left anterior descending; LCX, left circumflex; PFA, pulsed field ablation; TF, tunica (media) fibrosis. (*From* Higuchi S, Im SI, Stillson C, et al. Effect of Epicardial Pulsed Field Ablation Directly on Coronary Arteries. JACC Clin Electrophysiol. Dec 2022;8(12):1486-1496. https://doi.org/10.1016/j.jacep.2022.09.003.)

Aortic Wall Injury

Just like RFA, direct thermal injury of the aorta has been reported with PFA and is common when the aortic wall contacts the left atrium.[58] The mechanism of injury, though, may be distinct from thermal ablation. This results in less injury than for thermal ablation (33% vs 43%, $P = .52$).[59] This may also affect long-term outcomes, but there have been no clinical implications with either ablation modality to date.

Hemolysis and Hemolysis-related Renal Failure

Hemolysis—evidenced by low haptoglobin, high bilirubin, and lactate dehydrogenase—is a unique complication of PFA caused by electroporation of nearby erythrocytes, leading to cell rupture and release of intracellular contents (**Fig. 4**A). It may occur in up to 94% of patients undergoing PFA and remains an active research area.[60] The severity of hemolysis appears to increase with the number and intensity of applications and larger catheter surface area.[60,61] As such, procedural techniques like intracardiac ultrasound to

ensure better tissue contact, conservative energy application, and avoiding "bonus" applications may mitigate risk.

Hemolysis may also lead to AKI, especially in those with preexisting renal disease, due to oxidative stress and renal tubular damage (see **Fig. 4**B).[62] In the MANIFEST-17K study, creatinine levels doubled post-procedure in all patients, and 5 patients had acute renal failure.[6] Hydration is key to preventing and treating AKI, as dehydration is an independent predictor of injury.[63]

Autonomic Dysfunction

Neuronal cells have demonstrated greater susceptibility to electroporation than cardiomyocytes, and the nervous system is particularly susceptible to PFA.[64] AF ablation with any energy source can result in transient or permanent autonomic dysfunction, presenting as bradycardia, tachycardia, atrioventricular block, or changes in heart rate variability stemming from the destruction of the ganglionic plexi near the PV.[65–67] Even though early clinical studies suggested no change in heart rate variability or neural injury biomarkers, more recent data suggest high rates of quickly resolving

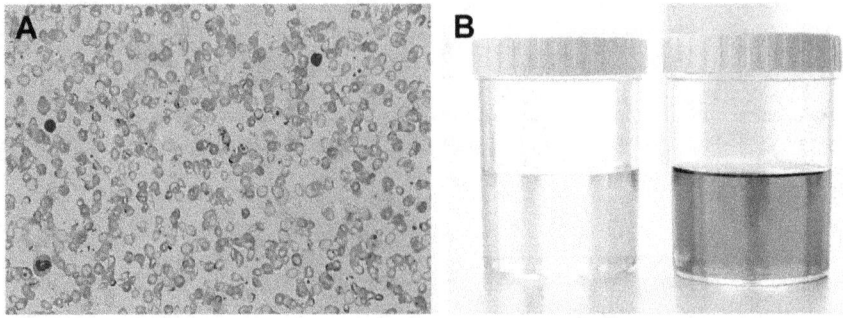

Fig. 4. Hemolysis and resulting hemoglobinuria. Pulsed-field ablation can cause hemolysis (*A*) and subsequent hemoglobinuria (*B*; *left:* normal urine, *right:* moderate hemoglobinuria) that can cause an acute kidney injury.

intraprocedural vagal reactions (70% vs 28%, $P = .001$).[68,69] Lowering field strength, voltage, and frequency may reduce risks, but concerns about long-term dysautonomia and impacts on nearby structures, like the stomach, remain. Furthermore, persistent dysfunction may require cardiac pacemaker implantation or cardio-neural ablation. Specific studies are needed to clarify the effects of PFA on autonomic function and surveillance of each PFA system.

Tropinemia

PFA, unlike thermal ablation, can cause a multiple-fold increase in myocardial cellular death, but significantly higher troponin levels (mean difference 470.28, 95% CI 18.89–921.67) greater than expected have been noted compared to conventional RFA and CRA systems.[70,71] This likely arises from the current large-profile single-shot PFA ablation systems, which require contact force for lesion durability. This suggests extensive atrial tissue electroporation, but its effects on short-term and long-term atrial dynamics and remodeling are unknown and require further study.

ADDITIONAL CONSIDERATIONS FOR PULSE FIELD VERSUS THERMAL ENERGY

PFA has shown promising efficacy and appears to have an improved safety profile compared to RFA and CRA. However, complications can still occur. Additionally, factors like the variety of catheters and resource utilization must be considered in evaluating its overall value, underscoring its benefits and limitations.

Advantages and Disadvantages

PFA offers advantages and disadvantages (**Table 3**) compared to thermal ablation. Studies suggest that PFA has significantly shorter procedural times than thermal ablation, resulting in considerably less radiographic exposure for patients and operators.[28] However, PFA also appears to be associated with higher sedation and analgesia requirements.[72]

While not associated with acute or subacute PV stenosis or esophageal injury, PFA poses unique risks to coronary arteries and may lead to more AKI. The sensitivity of neuronal cells also raises concerns about autonomic dysfunction. The extent of these adverse effects may be offset by the pre-procedural and periprocedural sinus rhythm, but further study is required. Thus, there is still a critical need to understand the long-term impact of PFA on outcomes and whether they differ from those with traditional tools; its ability to cause significant tissue injury, its effects on atrial function, and the risk of stiff atrial syndrome must be better understood. In certain high-risk patients, thermal ablation may still be preferable.

Catheter Selection

The safety risks of PAF are affected by the catheter selection. Whereas early animal studies often used circular multielectrode catheters, clinical trials primarily used the FaraPulse (Boston Scientific, Marlborough, MA) catheter, which creates circumferential lesions in a flower or basket arrangement. Other catheter designs, such as lattice tip, spiral, or focal arrangement of electrodes, and sizes have been evaluated.[40,73,74] Larger catheters also destroy more tissue. Risk profiles likely vary between these systems. No head-to-head trials comparing PFA technologies exist, but they are critically needed. Furthermore, each tool requires more preclinical data to optimize ablation parameters and improve long-term outcomes.

Lack of Standardization for Pulse Field Technologies

Many factors beyond conventional RFA catheter design influence the safety and efficacy of novel PFA catheters, adding significant complexity to

Table 3
Advantages and disadvantages of pulse field ablation

Advantages	Disadvantages
• Non-inferior to RFA and similar efficacy	• Increased costs
• Tissue selective mechanism	• No standardization between catheters
• Variety of PFA catheters and systems	• Additional, electroporation and tissue-specific complications
• No reports of esophageal injury or pulmonary vein stenosis	• Novel technology without long-term efficacy or safety data
• Avoid thermal injury to adjacent structures	

There are advantages and disadvantages to the technology. Currently, there is no way to assess these against each other.
   Abbreviations: PFA, pulse field ablation; RFA, radiofrequency ablation.

standardizing approval processes and comparing these technologies. The US Food and Drug Administration must establish new benchmarks to rigorously evaluate and approve PFA systems. While current comparisons are made against RFA catheters, developing updated standards tailored to PFA's unique characteristics is essential to ensure fair and accurate assessments.

Resource Utilization, Cost, and Inequalities of Access

Despite a favorable safety risk and shorter procedural times leading to lower staffing and laboratory costs, PFA procedures remain more expensive due to higher equipment costs. We have observed 3 to 4 times higher costs than RFA platforms. In an informal cost-effective analysis, Calvert and colleagues[75] suggest that the mean total procedural cost of PFA was 12% higher than RFA and 23% higher than CRA. These are conservative estimates and do not account for costs of adoption, such as new generators, workflows, and staff orientation; current technologies also require a dedicated operator that is currently required to administer PFA energy. As more manufacturers enter the market, costs may become more competitive, but the incremental value of this technology in its current form is not cost-effective. These high costs remain a limiting factor, disenfranchising those in underserved and resource-limited markets.

CURRENT CONTROVERSIES

The advent of PFA has been considered a significant technological advancement in CA. Nevertheless, many unmet needs remain. Our knowledge of optimizing ablation, improving durability, and lowering the risks of traditional and nontraditional risk factors is still evolving. Many of these have been discussed throughout this review (**Box 1**).

Box 1
Current controversies of pulse field ablation

Controversies

• Safety of PFA continues to be judged by evaluating its thermal complications. Does this underestimate the risk of PFA? Additionally, electrical injury will have unique early and late complications.

• Can we continue to call PFA tissue sensitive? Many of these complications discussed today are a result of electroporation on adjacent tissue. This includes coronary artery vasospasm, autonomic dysfunction, aortic wall injury.

• There are several varieties of PFA delivery. How do we optimally deliver PFA? How do we titrate PFA to make it more effective?

• There is a lack of post-procedural remapping data. Is there an increased propensity for recurrent atrial tachycardia?

• Is acute renal injury related to hemolysis or lack of hydration?

• What is the long-term efficacy of PFA? Have we truly eliminated esophageal injury and pulmonary vein stenosis? Does intimal hyperplasia result in subsequent coronary artery disease?

• Currently, the majority of the data arises from atrial arrhythmias. There is a chance that additional, previously undescribed complications may be noted as it is used for ventricular arrhythmias.

• PFA results in excessive, unwarranted atrial tissue destruction. This may have unbeknownst impact on atrial function and long-term remodeling.

There are also many controversies associated with technology. This highlights the future need for continued study. *Abbreviation:* PFA, pulse field ablation.

FUTURE DIRECTIONS

Over the last 3 decades, we have learned how to identify, mitigate, and manage complications of thermal ablation, particularly RFA, but there are many unknowns about PFA. While some of these gaps are due to PFA being a relatively new tool, others reflect a unique, nonthermal cell injury. Future studies will be crucial in identifying and addressing these gaps. This will also require added diligence in industry-sponsored studies moving forward.

SUMMARY

PFA is a novel and promising technology for the CA of AF. Current data suggest a favorable safety profile, with minimal complications specific to the technology and dependent on multiple factors. There is still much to be learned, and with the increasing use of PFA, the authors expect a better understanding of efficacy and complications in the future.

CLINICS CARE POINTS

- PFA eliminates the risk of PV stenosis and esophageal injury, but other procedural and traditional complications are still possible at a lower frequency.

- Energy-specific complications, including gaseous microbubble formation, CAS, aortic wall injury, hemolysis, hemolysis-related acute injury, and autonomic dysfunction, are still possible and may result in significant morbidity.

- Complications related to PFA and electroporation are further confounded by various systems by separate manufacturers. The energy levels, frequency of applications, and catheter design affect the severity and type of complications.

- The use of PFA may still require a health level of suspicion as long-term implications and outcomes of these complications are still unknown and need further study.

DISCLOSURES

Dr A. Katapadi has no disclosures. Dr T.J. Bunch received research grants from Alta Thera, Boehringer Ingelheim, United States, and Cardiva Medical. Dr R. Kabra is a consultant and/or receives research grants from Medtronic and Boston Scientific, United States. Dr T.F. Deering is a consultant for HearBeam, Omny Health, PaceMate, and Preventice. He has received research grants from Abbott, Biosense Webster, United States, Biotronik, Germany, and Medtronic. Dr D. Lakkireddy is a consultant to and/or receives research grants from Abbott Vascular, United States, AtriCure, United States, Biotrtonik, BioSense Webster, Boston Scientific, Medtronic, Northeast Scientific.

REFERENCES

1. Batista Napotnik T, Polajžer T, Miklavčič D. Cell death due to electroporation – a review. Bioelectrochemistry 2021;141:107871.
2. Reddy VY, Neuzil P, Koruth JS, et al. Pulsed field ablation for pulmonary vein isolation in atrial fibrillation. J Am Coll Cardiol 2019;74(3):315–26.
3. Ekanem E, Reddy VY, Schmidt B, et al. Multi-national survey on the methods, efficacy, and safety on the post-approval clinical use of pulsed field ablation (MANIFEST-PF). EP Europace 2022;24(8):1256–66.
4. Verma A, Haines DE, Boersma LV, et al. Pulsed field ablation for the treatment of atrial fibrillation: PULSED AF pivotal trial. Circulation 2023;147(19):1422–32.
5. Reddy Vivek Y, Gerstenfeld Edward P, Natale A, et al. Pulsed field or conventional thermal ablation for paroxysmal atrial fibrillation. N Engl J Med 2023;389(18):1660–71.
6. Ekanem E, Neuzil P, Reichlin T, et al. Safety of pulsed field ablation in more than 17,000 patients with atrial fibrillation in the MANIFEST-17K study. Nat Med 2024;30(7):2020–9.
7. Scheinman MM, Morady F, Hess DS, et al. Catheter-induced ablation of the atrioventricular junction to control refractory supraventricular arrhythmias. JAMA 1982;248(7):851–5.
8. Bardy GH, Coltorti F, Stewart RB, et al. Catheter-mediated electrical ablation: the relation between current and pulse width on voltage breakdown and shock-wave generation. Circ Res 1988;63(2):409–14.
9. Hauer RN, Robles de Medina EO, Borst C. Proarrhythmic effects of ventricular electrical catheter ablation in dogs. J Am Coll Cardiol 1987;10(6):1350–6.
10. Ahsan AJ, Cunningham D, Rowland E, et al. Catheter ablation without fulguration: design and performance of a new system. Pacing Clin Electrophysiol 1989;12(9):1557–61.
11. Di Monaco A, Vitulano N, Troisi F, et al. Pulsed field ablation to Treat atrial fibrillation: a review of the literature. J Cardiovasc Dev Dis 2022;9(4):94.
12. Song Y, Zheng J, Fan L. Nonthermal irreversible electroporation to the esophagus: evaluation of acute and long-term pathological effects in a rabbit model. J Am Heart Assoc 2021;10(22):e020731.
13. Sugrue A, Vaidya V, Witt C, et al. Irreversible electroporation for catheter-based cardiac ablation: a systematic review of the preclinical experience. J Interv Card Electrophysiol 2019;55(3):251–65.

14. Iyengar SK, Iyengar S, Srivathsan K. The promise of pulsed field ablation and the challenges ahead. Front Cardiovasc Med 2023;10:1235317.

15. Amin AM, Nazir A, Abuelazm MT, et al. Efficacy and safety of pulsed-field versus conventional thermal ablation for atrial fibrillation: a systematic review and meta-analysis. J Arrhythm 2024. https://doi.org/10.1002/joa3.13118.

16. Reddy VY, Koruth J, Jais P, et al. Ablation of atrial fibrillation with pulsed electric fields: an ultra-rapid, tissue-selective modality for cardiac ablation. JACC Clin Electrophysiol 2018;4(8):987–95.

17. Loh P, van Es R, Groen MHA, et al. Pulmonary vein isolation with single pulse irreversible electroporation. Circ Arrhythm Electrophysiol 2020;13(10):e008192.

18. Ekanem E, Reddy VY, Schmidt B, et al. Multi-national survey on the methods, efficacy, and safety on the post-approval clinical use of pulsed field ablation (MANIFEST-PF). Europace 2022;24(8):1256–66.

19. Shaheen N, Shaheen A, Ramadan A, et al. Efficacy and safety of novel pulsed field ablation (PFA) technique for atrial fibrillation: a systematic review and meta-analysis. Health Sci Rep 2023;6(1):e1079.

20. Aldaas OM, Malladi C, Aldaas AM, et al. Safety and acute efficacy of catheter ablation for atrial fibrillation with pulsed field ablation vs thermal energy ablation: a meta-analysis of single proportions. Heart Rhythm O2 2023;4(10):599–608.

21. Benali K, Khairy P, Hammache N, et al. Procedure-related complications of catheter ablation for atrial fibrillation. J Am Coll Cardiol 2023;81(21):2089–99.

22. Eckardt L, Doldi F, Anwar O, et al. Major in-hospital complications after catheter ablation of cardiac arrhythmias: individual case analysis of 43 031 procedures. EP Europace 2024;26(1):euad361.

23. Cappato R, Calkins H, Chen SA, et al. Worldwide survey on the methods, efficacy, and safety of catheter ablation for human atrial fibrillation. Circulation 2005;111(9):1100–5.

24. Holmes David R, Nishimura R, Fountain R, et al. Iatrogenic pericardial effusion and tamponade in the percutaneous intracardiac intervention era. JACC Cardiovasc Interv 2009;2(8):705–17.

25. Price MJ, Valderrábano M, Zimmerman S, et al. Periprocedural pericardial effusion complicating transcatheter left atrial appendage occlusion: a report from the NCDR LAAO Registry. Circ Cardiovasc Interv 2022;15(5):e011718.

26. von Olshausen G, Tabrizi F, Sigurjónsdóttir R, et al. Cardiac tamponades related to interventional electrophysiology procedures are associated with higher risk of short-term hospitalization for pericarditis but favourable long-term outcome. EP Europace 2023;25(6):euad140.

27. du Fay de Lavallaz J, Badertscher P, Ghannam M, et al. Severe periprocedural complications after ablation for atrial fibrillation: an International collaborative individual patient data Registry. Clin Electrophysiol 2024;10(7_Part_1):1353–64.

28. Della Rocca DG, Marcon L, Magnocavallo M, et al. Pulsed electric field, cryoballoon, and radiofrequency for paroxysmal atrial fibrillation ablation: a propensity score-matched comparison. Europace 2023;26(1). https://doi.org/10.1093/europace/euae016.

29. Scherr D, Sharma K, Dalal D, et al. Incidence and predictors of periprocedural cerebrovascular accident in patients undergoing catheter ablation of atrial fibrillation. J Cardiovasc Electrophysiol 2009;20(12):1357–63.

30. Di Biase L, Burkhardt JD, Santangeli P, et al. Periprocedural stroke and bleeding complications in patients undergoing catheter ablation of atrial fibrillation with different anticoagulation management. Circulation 2014;129(25):2638–44.

31. Page SP, Herring N, Hunter RJ, et al. Periprocedural stroke risk in patients undergoing catheter ablation for atrial fibrillation on uninterrupted warfarin. J Cardiovasc Electrophysiol 2014;25(6):585–90.

32. Patel C, Gerstenfeld EP, Gupta SK, et al. Comparison of cerebral safety after atrial fibrillation using pulsed field and thermal ablation: results of the neurological assessment subgroup in the ADVENT trial. Heart Rhythm 2024. https://doi.org/10.1016/j.hrthm.2024.05.048.

33. Schrickel JW, Lickfett L, Lewalter T, et al. Incidence and predictors of silent cerebral embolism during pulmonary vein catheter ablation for atrial fibrillation. EP Europace 2010;12(1):52–7.

34. Herrera Siklódy C, Deneke T, Hocini M, et al. Incidence of asymptomatic intracranial embolic events after pulmonary vein isolation: comparison of different atrial fibrillation ablation technologies in a multicenter study. J Am Coll Cardiol 2011;58(7):681–8.

35. Reinsch N, Füting A, Höwel D, et al. Cerebral safety after pulsed field ablation for paroxysmal atrial fibrillation. Heart Rhythm 2022;19(11):1813–8.

36. Calvert P, Kollias G, Pürerfellner H, et al. Silent cerebral lesions following catheter ablation for atrial fibrillation: a state-of-the-art review. Europace 2023;25(6). https://doi.org/10.1093/europace/euad151.

37. Bisignani A, Schiavone M, Solimene F, et al. National workflow experience with pulsed field ablation for atrial fibrillation: learning curve, efficiency, and safety. J Interv Card Electrophysiol 2024. https://doi.org/10.1007/s10840-024-01835-6.

38. Grosse Meininghaus D, Freund R, Koerber B, et al. Pulsed-field ablation does not induce esophageal and periesophageal injury—a new esophageal safety paradigm in catheter ablation of atrial fibrillation. J Cardiovasc Electrophysiol 2024;35(1):86–93.

39. Grosse Meininghaus D, Freund R, Koerber B, et al. Pulsed-field ablation does not induce esophageal

and periesophageal injury-A new esophageal safety paradigm in catheter ablation of atrial fibrillation. J Cardiovasc Electrophysiol 2024;35(1):86–93.

40. Aryana A, Ji SY, Hata C, et al. Preclinical evaluation of a novel single-shot pulsed field ablation system for pulmonary vein and atrial ablation. J Cardiovasc Electrophysiol 2023;34(11):2203–12.

41. Kirstein B, Heeger CH, Vogler J, et al. Impact of pulsed field ablation on intraluminal esophageal temperature. J Cardiovasc Electrophysiol 2024;35(1): 78–85.

42. Raeisi-Giglou P, Wazni OM, Saliba WI, et al. Outcomes and management of patients with severe pulmonary vein stenosis from prior atrial fibrillation ablation. Circ Arrhythm Electrophysiol 2018;11(5):e006001.

43. Kuroki K, Whang W, Eggert C, et al. Ostial dimensional changes after pulmonary vein isolation: pulsed field ablation vs radiofrequency ablation. Heart Rhythm 2020;17(9):1528–35.

44. Mansour M, Gerstenfeld EP, Patel C, et al. Pulmonary vein narrowing after pulsed field versus thermal ablation. Europace 2024;26(2). https://doi.org/10.1093/europace/euae038.

45. Mol D, Renskers L, Balt JC, et al. Persistent phrenic nerve palsy after atrial fibrillation ablation: follow-up data from The Netherlands Heart Registration. J Cardiovasc Electrophysiol 2022;33(3):559–64.

46. Pansera F, Bordignon S, Bologna F, et al. Catheter ablation induced phrenic nerve palsy by pulsed field ablation-completely impossible? A case series. Eur Heart J Case Rep 2022;6(9):ytac361.

47. Franceschi F, Koutbi L, Maille B, et al. First electromyographic monitoring of a progressive phrenic nerve palsy in a pulsed field ablation procedure. HeartRhythm Case Rep 2024;10(7):447–50.

48. Howard B, Haines DE, Verma A, et al. Characterization of phrenic nerve response to pulsed field ablation. Circ Arrhythm Electrophysiol 2022;15(6):e010127.

49. van Es R, Groen MHA, Stehouwer M, et al. In vitro analysis of the origin and characteristics of gaseous microemboli during catheter electroporation ablation. J Cardiovasc Electrophysiol 2019;30(10):2071–9.

50. Bruce GK, Bunch TJ, Milton MA, et al. Discrepancies between catheter tip and tissue temperature in cooled-tip ablation: relevance to guiding left atrial ablation. Circulation 2005;112(7):954–60.

51. Suzuki A, Lehmann HI, Konishi H, et al. Potential microemboli formation risk and its management during the heated saline-enhanced radiofrequency needle-tip catheter ablation. Heart Rhythm 2024. https://doi.org/10.1016/j.hrthm.2024.05.050.

52. Nakamura T, Takami M, Fukuzawa K, et al. Incidence and characteristics of coronary artery spasms related to atrial fibrillation ablation procedures — large-scale multicenter analysis. Circ J 2021;85(3):264–71.

53. Ishimura M, Yamamoto K, Yamamoto M, et al. Cardiac arrest due to late-onset coronary artery spasm after radiofrequency catheter ablation in a patient with an implantable cardioverter-defibrillator. J Cardiol Cases 2023;27(5):207–11.

54. Reddy VY, Petru J, Funasako M, et al. Coronary arterial spasm during pulsed field ablation to Treat atrial fibrillation. Circulation 2022;146(24):1808–19.

55. Zhang C, Neuzil P, Petru J, et al. Coronary artery spasm during pulsed field vs radiofrequency catheter ablation of the mitral isthmus. JAMA Cardiol 2024;9(1):72–7.

56. Malyshev Y, Neuzil P, Petru J, et al. Does acute coronary spasm from pulsed field ablation translate into chronic coronary arterial lesions? JACC Clin Electrophysiol 2024;10(5):970–2.

57. Higuchi S, Im SI, Stillson C, et al. Effect of epicardial pulsed field ablation directly on coronary arteries. JACC Clin Electrophysiol 2022;8(12):1486–96.

58. Tung P, Hong SN, Chan RH, et al. Aortic injury is common following pulmonary vein isolation. Heart Rhythm 2013;10(5):653–8.

59. Cochet H, Nakatani Y, Sridi-Cheniti S, et al. Pulsed field ablation selectively spares the oesophagus during pulmonary vein isolation for atrial fibrillation. Europace 2021;23(9):1391–9.

60. Popa MA, Venier S, Menè R, et al. Characterization and clinical significance of hemolysis after pulsed field ablation for atrial fibrillation: results of a multicenter analysis. Circ Arrhythm Electrophysiol 2024e012732. https://doi.org/10.1161/circep.124.012732.

61. Fiserova I, Fiser O, Novak M, et al. Significant hemolysis is present during irreversible electroporation of cardiomyocytes in vitro. Heart Rhythm 2024. https://doi.org/10.1016/j.hrthm.2024.08.019.

62. Venier S, Vaxelaire N, Jacon P, et al. Severe acute kidney injury related to haemolysis after pulsed field ablation for atrial fibrillation. Europace 2023;26(1). https://doi.org/10.1093/europace/euad371.

63. Mohanty S, Casella M, Compagnucci P, et al. Acute kidney injury resulting from hemoglobinuria after pulsed-field ablation in atrial fibrillation. JACC Clin Electrophysiol 2024;10(4):709–15.

64. Avazzadeh S, Dehkordi MH, Owens P, et al. Establishing electroporation thresholds for targeted cell specific cardiac ablation in a 2D culture model. J Cardiovasc Electrophysiol 2022;33(9):2050–61.

65. Friedman PL, Stevenson WG, Kocovic DZ. Autonomic dysfunction after catheter ablation. J Cardiovasc Electrophysiol 1996;7(5):450–9.

66. Bauer A, Deisenhofer I, Schneider R, et al. Effects of circumferential or segmental pulmonary vein ablation for paroxysmal atrial fibrillation on cardiac autonomic function. Heart Rhythm 2006;3(12):1428–35.

67. Tang LYW, Hawkins NM, Ho K, et al. Autonomic alterations after pulmonary vein isolation in the CIRCA-DOSE (cryoballoon vs irrigated radiofrequency catheter ablation) study. J Am Heart Assoc 2021;10(5):e018610.

68. Del Monte A, Cespón Fernández M, Vetta G, et al. Quantitative assessment of transient autonomic modulation after single-shot pulmonary vein isolation with pulsed-field ablation. J Cardiovasc Electrophysiol 2023;34(11):2393–7.

69. Guo F, Wang J, Deng Q, et al. Effects of pulsed field ablation on autonomic nervous system in paroxysmal atrial fibrillation: a pilot study. Heart Rhythm 2023;20(3):329–38.

70. Zhang H, Zhang H, Lu H, et al. Meta-analysis of pulsed-field ablation versus cryoablation for atrial fibrillation. Pacing Clin Electrophysiol 2024;47(5):603–13.

71. Osmancik P, Bacova B, Hozman M, et al. Myocardial damage, inflammation, coagulation, and platelet activity during catheter ablation using radiofrequency and pulsed-field energy. JACC Clin Electrophysiol 2024;10(3):463–74.

72. Wahedi R, Willems S, Feldhege J, et al. Pulsed-field versus cryoballoon ablation for atrial fibrillation-Impact of energy source on sedation and analgesia requirement. J Cardiovasc Electrophysiol 2024;35(1):162–70.

73. Yavin H, Shapira-Daniels A, Barkagan M, et al. Pulsed field ablation using a lattice electrode for focal energy delivery: biophysical characterization, lesion durability, and safety evaluation. Circ Arrhythm Electrophysiol 2020;13(6):e008580.

74. Anić A, Phlips T, Brešković T, et al. Pulsed field ablation using focal contact force-sensing catheters for treatment of atrial fibrillation: acute and 90-day invasive remapping results. Europace 2023;25(6). https://doi.org/10.1093/europace/euad147.

75. Calvert P, Mills MT, Xydis P, et al. Cost, efficiency, and outcomes of pulsed field ablation vs thermal ablation for atrial fibrillation: a real-world study. Heart Rhythm 2024;21(9):1537–44.

Pulsed Field Ablation Using a Lattice-Tip Catheter for Treatment of Ventricular Tachycardias

Moritz Nies, MD, Andreas Metzner, MD, Andreas Rillig, MD*

KEYWORDS

- Catheter ablation • Ventricular tachycardia • Electroporation • Myocardium

KEY POINTS

- Success rates of catheter ablation for ventricular arrhythmias remain limited due to several flaws of conventional ablation modalities in ventricular myocardium.
- Pulsed field ablation (PFA) has been established as a novel modality for atrial ablation. Several unique features make PFA an interesting option for ventricular ablation as well.
- A novel PFA system features a conformable, lattice-tip catheter that might prove particularly applicable for the ablation of ventricular myocardium.
- Preclinical porcine studies have shown that ventricular PFA using this system penetrated scar and fat tissue, created deep lesions, and successfully address difficult ablation targets.
- Initial clinical reports about ventricular PFA with the lattice-tip catheter have been published, but more data are needed to evaluate PFA as a true alternative to conventional ablation.

CATHETER ABLATION OF VENTRICULAR MYOCARDIUM: CURRENT PRACTICE AND LIMITATIONS

In current clinical practice, catheter ablation of ventricular arrhythmia is predominantly performed using radiofrequency current (RFC) but continues to have limited long-term success rates.[1–3] Compared to atrial tissue, ventricular myocardium poses several challenges for catheter ablation with RFC: (1) The increased wall thickness limits our ability to achieve transmural lesions and to target intramural substrates; (2) structural alterations in myocardium typically associated with arrhythmia impede lesion formation, and (3) for ablation of anatomically complex, mobile intracavitary structures (eg, papillary muscles or moderator bands), the prolonged catheter-tissue contact required for optimal energy transfer and thus high-quality lesions is difficult to achieve.[4–9] Modifications to RFC-delivery and alternative ablation modalities have been developed to tackle these challenges but ablation success rates remain suboptimal.[10–14]

PULSED FIELD ABLATION OF VENTRICULAR MYOCARDIUM: GENERAL CONSIDERATIONS

Pulsed field ablation (PFA) has been established for atrial ablation and has shown a superior safety profile as compared to thermal ablation modalities.[15] Several features of PFA might be advantageous for ventricular ablation as well: (1) PFA-applications are delivered in a shorter time than RFC-applications and are, therefore, less reliant on prolonged high-quality tissue contact.[16] This is advantageous for ablation of the contracting, mobile ventricular myocardium, especially for

Department of Cardiology, University Heart and Vascular Center, Martinistraße 52, Hamburg 20246, Germany
* Corresponding author.
E-mail address: a.rillig@uke.de

Card Electrophysiol Clin 17 (2025) 227–237
https://doi.org/10.1016/j.ccep.2025.02.010

mobile intracavitary structures. A recent preclinical study showed significantly deeper lesions after PFA of the papillary muscles and the left ventricular (LV) summit as compared to RFC-ablation using an investigational, focal ablation catheter.[17] (2) The ablative electric field does not seem to be significantly influenced by structural changes and subsequent impedance disparities in the targeted tissue. Therefore, ventricular PFA might overcome the limitation of impeded RFC-lesion formation in diseased myocardium (eg, heterogeneous postinfarction tissue/diffuse fibrosis in cardiomyopathies).[18] Indeed, PFA has been reported to penetrate nonmyocardial tissue better than thermal ablation.[19]

THE LARGE-FOCAL, LATTICE-TIP PULSED FIELD ABLATION CATHETER AND ABLATION SYSTEM

A novel ablation system features a deflectable, large focal lattice-tip catheter (Sphere-9, Medtronic, MN, USA). Its conformable, spherical, 9 mm nitinol-tip contains 9 mini-electrodes evenly distributed over its surface and 1 central electrode for three-dimensional electroanatomical mapping (Affera Mapping System, Medtronic). Monopolar PFA can be delivered from the entire lattice-tip using a PFAgenerator with a proprietary, biphasic waveform (HexaPulse, Medtronic).[16] Of note, the irrigated catheter can also be used to deliver RFC-ablation using an integrated RFC-generator (HexaGen, Medtronic) without the need to change the system setup.[20] The integration of PFA, RFC, and three-dimensional mapping capabilities into the same catheter makes the ablation system a versatile tool for catheter ablation. Focal lesions and the ability to toggle between RFC and PFA give the operator freedom to individualize lesion sets. Due to the comparatively large lesion size, linear ablation lesions can be created rapidly and with high success rates.[21]

The catheter design offers several advantages for ventricular ablation. (1) Its nitinol lattice-tip creates a certain degree of friction when it is in contact with myocardium (**Fig. 1**). When higher contact force is applied to the conformable tip, the area of catheter–tissue contact increases (**Fig. 2**), which further amplifies this friction and improves catheter stability.[22] (2) The ability to switch between RFC and PFA allows for tailored ablation lesions depending on the targeted area. While PFA might be used for heterogeneous scar tissue to overcome limitations of RFC in terms of lesion formation, titratable RFC might be the safer option when ablation is performed close to the coronary arteries or the conduction system to avoid coronary artery spasm or negative impact on

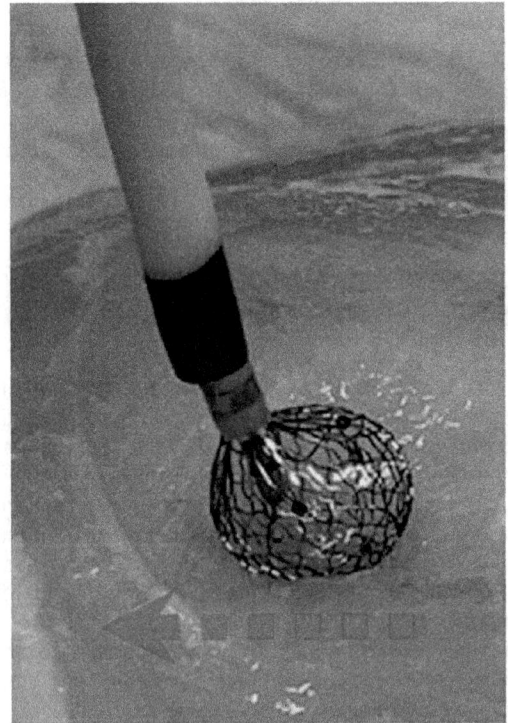

Fig. 1. Friction with catheter–tissue contact. The catheter shaft is moved leftward (*blue dotted arrow*) with the lattice-tip catheter in contact with muscle tissue. The friction caused by the lattice-tip design prevents the catheter from sliding on the muscle tissue. Instead, the catheter tip stays in place. (*From* Elad Anter et al., A Lattice-Tip Temperature-Controlled Radiofrequency Ablation Catheter for Wide Thermal Lesions: First-in-Human Experience With Atrial Fibrillation, JACC: Clinical Electrophysiology, 6 (5), 2020, 507-519, https://doi.org/10.1016/j.jacep.2019.12.015.)

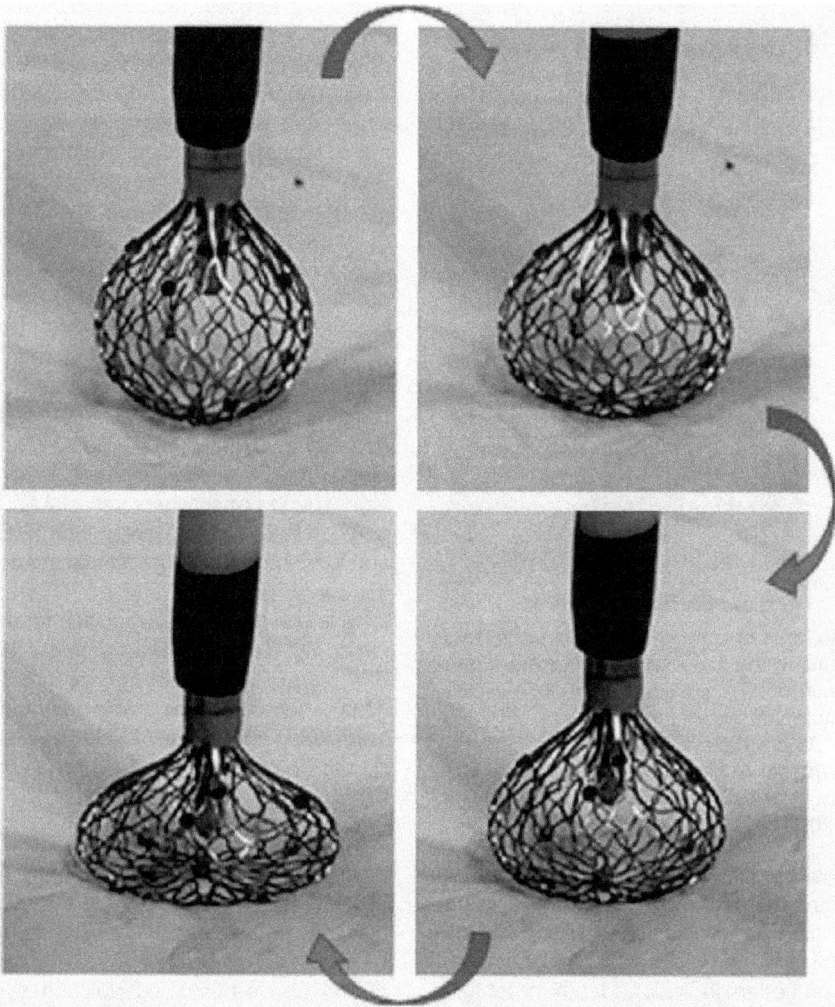

Fig. 2. Progressive change of the conformable lattice-tip with increasing pressure (*top left to bottom left*). Note how the area of contact increases with higher pressure (max. *bottom left*). (*From* Elad Anter et al., A Lattice-Tip Temperature-Controlled Radiofrequency Ablation Catheter for Wide Thermal Lesions: First-in-Human Experience With Atrial Fibrillation, JACC: Clinical Electrophysiology, 6 (5), 2020, 507-519, https://doi.org/10.1016/j.jacep.2019.12.015.)

conduction system properties. Furthermore, after PFA applications, electrical silence due to extensive reversible electroporation might occur, making signal interpretation more difficult. (3) This article will focus on PFA using the lattice-tip catheter. However, it should be noted that the large area of catheter–tissue contact compared to conventional focal catheters (**Fig. 3**) results in lower current density during RFC-ablation (**Fig. 4**).[22] This allows for more energy transfer and significantly larger lesions without excessive catheter heating and associated risks for charring or steam pop formation.[23] Therefore, even RFC-ablation using the lattice-tip catheter is a promising option to improve success rates of catheter ablation for ventricular arrhythmias.

VENTRICULAR PULSED FIELD ABLATION USING THE LATTICE-TIP CATHETER: PRECLINICAL EXPERIENCE

Several animal studies have evaluated ventricular PFA using the lattice-tip catheter: In an early preclinical evaluation, Younis and colleagues demonstrated that endocardial PFA of ventricular myocardium is feasible and that lesion size is dependent on application repetition. The maximum lesion depth observed in this study was approximately 9 mm.[24] Kawamura and colleagues[25] performed a porcine animal study with 11 swine in which PFA was delivered via the lattice-tip catheter endocardially in healthy myocardium, epicardially, and on the border zone of chronic ablation scar.

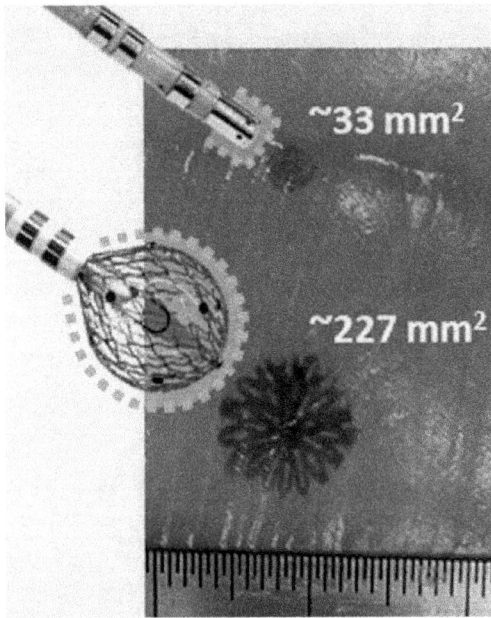

Fig. 3. Surface area of conventional, 3.5 mm tip focal catheter (*top*) and the 9 mm lattice-tip catheter (*bottom*) in comparison. (*From* Elad Anter et al., A Lattice-Tip Temperature-Controlled Radiofrequency Ablation Catheter for Wide Thermal Lesions: First-in-Human Experience With Atrial Fibrillation, JACC: Clinical Electrophysiology, 6 (5), 2020, 507-519, https://doi.org/10.1016/j.jacep.2019.12.015.)

They demonstrated that endocardial PFA achieved lesion depths of up to 6 mm, dependent on application repetition. PFA was also observed to penetrate epicardial fat and chronic ablation scar without significant reduction in lesion depth potentially impacting epicardial ablation. Younis and colleagues[26] employed an infarction model in 9 swine and compared lesion formation of RFC and PFA in chronic ventricular infarction tissue 8 to 10 weeks postinfarction. They demonstrated that in this heterogeneous tissue, PFA lesions were significantly larger and deeper compared to RFC lesions. A more recent study was performed to evaluate PFA using the lattice-tip catheter for the ablation of particularly challenging ablation targets. In a total of 14 swine, it was shown that mobile intracavitary structures like papillary muscles and moderator bands can be successfully ablated using the lattice-tip catheter. Using a bipolar approach with 2 ablation catheters (one of which acted as grounding electrode), LV myocardium could be transmurally ablated with a mean lesion depth of approximately 14 mm.[27] Typical features associated with PFA such as tissue-selectivity (morphologic sparing of coronary vessels) and nonthermal ablation lesions have been confirmed for this ablation system in these preclinical studies as well. In summary, preclinical studies have shown promising lesion formation capacities for PFA using the lattice-tip catheter while common advantages of PFA over RFC-ablation were retained. These data have sparked considerable enthusiasm for its application for clinical VT ablation.

CLINICAL EXPERIENCE

Whereas a certain amount of preclinical data have been obtained, only limited data exist on the clinical use of the novel ablation system for the treatment of ventricular arrhythmias. In part, this might be explained by the absence of regulatory approval of the above-described ablation system for VT ablation. However, the manufacturer announced Food and Drug Administration approval for an early

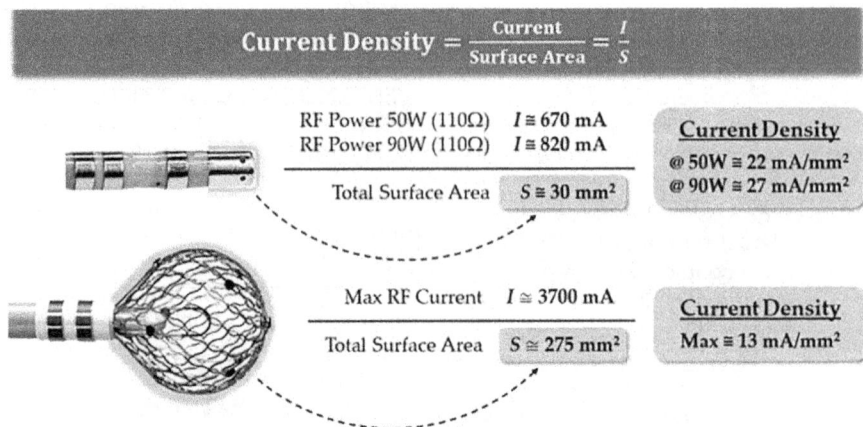

Fig. 4. Surface area and current density of a conventional 3.5 mm focal tip ablation catheter (*top*) and the 9 mm lattice-tip catheter (*bottom*). (*Data from* Anter E, Neužil P, Rackauskas G, et al. A lattice-tip temperature-controlled radiofrequency ablation catheter for wide thermal lesions. JACC Clin Electrophysiol 2020;6(5):507–19. https://doi.org/10.1016/j.jacep.2019.12.015.)

feasibility trial using the system for VT ablation in October 2024.[28] Besides several case reports for bailout ablation,[29-31] 2 series with larger patient numbers have been published to date, including patients with right ventricular (RV), LV, or epicardial VT ablation.

The first clinical use of the lattice-tip catheter for VT ablation was published in a case report on a patient with a septal intramural substrate with recurrent VT after several RFC-ablation attempts. A dual-energy approach using RFC followed by PFA led to durable suppression of VT.[29] More recently, a first case series was published by Pannone and colleagues[32] providing insights into the ablation procedures of 4 patients with different primary diseases (Brugada syndrome, arrhythmogenic right ventricular cardiomyopathy (ARVC), nonischemic heart disease, and ischemic heart disease). In the 2 patients with Brugada syndrome and ARVC, only right-sided ventricular ablation using PFA-only was performed, based on the assumption that lesion depth would be sufficient to create transmural lesions within the RV. For LV ablation in the 2 remaining patients, the primary strategy was high-power, temperature-controlled RFC ablation, followed by PFA. Considerations for this approach included potential alteration of intracardiac signal interpretation after PFA application. Electrical silence often occurs to a certain extent after PFA, making it more difficult to assess abolition of all critical areas. Based on preclinical experience, application of pulsed field (PF) energy in the ventricle might lead to ventricular arrhythmia, albeit in swine models that are notoriously susceptible for arrhythmia induction during ablation.[25,27] In none of the clinical cases, VT or ventricular fibrillation was induced during ventricular PFA, but irritative firing greater than 3 seconds postablation was observed in the patient with Brugada syndrome during 4 PF applications.[32]

Peichl and colleagues[33] published the largest series of patients with VT treated with the lattice-tip catheter, the majority of which had structural heart disease. All 18 patients were ablated within the LV, in 4 cases (22%) with a combined endocardial and epicardial approach. In this study, operators started with RFC ablation as the primary energy source and used PFA thereafter for lesion consolidation. Considerations were based on several aspects including long experience with RFC, optimized signal interpretation after initial applications, and the potential for larger lesion sets.[24] As 66% of the patients underwent redo-ablation, subsequent PFA offered the advantage of enhanced penetration of fibrotic or preablated tissue and thus was applied in all patients after RFC application.

ENERGY SETTINGS FOR VENTRICULAR PULSED FIELD ABLATION WITH THE SPHERE-9 CATHETER

Whereas for atrial ablation, recommended energy presets for RFC and PFA application are used by the majority of operators, the optimal mode for VT ablation is less clear. The optimal energy settings for PFA might differ both between RV and LV ablations and between endocardial and epicardial ablation depending on wall thickness and type of substrate. Duration and number of PF applications as well as interlesion distance have to be further evaluated. Pannone and colleagues[32] described the energy settings for PFA in the ventricles as follows: 1500 pulses/train, 12 trains/application, and 350 millisecond intertrain delay.

GENERAL ANESTHESIA VERSUS DEEP SEDATION

In both patient series, all VT ablation procedures were performed in general anesthesia (GA), and muscle relaxants were applied in some cases.[32,33] There is an ongoing debate, whether GA should be preferred over deep sedation when PFA with the lattice-tip catheter is performed. Based on the monopolar nature of PF application with this system, muscle contraction resulting in patient movement or map shifts might be expected. In patients with atrial fibrillation, one study has demonstrated that deep sedation appears to be feasible without map shifts or an increase in complication rates and results in shorter laboratory-occupancy times as compared to GA.[34] Although patients with VT might be treated in GA for several reasons, including optimized blood pressure control, fluid-management, and more stable conditions during ongoing VT, incessant VT, and electrical storm, deep sedation might be an attractive setting for patients with stable VT or premature ventricular contractions.

Irreversible electroporation is the goal of PFA, but reversible electroporation often occurs in adjacent areas.[35] Although PF application might lead to difficulties in subsequent signal interpretation, so-called pulsed-field mapping using low-dose PF applications could be a reasonable approach to test whether PFA at a distinct area might result in damage of critical adjacent structures such as the cardiac conduction system, or help to identify the critical isthmus of VT without permanent damage.[29,36]

Epicardial ablation is still mandatory in a significant number of patients with VT and is usually considered after failure of initial endocardial ablation or based on electrocardiographic features.[37]

Epicardial fat is one of the major determinants of epicardial ablation failure, in particular at regions of RV or RV outflow tract (RVOT). As mentioned earlier, this limitation might be overcome with PFA. According to several reports,[31] epicardial PF application might enhance ablation success in patients with VT, although transmurality of epicardial lesions could not be confirmed by endocardial remapping in one study with a limited number of patients.[33] Bipolar ablation might be helpful for patients in which even epicardial ablation is ineffective for modification of the VT re-entrant circuit, or if intramural substrate is likely.[27,38]

POTENTIAL RISKS DURING VENTRICULAR TACHYCARDIA ABLATION WITH PULSED FIELD ABLATION

One of the most feared complications during ventricular RFC application is cardiac tamponade resulting either from perforation of the cardiac wall with the rather stiff and thin catheter tip of conventional ablation catheters or from steam pops.[39] The risk for a steam pop is reduced by PF application with the lattice-tip catheter as temperature rise measured via the 9 mini-electrodes with thermocouples at the catheter tip is not observed to exceed 2°C to 3°C during PFA, and therefore, excessive tissue heating is unlikely. In addition, the central lumen for catheter irrigation is surrounded by the rather large lattice tip, making ineffective cooling during RFC applications with this catheter unlikely. Moreover, the flexible and compressible tip of the lattice-tip catheter might prevent excessive contact force applied to the cardiac wall during both mapping and ablation, keeping the risk for perforation low. [22]

Coronary artery spasm has been described after PFA in close vicinity to the coronary arteries.[40,41] Whether PF application can induce coronary artery spasm during endocardial VT ablation has not been demonstrated yet. However, epicardial VT ablation might result in clinical (electrocardiogram changes) or subclinical coronary artery spasm, which is sensitive to nitroglycerin administration, as observed during coronary angiography before and after epicardial PF ablation.[33] Even though coronary artery spasm usually resolves within minutes after intravenous or intracoronary nitroglycerin application, the long-term consequences of coronary artery spasms after PFA are not fully understood. Neointimal neoplasia in preclinical data gives rise to concerns about late coronary narrowing.[42] This finding warrants further research to better understand whether coronary angiography should become a standard during or after epicardial PFA in close proximity (<20 mm) to the coronary arteries. Considering the relevant risk for permanent coronary artery damage with RFC ablation,[43] PFA might still be a viable alternative for ablation close to epicardial vessels despite the risk for acute coronary spasm.

PFA for atrial fibrillation appears to carry at least a very low risk for transient phrenic nerve palsy.[15,44] In contrast, phrenic nerve palsy was not observed during epicardial PFA with the lattice-tip catheter, even when PFA was applied in areas with left phrenic nerve capture.[33] Recent reports on hemolysis after PFA have identified a high number of applications, imperfect tissue contact as well as renal insufficiency as risk factors for kidney injury after PFA, albeit with a different ablation system.[45–48] In the VT cases published to date, no relevant signs of hemolysis have been reported.[32,33]

MAPPING OPPORTUNITIES AND CATHETER CONTACT DURING ABLATION

The lattice-tip catheter with its 9 mini-electrodes provides rapid high-density mapping in the atria,[21,44] but also in the ventricles, allowing for fast and accurate identification of substrate and ablation targets (**Fig. 5**).[32,33] Whereas some operators report on difficulties to capture ventricular myocardium for pace mapping or arrhythmia induction (potentially due to the small extent of the mini-electrodes)[33] others describe reasonable feasibility of the system for activation and entrainment mapping.[32] Besides high-quality mapping, the lattice-tip catheter might offer enhanced catheter–tissue contact due to its large, conformable tip, which provides more friction based on its nitinol cage structure. Whether significant patient movement occurs during VT ablation with this monopolar system in deep sedation has to be evaluated in larger clinical case series without GA (see also "General anesthesia versus deep sedation" section). Since the large lattice tip of the Sphere-9 catheter can be easily visualized via ultrasound within the cardiac chambers even at more difficult ablation sites such as the papillary muscles, ICE-guided nonfluoroscopic navigation might be an attractive option to facilitate VT ablation procedures (**Fig. 6**).[29,27,33]

The impact of catheter-tissue contact for ablation using thermal energy sources has been investigated intensively.[49] For PFA, the impact of contact force on lesion creation is not fully understood.[35] There are several reports on how to increase lesion depth and size during PF application. Besides a higher number of train repetitions[24,25] and the stability of catheter–tissue contact,[27] a higher contact

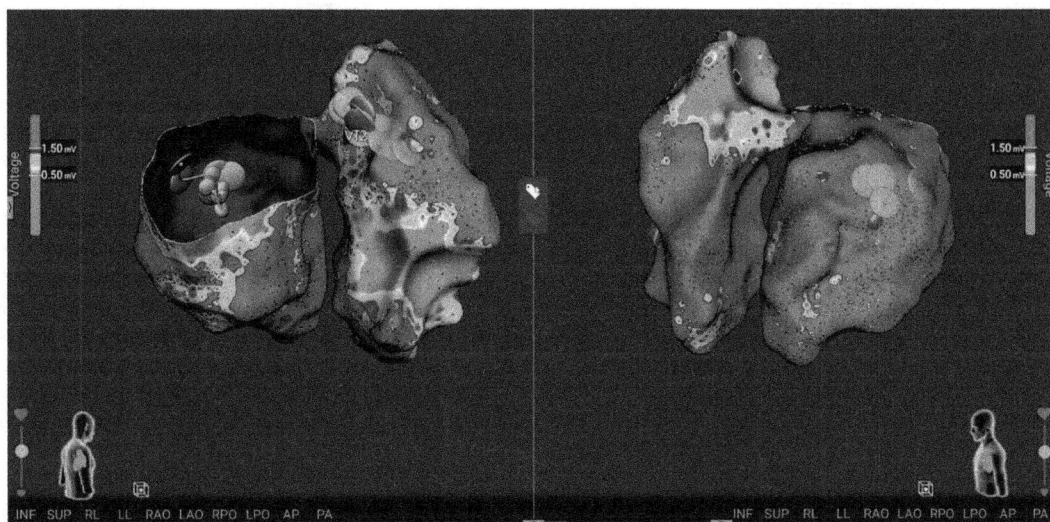

Fig. 5. High-density voltage map of right and left ventricle during VT ablation using the Affera system with the Sphere-9 lattice tip catheter. Red dots indicate RF application, and green dots PFA application.

force per se has been shown to enhance lesion formation.[50]

The bidirectional design of the lattice-tip catheter facilitates the use of 2 differently shaped curves within one ablation tool. This might improve navigation in challenging anatomies and provide the opportunity to adjust between better steerability (small curve 35 mm) and increased accessibility (larger curve 50 mm).

EXTENT OF MYOCARDIAL DAMAGE

Troponin release is regularly observed after catheter ablation.[51] Troponin T levels after VT ablation using a combined approach of both RFC and PFA with the lattice-tip catheter were not excessively high.[33] It, therefore, appears reasonable to assume that PFA in the ventricles is not associated with disproportionate tissue damage when compared to thermal ablation.

FUTURE DIRECTIONS AND UNANSWERED QUESTIONS

The lattice-tip catheter with its unique design in combination with the specific option to toggle between RFC and PFA offers the attractive option to choose between energy sources, depending on the underlying substrate. Especially in preablated patients, larger low-voltage areas, or intramural foci, the additional application of PFA in the ventricles might be of value. It will require further studies to better understand at which locations RFC or PFA might be the preferable energy source to start VT

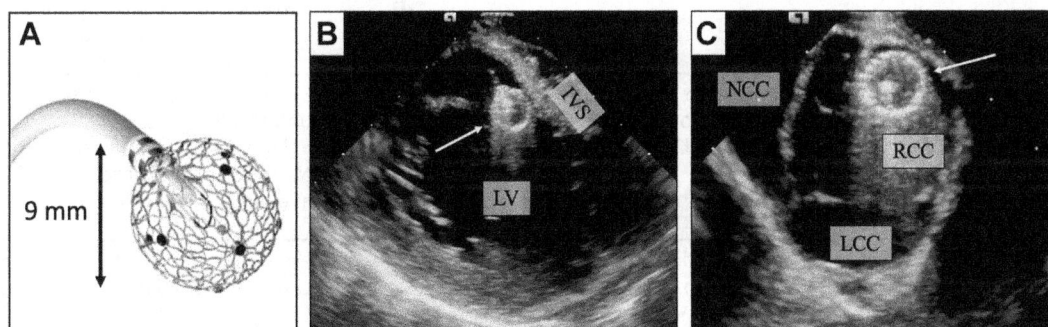

Fig. 6. (*A*) Lattice-tip catheter (Sphere-9, Medtronic). (*B*) Intracardiac echocardiography (ICE) view of the catheter tip (*arrow*) in the left ventricle (LV) at LV septum. (*C*) ICE-view of the catheter before ICE-guided passing of the aortic valve for retrograde access to the LV. IVS, interventricular septum; LCC, left coronary cusp; NCC, noncoronary cusp; RCC, right coronary cusp. (*Data from* Nies M, Koruth JS, Musikantow DR, et al. Pulsed field mapping of ventricular tachycardia: verifying the ablation target at a critical location, J Am Coll Cardiol, **10** (3), 2024, 630–6.)

ablation procedures. PFA offers the opportunity to deliver applications with very short duration, which might be helpful at difficult ablation sites such as papillary muscles or the moderator band, as shorter periods of stable contact are required.

Long-term outcomes of VT ablation using the lattice-tip catheter with PFA for VT are lacking. The longest follow-up reported in larger case series was 3 to 5 months and is, therefore, still limited.[32,33] Significant recurrence rates have been observed after VT ablation with PFA systems using a conventional 4 mm single-tip catheter,[52] potentially based on extensive reversible electroporation, resulting in nondurable lesions. Therefore, data on long-term outcomes after VT ablation with the lattice-tip catheter using PFA are needed. Although ganglionated plexuses and nerves appear to be less sensitive to this novel energy source,[53] safety of PFA application in proximity of the cardiac conduction system warrants further evaluation. One preclinical report described viable Purkinje fibers within an ablated area, suggesting a lower susceptibility for PFA.[54] However, PFA application close to the conduction system can result at least in a transient atrioventricular (AV) block and elimination of Purkinje potentials.[36,55,56] Low-dose PFA might help to titrate PFA in corresponding regions.

PFA for substrate modification to a larger extent in the ventricles might result in stunning of larger areas of vital myocardium with further deterioration of pre-existing reduced LV ejection fraction leading to hemodynamic instability or progressive heart failure. Although no significant compromise has been observed in the limited number of clinical VT ablations so far, this issue needs further clarification. **Table 1** shows pros and cons of the lattice-tip ablation catheter and ablation system for VT ablation.

The majority of VT treatments has been described in patients with structural heart disease.[57,58] More experience is needed for the treatment of patients with idiopathic ventricular arrhythmias and outflow tract tachycardia.

Table 1
Pros and cons of the lattice-tip ablation catheter and ablation system for ventricular tachycardia ablation

	+	−

Safety	• No steam pops reported so far
	• Nonthermal ablation
	• Low perforation risk (conformable tip)
	• Only single transseptal access required
		• Coronary spasm
		• Limited safety data available, open questions:
		  ○ Extent of hemolysis
		  ○ Arrhythmogenic effects
		  ○ Effects on the conduction system
		  ○ Effects of stunning on left ventricular function

Efficacy	• Penetration of fibrotic and fatty tissue
	• Bipolar ablation using 2 catheters feasible
	  ○ Transmural LV ablation possible (animal studies)
	• Only short stable catheter–tissue contact necessary
		• Extent of reversible effects unknown
		  ○ Endpoints undefined
		• No long-term efficacy data available

Workflow/ applicability	• Short application time • RF and PFA possible • HD 3D-mapping capabilities • Offers pulsed field mapping • High echogenicity ○ ICE-guiding facilitated	• High cost • Limited availability

Abbreviations: HD, High-density; ICE, intracardiac echocardiography; LV, left ventricular; PFA, pulsed field ablation; RF, radiofrequency.

SUMMARY

The 9 mm lattice-tip catheter with its unique design combined with the specific opportunity to toggle between RFC and PFA offers an attractive option to choose between energy sources, depending on underlying substrate. Especially in preablated patients, larger low-voltage areas or intramural foci, the additional application of PFA in the ventricles might be of value. Larger studies with long-term follow-up are needed.

CLINICS CARE POINTS

- The lattice-tip mapping and ablation catheter has a unique tip design that promotes catheter stability and provides a large area of catheter–tissue contact. Conceptually, these features offer significant advantages over established catheter technologies for the ablation of ventricular myocardium.

- PFA using the lattice-tip catheter has demonstrated promising lesion formation capacities in preclinical studies, and it might offer the potential to overcome limitations of radiofrequency ablation with conventional ablation catheters.

- Clinical experience using the lattice-tip catheter for VT ablation remains limited. Long-term safety and efficacy data with large patient cohorts are needed.

DISCLOSURE

Dr M. Nies has received a scholarship from the German Research Foundation (Deutsche Forschungsgemeinschaft). Dr A. Metzner received consultant fees from Medtronic, Biosense Webster, Boston Scientific, Abbott, and travel grants and lecture fees from Medtronic, Biosense Webster, Boston Scientific, Abbott, Lifetech, Bristol-Myers-Squibb, Bayer, KODEX-EPD. Dr A. Rillig received consultant fees from Medtronic, KODEX-EPD, Biosense Webster, Boston Scientific, and travel grants and lecture fees or compensation for advisory board from Medtronic, Cardiofocus, Biosense Webster, Abbott, Boehringer Ingelheim, Philips KODEX-EPD, Ablamap, Bayer, Novartis, Lifetech, Boston Scientific, Atricure, and Lilly.

REFERENCES

1. Della Bella P, Baratto F, Tsiachris D, et al. Management of ventricular tachycardia in the setting of a dedicated unit for the treatment of complex ventricular arrhythmias: long-term outcome after ablation. Circulation 2013;127(13):1359–68.

2. Wasmer K, Reinecke H, Heitmann M, et al. Clinical, procedural and long-term outcome of ischemic VT ablation in patients with previous anterior versus inferior myocardial infarction. Clin Res Cardiol 2020;109(10):1282–91.

3. Yamashita S, Cochet H, Sacher F, et al. Impact of new technologies and approaches for post-myocardial infarction ventricular tachycardia ablation during long-term follow-up. Circ Arrhythm Electrophysiol 2016; 9(7). https://doi.org/10.1161/CIRCEP.116.003901.

4. Latchamsetty R, Yokokawa M, Morady F, et al. Multicenter outcomes for catheter ablation of idiopathic premature ventricular complexes. JACC Clin Electrophysiol 2015;1(3):116–23.

5. Schwartzman D, Chang I, Michele JJ, et al. Electrical impedance properties of normal and chronically infarcted left ventricular myocardium. J Interv Card Electrophysiol 1999;3(3):213–24.

6. Barkagan M, Leshem E, Shapira-Daniels A, et al. Histopathological characterization of radiofrequency ablation in ventricular scar tissue. JACC Clin Electrophysiol 2019;5(8):920–31.

7. Rivera S, Ricapito Mde L, Tomas L, et al. Results of cryoenergy and radiofrequency-based catheter ablation for treating ventricular arrhythmias arising from the papillary muscles of the left ventricle, guided by intracardiac echocardiography and image integration. Circ Arrhythm Electrophysiol 2016; 9(4):e003874.

8. Mariani MV, Piro A, Magnocavallo M, et al. Catheter ablation for papillary muscle arrhythmias: a systematic review. Pacing Clin Electrophysiol 2022;45(4): 519–31.

9. Yokokawa M, Good E, Desjardins B, et al. Predictors of successful catheter ablation of ventricular arrhythmias arising from the papillary muscles. Heart Rhythm 2010;7(11):1654–9.

10. Brugada P, de Swart H, Smeets JL, et al. Transcoronary chemical ablation of ventricular tachycardia. Circulation 1989;79(3):475–82.

11. Loo BW Jr, Soltys SG, Wang L, et al. Stereotactic ablative radiotherapy for the treatment of refractory cardiac ventricular arrhythmia. Circ Arrhythm Electrophysiol 2015;8(3):748–50.

12. Timmermans C, Manusama R, Alzand B, et al. Catheter-based cryoablation of postinfarction and idiopathic ventricular tachycardia: initial experience in a selected population. J Cardiovasc Electrophysiol 2010;21(3):255–61.

13. Koruth JS, Dukkipati S, Miller MA, et al. Bipolar irrigated radiofrequency ablation: a therapeutic option for refractory intramural atrial and ventricular tachycardia circuits. Heart Rhythm 2012;9(12): 1932–41.

14. Nguyen DT, Tzou WS, Sandhu A, et al. Prospective multicenter experience with cooled radiofrequency ablation using high impedance irrigant to target deep

myocardial substrate refractory to standard ablation. JACC Clin Electrophysiol 2018;4(9):1176–85.

15. Ekanem E, Neuzil P, Reichlin T, et al. Safety of pulsed field ablation in more than 17,000 patients with atrial fibrillation in the MANIFEST-17K study. Nat Med 2024;30(7):2020–9.

16. Koruth JS, Kuroki K, Kawamura I, et al. Focal pulsed field ablation for pulmonary vein isolation and linear atrial lesions: a preclinical assessment of safety and durability. Circ Arrhythm Electrophysiol 2020;13(6):e008716.

17. Younis A, Tabaja C, Kleve R, et al. Comparative efficacy and safety of pulsed field ablation versus radiofrequency ablation of idiopathic LV arrhythmias. J Am Coll Cardiol 2024;10(9):1998–2009.

18. Kawamura I, Reddy VY, Santos-Gallego CG, et al. Electrophysiology, pathology, and imaging of pulsed field ablation of scarred and healthy ventricles in Swine. Circ Arrhythm Electrophysiol 2023;16(1):e011369.

19. Im SI, Higuchi S, Lee A, et al. Pulsed field ablation of left ventricular myocardium in a swine infarct model. JACC Clin Electrophysiol 2022;8(6):722–31.

20. Reddy VY, Anter E, Rackauskas G, et al. Lattice-tip focal ablation catheter that toggles between radiofrequency and pulsed field energy to treat atrial fibrillation: a first-in-human trial. Circ Arrhythm Electrophysiol 2020;13(6):e008718.

21. Metzner A, Rottner L, Moser F, et al. A novel platform allowing for pulsed field and radiofrequency ablation: first commercial atrial fibrillation ablation procedures worldwide with and without general anesthesia. Heart Rhythm 2024;21(4):497–8.

22. Anter E, Neuzil P, Rackauskas G, et al. A lattice-tip temperature-controlled radiofrequency ablation catheter for wide thermal lesions. J Am Coll Cardiol 2020;6(5):507–19.

23. Shapira-Daniels A, Barkagan M, Yavin H, et al. Novel irrigated temperature-controlled lattice ablation catheter for ventricular ablation: a preclinical multimodality biophysical characterization. Circ Arrhythm Electrophysiol 2019;12(11):e007661.

24. Yavin HD, Higuchi K, Sroubek J, et al. Pulsed-field ablation in ventricular myocardium using a focal catheter: the impact of application repetition on lesion dimensions. Circ Arrhythm Electrophysiol 2021;14(9):e010375.

25. Kawamura I, Reddy VY, Wang BJ, et al. Pulsed field ablation of the porcine ventricle using a focal lattice-tip catheter. Circ Arrhythm Electrophysiol 2022;15(9):e011120.

26. Younis A, Zilberman I, Krywanczyk A, et al. Effect of pulsed-field and radiofrequency ablation on heterogeneous ventricular scar in a swine model of healed myocardial infarction. Circ Arrhythm Electrophysiol 2022;15(10):e011209.

27. Nies M, Watanabe K, Kawamura I, et al. Preclinical study of pulsed field ablation of difficult ventricular targets: intracavitary mobile structures, interventricular septum, and left ventricular free wall. Circ Arrhythm Electrophysiol 2024;17(6):e012734.

28. Medtronic. Medtronic announces FDA approval for early feasibility trial of Affera™ Mapping and Ablation System with Sphere-9™ Catheter for the treatment of ventricular tachycardia. Available at: https://news.medtronic.com/Medtronic-announces-FDA-approval-for-early-feasibility-trial-of-Affera-TM-Mapping-and-Ablation-System-with-Sphere-9-TM-Catheter-for-the-treatment-of-ventricular-tachycardia. Accessed November 5, 2024.

29. Nies M, Koruth JS, Musikantow DR, et al. Pulsed field mapping of ventricular tachycardia: verifying the ablation target at a critical location. J Am Coll Cardiol 2024;10(3):630–6.

30. Benali K, Monaco C, Jais P, et al. Pulsed field ablation for refractory ventricular arrhythmias in patients with left ventricular assist devices. JACC Clin Electrophysiol 2024. https://doi.org/10.1016/j.jacep.2024.08.012.

31. Yokoyama M, Vlachos K, Duchateau J, et al. Pulsed field epicardial ablation for VT storm: a case report of bailout therapy. Heart Rhythm 2024. https://doi.org/10.1016/j.hrthm.2024.08.021.

32. Pannone L, Doundoulakis I, Cespón-Fernández M, et al. A large footprint focal catheter toggling between pulsed field and radiofrequency energy: first clinical experience for ventricular tachycardia ablation. EP Europace 2024;26(7). https://doi.org/10.1093/europace/euae193.

33. Peichl P, Wichterle D, Schlosser F, et al. Mapping and ablation of ventricular tachycardia using dual-energy lattice-tip focal catheter: early feasibility and safety study. EP Europace 2024. https://doi.org/10.1093/europace/euae275.

34. Rillig A, Hirokami J, Moser F, et al. General anaesthesia and deep sedation for monopolar pulsed field ablation using a lattice-tip catheter combined with a novel three-dimensional mapping system. EP Europace 2024;26(11). https://doi.org/10.1093/europace/euae270.

35. Chun K-RJ, Miklavčič D, Vlachos K, et al. State-of-the-art pulsed field ablation for cardiac arrhythmias: ongoing evolution and future perspective. EP Europace 2024;26(6). https://doi.org/10.1093/europace/euae134.

36. Koruth JS, Neuzil P, Kawamura I, et al. Reversible pulsed electrical fields as an in vivo tool to study cardiac electrophysiology: the advent of pulsed field mapping. Circ Arrhythm Electrophysiol 2023e012018. https://doi.org/10.1161/CIRCEP.123.012018.

37. Sultan A, Futyma P, Metzner A, et al. Management of ventricular tachycardias: insights on centre settings, procedural workflow, endpoints, and implementation of guidelines-results from an EHRA survey. Europace 2024;26(2). https://doi.org/10.1093/europace/euae030.

38. Futyma P, Sultan A, Zarębski Ł, et al. Bipolar radiofrequency ablation of refractory ventricular arrhythmias: results from a multicentre network. Europace 2024; 26(10). https://doi.org/10.1093/europace/euae248.

39. Seiler J, Roberts-Thomson KC, Raymond J-M, et al. Steam pops during irrigated radiofrequency ablation: feasibility of impedance monitoring for prevention. Heart Rhythm 2008;5(10):1411–6.

40. Reddy VY, Petru J, Funasako M, et al. Coronary arterial spasm during pulsed field ablation to treat atrial fibrillation. Circulation 2022;146(24):1808–19.

41. Gunawardene MA, Schaeffer BN, Jularic M, et al. Coronary spasm during pulsed field ablation of the mitral isthmus line. JACC Clin Electrophysiol 2021; 7(12):1618–20.

42. Higuchi S, Im SI, Stillson C, et al. Effect of epicardial pulsed field ablation directly on coronary arteries. JACC Clin Electrophysiol 2022;8(12):1486–96.

43. Wong KCK, Lim C, Sadarmin PP, et al. High incidence of acute sub-clinical circumflex artery 'injury' following mitral isthmus ablation. Eur Heart J 2011; 32(15):1881–90.

44. Anter E, Mansour M, Nair DG, et al. Dual-energy lattice-tip ablation system for persistent atrial fibrillation: a randomized trial. Nat Med 2024;30(8): 2303–10.

45. Popa MA, Venier S, Menè R, et al. Characterization and clinical significance of hemolysis after pulsed field ablation for atrial fibrillation: results of a multicenter analysis. Circulation 2024;17(10):e012732.

46. Osmancik P, Bacova B, Herman D, et al. Periprocedural intravascular hemolysis during atrial fibrillation ablation. JACC (J Am Coll Cardiol) 2024;10(7_Part_2):1660–71.

47. Venier S, Vaxelaire N, Jacon P, et al. Severe acute kidney injury related to haemolysis after pulsed field ablation for atrial fibrillation. Europace 2023;26(1).

48. Nies M, Koruth JS, Mlček M, et al. Hemolysis after pulsed field ablation: impact of lesion number and catheter-tissue contact. Circ Arrhythm Electrophysiol 2024;17(6):e012765.

49. Nakagawa H, Jackman WM. The role of contact force in atrial fibrillation ablation. J Atr Fibrillation 2014;7(1):1027.

50. Di Biase L, Marazzato J, Govari A, et al. Pulsed field ablation index-guided ablation for lesion formation: impact of contact force and number of applications in the ventricular model. Circ Arrhythm Electrophysiol 2024;17(4):e012717.

51. Popa MA, Bahlke F, Kottmaier M, et al. Myocardial injury and inflammation following pulsed-field ablation and very high-power short-duration ablation for atrial fibrillation. J Cardiovasc Electrophysiol 2024;35(2):317–27.

52. Peichl P, Bulava A, Wichterle D, et al. Efficacy and safety of focal pulsed-field ablation for ventricular arrhythmias: two-centre experience. EP Europace 2024;26(7).

53. Lemoine MD, Mencke C, Nies M, et al. Pulmonary vein isolation by pulsed-field ablation induces less neurocardiac damage than cryoballoon ablation. Circ Arrhythm Electrophysiol 2023;16(4):e011598.

54. Koruth JS, Kawamura I, Reddy VY. Selective sparing of Purkinje fibres with pulsed-field myocardial ablation. Europace 2023;25(2):330.

55. Livia C, Sugrue A, Witt T, et al. Elimination of purkinje fibers by electroporation reduces ventricular fibrillation vulnerability. J Am Heart Assoc 2018;7(15): e009070.

56. Sugrue A, Vaidya VR, Livia C, et al. Feasibility of selective cardiac ventricular electroporation. PLoS One 2020;15(2):e0229214.

57. Pannone L, Doundoulakis I, Cespon-Fernandez M, et al. A large footprint focal catheter toggling between pulsed field and radiofrequency energy: first clinical experience for ventricular tachycardia ablation. Europace 2024;26(7).

58. Peichl P, Bulava A, Wichterle D, et al. Efficacy and safety of focal pulsed-field ablation for ventricular arrhythmias: two-centre experience. Europace 2024; 26(7).

Catheters and Tools with Pulsed Field Ablation— Pulmonary Vein Isolation with Focal Lattice-Tip Affera Sphere 9

María Cespón-Fernández, MD, PhD[a], Andrea Sarkozy, MD, PhD, FEHRA[b],*

KEYWORDS

- Lattice-tip catheter • Pulsed-field ablacion • Atrial fibrillation • Pulmonary veins • Catheter ablation

KEY POINTS

- The Affera system integrates radiofrequency and pulsed-field energy delivery through a versatile catheter design, offering flexibility for tailored ablation strategies in the treatment of atrial fibrillation.
- Preclinical and clinical studies have shown high acute success rates and durable lesion formation with excellent safety profile, with real-world data further supporting these favorable outcomes.
- The system's large ablation footprint, combined with precise mapping capabilities, enhances both efficacy and efficiency, leading to improved ablation results and reduced procedural times, particularly for pulmonary vein isolation.

INTRODUCTION

Pulsed field ablation (PFA) has emerged as a promising tool for the treatment of atrial fibrillation (AF), offering high efficacy and an improved safety profile due to its unique tissue-selectivity. By utilizing ultra-rapid electrical fields, PFA selectively targets cardiac tissue while minimizing damage to surrounding structures, such as the esophagus or phrenic nerves, a common concern in thermal ablation techniques. This distinct advantage has led to the development of various PFA-based tools, primarily designed for pulmonary vein isolation (PVI) in a single-shot manner. These tools are particularly effective for PVI, achieving fast and durable results.[1,2]

However, despite the advantages of single-shot PFA devices for PVI, they are often limited by a lack of flexibility, especially when addressing more complex ablation targets. This includes the need for more proximal antral isolation or for a more tailored ablation by creating linear lesions, both of which are essential for treating more extensive arrhythmogenic substrates. In this regard, the "point-by-point" ablation strategy, guided by 3D electroanatomical mapping (EAM), has traditionally dominated AF ablation, offering greater flexibility in lesion creation and aligning with operator preferences. To overcome this limitation, focal PFA catheters have been developed, offering a solution for both PVI and linear ablation.

[a] Department of Cardiology, Heart Rhythm Management Centre, European Reference Networks Guard-Heart, Universitair Ziekenhuis Brussel Heart Rhythm Research Brussels, Postgraduate Program in Cardiac Electrophysiology and Pacing, Vrije Universiteit Brussel, Av. du Laerbeek 101, Brussels, Jette 1090, Belgium; [b] Department of Cardiology, Ventricular Arhythmia and Sudden Cardiac Death Unit Heart, Rhythm Management Centre, European Reference Networks Guard-Heart, Universitair Ziekenhuis Brussel Heart Rhythm Research Brussels, Postgraduate Program in Cardiac Electrophysiology and Pacing, Vrije Universiteit Brussel, Brussels, Jette 1090, Belgium
* Corresponding author.
E-mail address: andreasarkozy@yahoo.ca

Card Electrophysiol Clin 17 (2025) 239–249
https://doi.org/10.1016/j.ccep.2025.02.011
1877-9182/25/© 2025 Elsevier Inc. All rights reserved, including those for text and data mining, AI training, and similar technologies.

cardiacEP.theclinics.com

Abbreviations	
AF	Atrial fibrillation
ACT	Activated clotting time
CTI	Cavotricuspid isthmus
EAM	Electroanatomical mapping
LA	Left atrium
LAA	Left atrial appendage
MI	Mitral isthmus
PFA	Pulsed field ablation
PF	Pulsed-field
PV	Pulmonary veins
PVI	Pulmonary vein isolation
RA	Right atrium
RF	Radiofrequency

There are currently 2 focal PFA systems dedicated for AF ablation, both with the capability of toggling between PFA and radiofrequency (RF) energies.

Recently, the Affera system (Medtronic, Minneapolis) has obtained the Conformité Européenne (CE) mark approval and clearance from the Food and Drug Administration (FDA) for its use as an ablation tool for atrial tachyarrhythmias. It consists of a large footprint combined ablation and mapping catheter, with a 9-mm compressible spherical tip that was developed to facilitate the use of both RF and pulsed-field (PF).[3]

DISCUSSION
Ablation System

Lattice-tip catheter
The Affera system features a 9-mm expandable spherical nitinol lattice-tip catheter (Sphere9), which serves both for mapping and ablation functions. It contains 9 mini-electrodes, each 0.7 mm diameter, spaced approximately 5 mm apart, which are uniformly distributed across the surface of the sphere. Each mini-electrode is equipped with a thermal sensor.

For mapping purposes, bipolar electrograms are configured between each mini-electrode and a central floating indifferent electrode. Continuous impedance monitoring between each mini-electrode and the central electrode enables tissue-contact assessment.

A central nozzle within the expandable electrode provides homogeneous saline irrigation both during mapping (4 mL/min) and ablation (15 mL/min–30 mL/min during PFA and 15 mL/min during RF delivery), all controlled by a peristaltic pump (HexaFLOW, Affera, Inc).

The catheter incorporates a 7.5 Fr bidirectional steerable shaft, which enhances catheter stability and tissue engagement. Additionally, there are 2 ring electrodes displayed on the shaft, proximal

to the sphere, for its visualization at the EAM system.

Energy sources
The Affera system displays a dual-generator design, enabling seamless switching between RF and PF energy.

Regarding RF energy, the Sphere9 catheter operates in monopolar mode, with the lattice struts functioning as a solid electrode. This large surface area allows for higher current delivery at a relatively low density, compared to standard 3.5 mm irrigated-tip catheters, resulting in resistive heating spreading across a substantially broader and deeper area than occurs with traditional systems. This may be particularly useful for thicker and tissue targets while reducing the risk of steam pops occurrence.[4–6]

Power titration is managed through the RF generator (HexaGEN, Affera, Inc) in a temperature-controlled mode, aiming for a surface temperature of 73°C, using up to 80% to 90% of a maximum current of 3.7 A for 5 seconds.

With respect to PF energy, the Affera system delivers a proprietary biphasic PF waveform through a programmable generator module (HexaPULSE, Affera, Inc) from the entire lattice-tip. The PF waveforms consist of a train of microsecond-scaled non-electrocardiogram-synchronized pulses. For right atrial (RA) and left atrial (LA) ablation, a predefined optimal energy setting (PULSE3) is applied, delivering 12 trains of 1500 pulses, using 95% of the maximum current output limit over 4 seconds. Unlike RF mode, in which temperature feedback is used for power titration, the thermocouples do not play a role in PF energy modulation or titration. However, although PFA is considered a nonthermal ablation modality, it is known to cause a small rise in tissue temperature.[7] The temperature rise detected by the thermocouples surrounding the lattice sphere serves as a surrogate marker of real-time assessment of tissue contact.

Mapping system
The Affera system allows multielectrode electrogram acquisition for magnetic-based EAM (Prism-1, HexaMAP; Affera, Inc), using a magnetic sensor integrated within the lattice-tip. To enhance mapping precision, anatomy acquisition is performed during a predefined respiratory phase using respiratory gating. Both voltage and activation maps are created simultaneously with anatomical acquisition. During activation mapping, a real-time vector is displayed alongside the catheter to represent the direction of the activation wavefront.

For the left pulmonary vein (PVs) mapping, the system offers a specialized "vein mode" feature. This mode focuses on more precise delineation of the ridge between left atrial appendage (LAA) and PVs by creating a repeat three-dimensional map edited to emphasize the critical area.

Additionally, continuous tissue-contact monitoring is achieved through real-time impedance tracking, with electrodes that exhibit elevated local impedance highlighted on the system screen, providing instant feedback on electrode-tissue contact.

Workflow description

In addition to the settings traditionally followed for AF ablation, there are some specific procedural steps that warrant mention when using the Affera system.

In terms of patient preparation, general anesthesia combined with muscle relaxants is recommended to enhance stability and improve tissue-catheter engagement during PF applications. However, recent data indicates that ablation may also be performed under deep sedation utilizing intravenous agents such as propofol, midazolam, and fentanyl.[8] Concerning anticoagulation management, the activated clotting time (ACT) must exceed 300 seconds prior to the insertion of the Sphere9 catheter into the blood pool.

In clinical practice, circumferential lesions around the PVs can be created using either exclusively PF energy or a combination of RF and PF approaches. While early studies using the Affera system have demonstrated the efficacy of RF alone for PVI,[9,10] the use of PF energy for lesions in the posterior LA is recommended due to its superior safety profile. Conversely, either PF or RF energy may be utilized for ablation in other regions. However, if there is evidence of phrenic nerve capture when targeting the anterior region of the right veins, PF should be preferred due to its safer profile in avoiding phrenic nerve injury.

Finally, a center-to-center interlesion spacing of less than 6 mm for both PF and less than 7 mm for RF lesions is recommended, based on prior preclinical evaluations that demonstrated consistent lesion overlap.[11]

Illustrative examples of 2 PVI procedures performed with the Affera system, using either PF exclusively or a combined RF and PF approach, are displayed in **Fig. 1**, with lesion graphs for both energy types below each panel. **Fig. 2** presents an index PVI and posterior wall isolation procedure with Affera system, alongside the voltage map from the subsequent redo procedure.

Preclinical Data

Efficacy and efficiency in preclinical in vivo studies

The aforementioned characteristics of the Sphere9 catheter offer significant advantages in ensuring durable lesions when using both RF and PF energy.

Several studies have evaluated the durability of lesions created by the Affera system with RF energy, showing promising results. In swine atrial models, lesion line durability at 30 days ranged from 85.7% to 100%. Notably, this durability was significantly higher when compared to standard RF catheters, where lesion line durability was found to be less than 40%.[3,6,11]

Specifically, only 1 study[11] has assessed the efficacy of RF lesions created by the Affera system for PVI in a preclinical in vivo model (swine). The study reported first-pass isolation in all 6 PVs (4 right superior PV and 2 inferior common PV) using a 5-second RF application. The average number of lesions per vein was 16.3 ± 5.2, with a mean total RF time per vein of 81.3 ± 25.9 seconds. This represents a 50% reduction in lesion count and 92% decrease in RF time compared to conventional RF ablation using a 3.5 mm catheter. Four-week remapping confirmed durable isolation in all 6 veins.

The Affera RF energy delivery system is capable of producing significantly larger lesions with greater continuity along the ablation line, requiring fewer applications and shorter overall radiofrequency time compared to conventional RF catheters. This advantage is primarily due to its substantially larger surface area (approximately 275 mm^2), which is around 10 times larger than that of standard RF catheters (around 28 mm^2).[6]

Regarding efficacy and durability with PF energy, the Sphere9 lattice-tip catheter has demonstrated excellent results in achieving both acute and durable linear lesion block targeting various sites in both atria and at different PF doses.[12]

In relation to PVI, Koruth and colleagues[12] conducted a comparative preclinical in vivo study to assess low-dose versus high-dose PFA. Both groups achieved a 100% success rate in first-pass isolation of the PVs (6/6 veins in each group). During chronic reassessment (after 2–4 weeks), persistent isolation was observed in 83.3% (5/6 veins) in the low-dose group and 100% (6/6 veins) in the high-dose group. The reconnection observed in the low-dose group was localized, with a narrow gap affecting only 2 to 3 mini-electrodes, indicating a limited area of potential recurrence.

Fig. 3 provides an overview of the Affera system's acute and chronic efficacy for PVI in preclinical in vivo studies.

Macroscopic and histologic characteristics of lesions

Preclinical necropsy data from swine models demonstrated complete transmurality of RF lesions

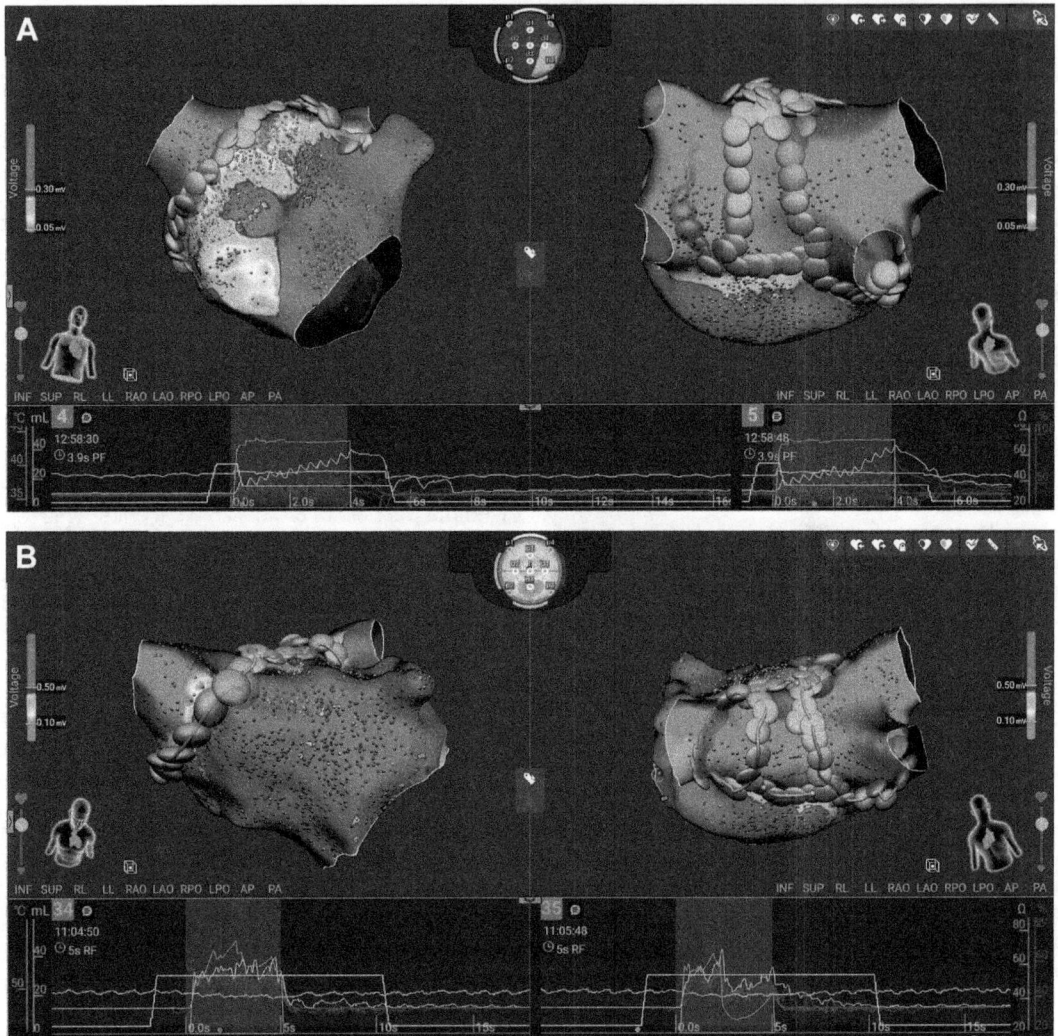

Fig. 1. PVI procedures performed with the Affera system. (A) PVI and posterior wall ablation performed exclusively with PF energy. PF lesion graph shows adequate temperature rise, indicating good contact and effective lesion formation. (B) Combined PVI approach with RF applied to the anterior PV region and PF to the posterior PV region and posterior wall. RF lesion graph displays temperature-controlled energy delivery.

delivered to various anatomical regions, including the PVs, posterior RA, cavotricuspid isthmus (CTI), and mitral isthmus (MI). Lesion depths measured at the MI and CTI were up to 2.3 ± 0.3 mm and 1.3 ± 0.2 mm, respectively.[11]

Additionally, gross necropsy of PF lesions delivered to the PVs demonstrated transmurality rates between 91% and 96%, depending on the PF settings used (low or high dose). The maximum depth of PF lesions ranged from 1.8 mm in PV ablations to over 3 mm when targeting the MI or posterior RA.[12]

Histological evaluation comparing PFA and radiofrequency ablation revealed that PF lesions were predominantly replaced by homogeneous fibrosis, which appeared relatively mature at as early as the 2-week time point. In contrast, RF lesions were characterized by extensive coagulative necrosis, accompanied by mild-to-moderate chronic inflammation, including lymphocytes, plasma cells, and occasional neutrophils and eosinophils. Additionally, multifocal areas of mild hemorrhage were observed in RF lesions, whereas these were minimal in PF lesions.[11–13]

Safety data

One of the primary concerns during AF ablation is the risk of inadvertently damaging adjacent structures and organs. To address this issue, a comprehensive investigation into potential injuries to these

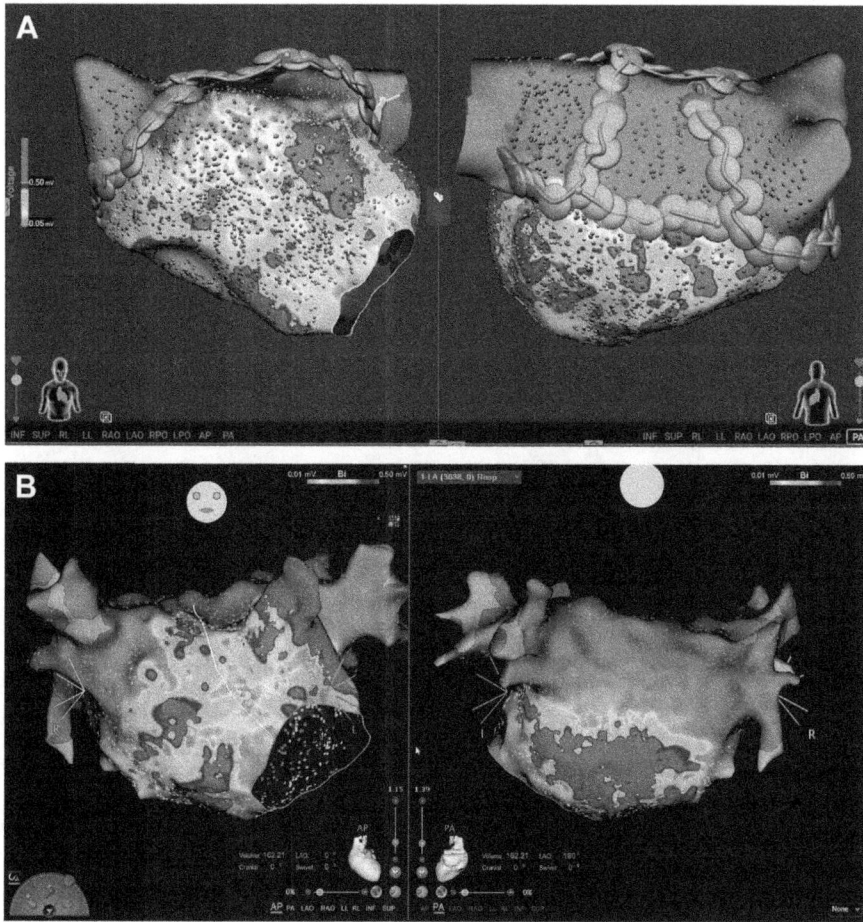

Fig. 2. Initial PVI procedure performed with the Affera system, and redo procedure using CARTO mapping system. (*A*) PVI and posterior wall ablation performed using PF energy. (*B*) Voltage map performed from the redo procedure 9 months later, showing durable PV and posterior wall isolation.

organs has been conducted in preclinical models using the lattice-tip catheter with various energy sources.

Following PVI and the creation of linear lesions in areas such as the posterior RA, CTI, and MI, no visible injury to the lungs or pericardium was observed in any of the studies, regardless of whether RF or PF energy was used. While phrenic nerve activation occurred during PF energy delivery, no subsequent damage was detected after either PF or RF ablation.[11,12]

Regarding the incidence of PV stenosis, there is extensive evidence supporting the virtual elimination of the risk of PV diameter reduction with the use of various PFA devices. In the case of the Affera system, no venous stenosis was observed with the use of PF energy in either the low-dose or high-dose cohorts in preclinical studies.[14–16]

Additionally, no esophageal injury was observed with either PF or RF energy during PV ablation in

in vivo swine models, even when a deviation balloon system was used to approximate the esophagus to the LA.[6,11,12] When PF energy was directly applied to the esophagus using the Affera system in these models, no macroscopic lesions were identified.[12] However, histologically, mild inflammation, edema, and focal necrosis were observed, although the epicardial fat overlying the PF lesions, along with arteries, veins, and nerves, were typically spared.[6] In contrast, direct RF application to the esophagus resulted in overt necrosis and hemorrhage, affecting the tissue from the superficial epithelium to the deep muscularis layer, including damage to nerves and vessels beyond the RF lesions.[11]

Finally, Koruth and colleagues[11] reported a single audible steam pop in a cohort of 5 swine models during RF energy delivery. This event was accompanied by a brief rise in impedance but did not result in cardiac perforation or char formation on the catheter tip.

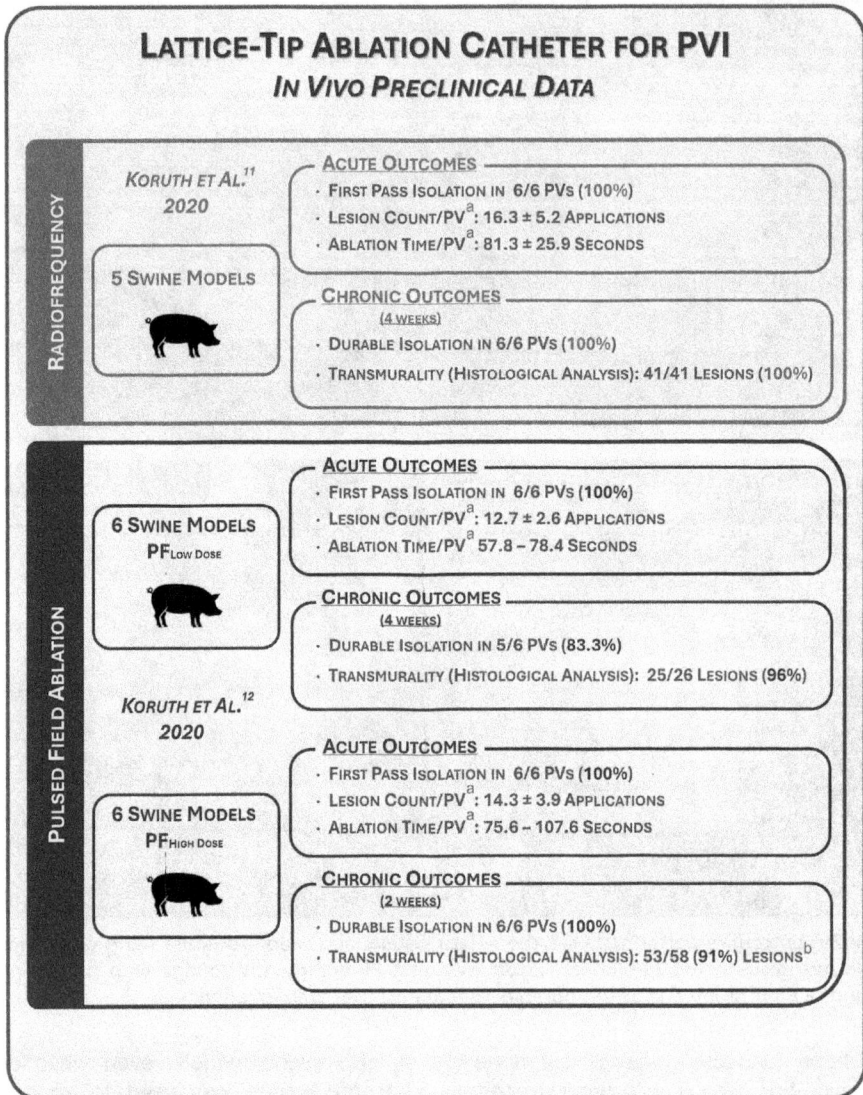

Fig. 3. Summary of the key characteristics and outcomes on acute and chronic efficacy for PVI of preclinical in vivo studies conducted with the Affera system. [a]Only data of right superior pulmonary vein is displayed. [b]Data of right superior vein was partially contaminated with PF and RF lesions on the left atrial roof.

Clinical Data on Pulmonary Vein Isolation Using the Affera System

Efficacy of pulmonary vein isolation and clinical outcomes

Early studies have demonstrated an excellent acute efficacy in both PVI and extra-PVI lesions, achieving success rates of approximately 99% when using either RF energy alone or a combination of RF and PF approaches for the anterior and posterior regions of the PVs.[3,12,17,18] Furthermore, a recent investigation by Reddy and colleagues[17] revealed that the Sphere-9 exhibited remarkable durability of lesions in a cohort of 178 patients with paroxysmal and persistent AF combining RF and PFA.

Following optimization of the PF waveform, the rate of isolation durability significantly increased from 51% with the initial waveform to 97% isolation durability at 3 months postprocedure using the optimized waveform. Similarly, Anter and colleagues[9] reported comparable results when PVI was approached exclusively using RF from the lattice-tip catheter, reaching 99.1% isolation durability at 3 months.

The isolation durability achieved with the Sphere9 catheter using the optimized PULSE3 waveform is comparable to that reported with other PFA systems, such as the pentaspline catheter (Farapulse, Boston Scientific, Marlborough, Massachusetts),[2] other focal PFA catheters

(CENTAURI, Galvanize Therapeutics Inc, San Carlos, California),[19] or the novel single-shot PFA catheter (Sphere-360, Medtronic, Inc).[20] These technologies consistently demonstrated durable PVI rates ranging from 84% to 99% on a per-vein basis.

Durability outcomes appear to be more favorable with PFA, compared to those achieved with other traditional ablation energy modalities, such as RF, cryothermal energy, and LASER ablation. In studies evaluating these energy sources, invasive remapping conducted several months after the initial procedure demonstrated durable PVI rates ranging from 76% to 91%.[21–26] This suggests that PFA may offer an at least similar long-term efficacy for maintaining vein isolation compared to the previous ablation techniques.

Long-term clinical efficacy

Several prospective studies have evaluated the clinical outcomes of PVI performed using the lattice-tip catheter over a 12-month follow-up period. In 1 study in which PVI using Affera system was exclusively performed using RF energy, Reddy and colleagues[10] reported a $94.4 \pm 3.2\%$ rate of freedom from any atrial arrhythmia at 12 month. More recently, the same group published data showing a 12-month atrial arrhythmia-free rate of $78.1 \pm 3.2\%$ when using either a combined RF and PF approach or PF exclusively. Importantly, there were no significant differences in outcomes between the RF/PF and PF-only subgroups, which showed $79.1 \pm 4.6\%$ and $77.3 \pm 4.3\%$ freedom from arrhythmias respectively.[17]

It should be noted that the higher rate of Holter monitoring compliance in the RF/PF and PF-only study (97.2%) compared to the RF-only study (66%) may account for some of the variations in the reported outcomes, as more consistent follow-up allows for a more accurate assessment of arrhythmia recurrence.

The 12-month efficacy outcomes achieved with the Affera system are once again comparable to those observed with other PFA technologies,[2] as well as with traditional ablation modalities.[1] This consistency in results highlights the effectiveness of the Affera system, positioning it as an alternative option for achieving durable arrhythmia control over the long term.

Real-world data have further validated the positive outcomes demonstrated in controlled studies. Tohoku and colleagues[8] reported on the acute and short-term follow-up results from a real-world cohort of 28 persistent AF patients, where PF energy was exclusively used for achieving PVI. The authors documented a 100% first-pass isolation

rate with no acute reconnections observed and low ablation times, consistent with previously reported data. Importantly, there were no critical procedural complications. In terms of clinical outcomes, the reported AF recurrence rate at 3 months was 15%.

Fig. 4 provides a comprehensive summary of all clinical studies on PVI using the Affera system. This includes both prospective cohort studies and real-world clinical data.

Recently, the results of the SPHERE PER-AF randomized multicenter clinical trial comparing the Affera system (employing a combined RF and PF approach) with traditional RF ablation techniques using a 3.5 mm irrigated, contact-force catheter have been published.[27] This study included a total of 400 patients with persistent AF. The primary effectiveness endpoint, which combined failure of acute isolation, recurrence of any atrial arrhythmia, repeated ablation, initiation or escalation of anti-arrhythmic drugs, or cardioversion over a 12-month follow-up, demonstrated noninferiority for the dual-energy catheter in treating persistent AF. Additionally, the safety endpoint, defined as the occurrence of procedure-related serious adverse events, also supported the noninferiority of the dual-energy approach. Notably, a secondary analysis revealed that the investigational device arm was associated with significantly shorter procedural times.

Fig. 5 illustrates the key characteristics and significant findings of this randomized trial.

Safety data

Several studies have investigated the incidence of silent cerebral events following PVI procedures using the Affera system, through postprocedural brain MRI examinations. Reported rates of silent cerebral events and lesions range between 14.6% and 15.7%.[17,18] Importantly, the authors noted that patients who developed cerebral lesions had significantly lower initial ACT compared to those without lesions (266 ± 41 seconds vs 335 ± 67 seconds). In fact, only 7.1% patients with initial ACT values above 300 seconds showed MRI-positive lesions.[18] This finding emphasizes the critical importance of achieving optimal anticoagulation levels, specifically maintaining an ACT above 300 seconds, before introducing the Sphere9 catheter into the LA to minimize the risk of silent cerebral events.

Concerning the change in the diameter of the PVs following PVI performed with the Affera system, clinical data corroborate the findings observed in preclinical studies and other investigations using other PF-based tools. Both EAM and CT scans have verified the absence of any

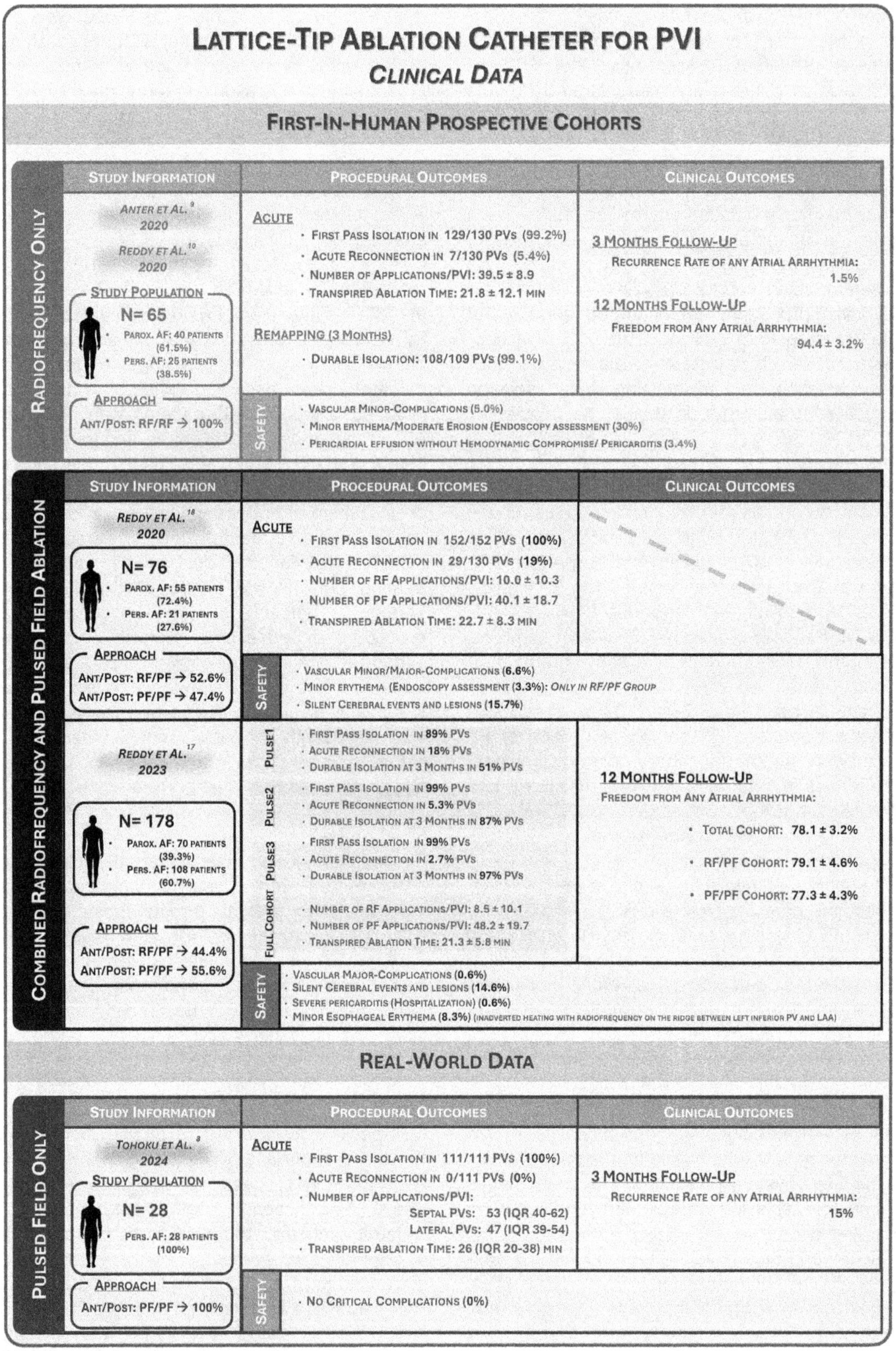

Fig. 4. Summary of the evidence from clinical studies reporting acute and long-term outcomes of PVI using the Affera system. ANT, anterior; POST, posterior.

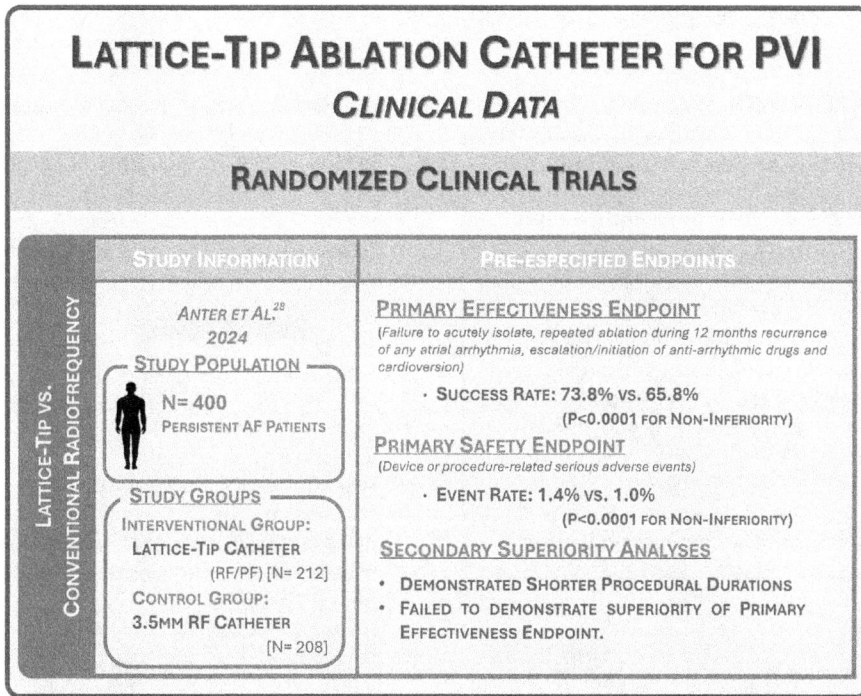

LATTICE-TIP ABLATION CATHETER FOR PVI
CLINICAL DATA

RANDOMIZED CLINICAL TRIALS

LATTICE-TIP VS. CONVENTIONAL RADIOFREQUENCY

STUDY INFORMATION	PRE-ESPECIFIED ENDPOINTS
ANTER ET AL.[28] 2024	**PRIMARY EFFECTIVENESS ENDPOINT** *(Failure to acutely isolate, repeated ablation during 12 months recurrence of any atrial arrhythmia, escalation/initiation of anti-arrhythmic drugs and cardioversion)*
STUDY POPULATION N= 400 PERSISTENT AF PATIENTS	• SUCCESS RATE: 73.8% VS. 65.8% (P<0.0001 FOR NON-INFERIORITY)
	PRIMARY SAFETY ENDPOINT *(Device or procedure-related serious adverse events)*
STUDY GROUPS INTERVENTIONAL GROUP: **LATTICE-TIP CATHETER** (RF/PF) [N= 212] CONTROL GROUP: **3.5MM RF CATHETER** [N= 208]	• EVENT RATE: 1.4% VS. 1.0% (P<0.0001 FOR NON-INFERIORITY) **SECONDARY SUPERIORITY ANALYSES** • DEMONSTRATED SHORTER PROCEDURAL DURATIONS • FAILED TO DEMONSTRATE SUPERIORITY OF PRIMARY EFFECTIVENESS ENDPOINT.

Fig. 5. Key features and summary of outcomes from the only randomized study comparing the Affera system to traditional RF ablation approach.

stenosis, even in instances where RF energy was partially employed for PVI, thereby supporting the safety profile of the system.[17,18]

Finally, concerning esophageal damage, it is known that low-level heating of the esophagus, typically in the range of 2° C to 3o C, can occur during PFA delivery of the posterior wall of the LA. However, it is important to note that no clinical consequences or esophageal lesions were observed in patient cohorts that underwent ablation using exclusively PF energy.[17] Notably, Reddy and colleagues documented cases of inadvertent heating of both the posterior LA and the esophagus while targeting the ridge between the LAA and the left inferior PV using RF energy. This unintended heating may be attributed to the bigger size or width of the lattice-tip catheter. Prior to recognizing this issue, the authors reported an occurrence rate of 8.3% for asymptomatic minor mucosal thermal injuries, a complication that was entirely eliminated when targeting this site exclusively with PF. Additionally, there was evidence indicating low-level heating associated with RF ablation of the anterior wall, resulting in a 3.3% incidence of minor erythema in the esophagus, which did not lead to any clinical consequences.[18]

Conversely, in studies where RF energy was the sole modality used to complete the PVI procedure, the incidence of minor and moderate thermal injuries to the esophagus significantly increased.[9] Remarkably, when RF was the exclusive energy source for PVI, including lesions delivered to the posterior regions of the PVs, endoscopic assessments revealed a notable prevalence of erythema and moderate erosion, with an overall occurrence rate of 30%. Specifically, 38% of patients experienced these complications following RF applications lasting 4 to 5 seconds, while 25% experienced them with shorter applications of up to 3.5 seconds. Although these injuries resolved completely within 2 weeks, this data emphasizes the need to carefully consider the benefits of PF over RF when addressing lesions in the posterior regions.

SUMMARY

In conclusion, the Affera system demonstrates a promising approach to PVI for AF, with clinical data supporting its efficacy and safety. The system exhibits comparable efficacy outcomes to traditional energy sources and other PFA systems while providing a superior safety profile over RF and cryoablation techniques. The versatility inherent to the focal catheter, combined with the efficiency advantages of a large footprint device, and the efficacy and safety profile of a PFA-based system, makes it a valuable tool for addressing AF catheter ablation.

CLINICS CARE POINTS

- The Affera system features a versatile catheter with a lattice-tip design, capable of mapping and delivering both RF and PF energy.
- This system combines the versatility of a focal catheter with the efficiency of a large footprint, enabling precise mapping and ablation across different atrial regions with fewer complications.
- Both preclinical and clinical studies reinforce the system's efficacy, safety, and procedural efficiency, positioning the Affera system as a reliable tool for addressing AF.
- However, clinical data on long-term efficacy and safety for this system remain limited.

DISCLOSURES

A. Sarkozy is a consultant for Biosense-Webster, Abbott, and Medtronic and received teaching compensation from Biosense Webster, Abbott, and Medtronic.

FUNDING

MCF is supported by a Juan Rodés postdoctoral fellowship from Carlos III Health Institute (JR24/00041).

REFERENCES

1. Della Rocca DG, Marcon L, Magnocavallo M, et al. Pulsed electric field, cryoballoon, and radiofrequency for paroxysmal atrial fibrillation ablation: a propensity score-matched comparison. Europace 2023;26(1):euae016.
2. Reddy VY, Dukkipati SR, Neuzil P, et al. Pulsed field ablation of paroxysmal atrial fibrillation: 1-year outcomes of IMPULSE, PEFCAT, and PEFCAT II. JACC Clin Electrophysiol 2021;7:614–27.
3. Yavin H, Shapira-Daniels A, Barkagan M, et al. Pulsed field ablation using a lattice electrode for focal energy delivery: biophysical characterization, lesion durability, and safety evaluation. Circ Arrhythm Electrophysiol 2020;13:e008580.
4. Shapira-Daniels A, Barkagan M, Yavin H, et al. Novel irrigated temperature-controlled lattice ablation catheter for ventricular ablation: a preclinical multimodality biophysical characterization. Circ Arrhythm Electrophysiol 2019;12:e007661.
5. Leshem E, Zilberman I, Barkagan M, et al. Temperature-controlled radiofrequency ablation using irrigated catheters: maximizing ventricular lesion dimensions while reducing steam-pop formation. JACC Clin Electrophysiol 2020;6:83–93.
6. Barkagan M, Leshem E, Rottmann M, et al. Expandable lattice electrode ablation catheter: a novel radiofrequency platform allowing high current at low density for rapid, titratable, and durable lesions. Circ Arrhythm Electrophysiol 2019;12:e007090.
7. Verma A, Asivatham SJ, Deneke T, et al. Primer on pulsed electrical field ablation: understanding the benefits and limitations. Circ Arrhythm Electrophysiol 2021;14:e010086.
8. Tohoku S, Bordignon S, Schaack D, et al. Initial real-world data on catheter ablation in patients with persistent atrial fibrillation using the novel lattice-tip focal pulsed-field ablation catheter. Europace 2024;26:euae129.
9. Anter E, Neužil P, Rackauskas G, et al. A lattice-tip temperature-controlled radiofrequency ablation catheter for wide thermal lesions: first-in-human experience with atrial fibrillation. JACC Clin Electrophysiol 2020;6:507–19.
10. Reddy VY, Neužil P, Peichl P, et al. A lattice-tip temperature-controlled radiofrequency ablation catheter: durability of pulmonary vein isolation and linear lesion block. JACC Clin Electrophysiol 2020;6:623–35.
11. Koruth JS, Kuroki K, Iwasawa J, et al. Feasibility, safety, and durability of porcine atrial ablation using a lattice-tip temperature-controlled radiofrequency ablation catheter. J Cardiovasc Electrophysiol 2020;31:1323–31.
12. Koruth JS, Kuroki K, Kawamura I, et al. Focal pulsed field ablation for pulmonary vein isolation and linear atrial lesions: a preclinical assessment of safety and durability. Circ Arrhythm Electrophysiol 2020;13:e008716.
13. Nakagawa H, Castellvi Q, Neal R, et al. Effects of contact force on lesion size during pulsed field catheter ablation: histochemical characterization of ventricular lesion boundaries. Circ Arrhythm Electrophysiol 2024;17.
14. Mansour M, Gerstenfeld EP, Patel C, et al. Pulmonary vein narrowing after pulsed field versus thermal ablation. Europace 2024;26:euae038.
15. Kuroki K, Whang W, Eggert C, et al. Ostial dimensional changes after pulmonary vein isolation: pulsed field ablation vs radiofrequency ablation. Heart Rhythm 2020;17:1528–35.
16. Yu F, Dong X, Ding L, et al. Pulsed field ablation for pulmonary vein isolation: preclinical safety and effectiveness of a novel hexaspline ablation catheter. J Cardiovasc Electrophysiol 2023;34:2195–202.
17. Reddy VY, Peichl P, Anter E, et al. A focal ablation catheter toggling between radiofrequency and pulsed field energy to treat atrial fibrillation. JACC Clin Electrophysiol 2023;9:1786–801.

18. Reddy VY, Anter E, Rackauskas G, et al. Lattice-tip focal ablation catheter that toggles between radiofrequency and pulsed field energy to treat atrial fibrillation: a first-in-human trial. Circ Arrhythm Electrophysiol 2020;13:e008718.

19. Anić A, Phlips T, Brešković T, et al. Pulsed field ablation using focal contact force-sensing catheters for treatment of atrial fibrillation: acute and 90-day invasive remapping results. Europace 2023;25:euad147.

20. Reddy VY, Anter E, Peichl P, et al. First-in-human clinical series of a novel conformable large-lattice pulsed field ablation catheter for pulmonary vein isolation. Europace 2024;26:euae090.

21. Iwasawa J, Koruth JS, Petru J, et al. Temperature-controlled radiofrequency ablation for pulmonary vein isolation in patients with atrial fibrillation. J Am Coll Cardiol 2017;70:542–53.

22. Galuszka OM, Baldinger SH, Servatius H, et al. Durability of CLOSE-guided pulmonary vein isolation in persistent atrial fibrillation: a prospective remapping study. JACC Clin Electrophysiol 2024;10:1090–100.

23. Hussein A, Das M, Riva S, et al. Use of ablation index-guided ablation results in high rates of durable pulmonary vein isolation and freedom from arrhythmia in persistent atrial fibrillation patients: the PRAISE study results. Circ Arrhythm Electrophysiol 2018;11:e006576.

24. Reddy VY, Sediva L, Petru J, et al. Durability of pulmonary vein isolation with cryoballoon ablation: results from the sustained PV isolation with arctic front advance (SUPIR) study. J Cardiovasc Electrophysiol 2015;26:493–500.

25. Miyazaki S, Taniguchi H, Hachiya H, et al. Quantitative analysis of the isolation area during the chronic phase after a 28-mm second-generation cryoballoon ablation demarcated by high-resolution electroanatomic mapping. Circ Arrhythm Electrophysiol 2016;9:e003879.

26. Dukkipati SR, Neuzil P, Kautzner J, et al. The durability of pulmonary vein isolation using the visually guided laser balloon catheter: multicenter results of pulmonary vein remapping studies. Heart Rhythm 2012;9:919–25.

27. Anter E, Mansour M, Nair DG, et al. Dual-energy lattice-tip ablation system for persistent atrial fibrillation: a randomized trial. Nat Med 2024. https://doi.org/10.1038/s41591-024-03022-6.

Safety, Effectiveness, and Clinical Workflow with a Balloon-Based Pulsed Field Ablation System
A Single-Center Experience

Monica Lo, MD, FHRS, FACC[a],*, Amber Miller, PhD[b], Kerri Leverence, BA[b]

KEYWORDS

- Pulsed field ablation • Clinical trial • Balloon-based catheter • Tissue proximity
- Paroxysmal atrial fibrillation • Persistent atrial fibrillation

KEY POINTS

- Balloon-based pulsed field ablation (PFA) catheter with tissue proximity and mapping integration has a quick learning curve for new users.
- Case series identifies procedural workflow for efficient translation of new PFA technology.
- Single-center, single operator experience demonstrates that the Volt PFA system is safe and effective for the treatment of paroxysmal atrial fibrillation and persistent atrial fibrillation.

INTRODUCTION

Cardiac ablation has been established as a beneficial therapy for the treatment of drug refractory paroxysmal or persistent atrial fibrillation (AF).[1] The use of pulsed field ablation (PFA) for cardiac ablation is being widely studied in the clinical setting due to the potential for improved safety profile and enhanced procedural efficiencies. The field of PFA for the treatment of AF has seen dramatic growth since the first feasibility studies were performed in humans less than 10 years ago, and first-generation PFA technologies are now becoming commercially available.[2–12] With the development of PFA, which utilizes a new ablation energy relative to the traditional thermal modalities such as radiofrequency (RF) and cryothermy, has come the opportunity to develop new and optimized ablation systems relative to traditional technologies. This includes the evaluation of new catheter form factors and procedural workflows. The translation of preclinical lessons with clinical study is critical during this time of substantial development and clinical trial. This review presents a single-operator experience with a novel form-factor PFA catheter during clinical study to demonstrate the translation of the PFA technology from its development, with preclinical learnings directly applied through physician training, to result in a safe and effective PFA solution that is easy to use and transition into the electrophysiology (EP) practice.

DEVICE TECHNOLOGY

The Volt PFA system (Abbott, USA) is a novel PFA solution currently under development and clinical study. The Volt PFA system is composed of the Volt PFA Catheter, Sensor Enabled, the Volt PFA Generator, Agilis NxT Steerable Introducer Dual-Reach, and EnSite X EP System EnSite Pulsed Field Ablation Module.

a Department of Electrophysiology, Arkansas Heart Hospital, 1701 South Shackleford Road, Little Rock, AR 72211, USA; b Abbott, 5050 Nathan Lane North, Plymouth, MN 55442, USA
* Corresponding author.
E-mail address: monica.lo@arheart.com

Card Electrophysiol Clin 17 (2025) 251–257
https://doi.org/10.1016/j.ccep.2025.02.012
1877-9182/25/© 2025 Elsevier Inc. All rights are reserved, including those for text and data mining, AI training, and similar technologies.

Abbreviations

3D	3 dimensional
AF	atrial fibrillation
CT	computerized topography
ICE	intracardiac echocardiography
LA	left atrium
LSPV	left superior pulmonary vein
PAF	paroxysmal atrial fibrillation
PersAF	persistent atrial fibrillation
PFA	pulsed field ablation
PV	pulmonary vein
RA	right atrium
RF	radiofrequency
RIPV	right inferior pulmonary vein
SL1	long transseptal sheath
TEE	transesophageal echo

The Volt PFA system is a fully integrated PFA solution that offers a unique and purpose-built catheter form factor and PFA generator with discreet therapeutic waveforms that integrate with the widely used EnSite X EP System to allow visualization of the catheter, tissue proximity feedback, and ablation location tracking. The Volt PFA Catheter Sensor Enabled is a 12.5 French, over the wire, balloon-in-basket bidirectional catheter. The balloon serves to insulate the interior of the 8 nitinol splines that have an active electrode region designed to deliver energy. Computational modeling was used during development and demonstrated the value of the balloon in driving energy delivery into the tissue and away from the blood pool.[13]

The balloon can also be filled with a saline/contrast mixture to allow visualization on fluoroscopy and intracardiac echocardiography (ICE). Along with the active electrodes, the catheter also has 3 magnetic sensors, 1 distal and 2 proximal to the basket, and 2 electrodes on the shaft that allow the catheter to be visualized on the EnSite X EP system.

The catheter connects to the Volt PFA Generator, which delivers PFA therapy and allows assessment of each electrode's proximity to cardiac tissue using the LivePoint display. Tissue proximity has been shown to be correlated with PFA lesion depth and, therefore, plays a critical role in lesion formation.[14] The system measures and displays dynamic tissue proximity based on changes in measured impedance relative to a baseline state. This dynamic measure of proximity is displayed on the generator and EnSite X mapping system in both a 2 dimensional and 3 dimensional (3D) displays that can assist in ensuring the desired positioning of the catheter prior to energy delivery. The PFA therapy is delivered as a bipolar biphasic pulsed electrical field through the active electrodes around the basket in sequential electrode pairs using R-wave gated pulse trains per therapy application. Baseline therapy consists of 2 applications of a nominal waveform or 3 applications of a low-voltage waveform developed for locations where phrenic nerve capture cannot be avoided. Additional applications beyond baseline have proven to be effective in creating safe, durable lesions when variation in pulmonary vein (PV) anatomy or challenges in positioning the catheter coaxial to the targeted vein are encountered.[15]

The lessons learned during preclinical testing of the system were used to inform the general procedural workflow with the Volt PFA system for clinical study. While clinical study protocol dictates specifics related to investigational system use and procedural workflow, many aspects are left to operator discretion. From the VOLT-AF IDE study (NCT06223789), which included 38 enrolling sites, the following discussion summarizes the general procedural workflow, including clinical study-specific requirements, procedural characteristics, and clinical outcomes from a single site and single operator experience to provide insight into the clinical translation and adoption of the Volt PFA system.

CLINICAL CASE SERIES
Procedural Workflow

A preprocedural computerized topography (CT) scan for each patient was acquired to help identify patient anatomy, vein branching, and evaluate procedural strategy ahead of time. General anesthesia was used for all procedures. Transesophageal echo (TEE) was performed at the start of the procedure to exclude the presence of thrombus and evaluate the baseline pericardial effusion status. The TEE probe was left in place to help with transseptal puncture if needed. Ultrasound guidance was used to gain vascular access and preclosure with Perclose was done for the access site due to the large bore sheath. An ICE and a coronary sinus catheter were placed. A multipolar mapping catheter (HD Grid, Abbott, USA) was advanced into the right atrium (RA) to the superior vena cava to assess the phrenic nerve. Per the study protocol, high output pacing stimulation was delivered through the multipolar mapping catheter to map the phrenic nerve location and mark it on the mapping system for assistance with postprocedure testing. Transseptal puncture was then performed using a long transseptal sheath (SL1) and transeptal (BRK XS, Abbott, USA) needle under ICE guidance. The multipolar mapping catheter was inserted into the left atrium (LA) and a preablation voltage map was acquired.

The SL1 sheath was exchanged for the investigational Agilis sheath. Due to the larger size, 13 F, the large bore sheath was aspirated and connected to a continuous flow pressure bag with heparinized saline. The Volt catheter was placed over the wire into the LA. The wire was connected to the EnSite X system to help visualize the distal tip of the wire within the heart on the electroanatomical map. Baseline impedance was acquired by maneuvering the Volt catheter splines in and out of contact with tissue to activate the LivePoint feature of the generator to detect tissue proximity. The Volt catheter was navigated to the left superior PV using a combination of the EnSite X system, fluoroscopy, LivePoint tissue proximity feedback, and ICE (**Fig. 1**). Once the Volt catheter location was confirmed to be aligned to the vein and in contact, the generator was used to deliver therapy with a baseline therapy of 2 nominal applications. Once a therapy has been completed, the EnSite X system will display AutoMarks to represent delivered treatment colored to correspond with tissue proximity feedback. For the second and any subsequent applications of the therapy, the Volt catheter was rotated so the splines were positioned in-between the previous lesions. This rotation is clearly visualized with the AutoMark lesion placement after each therapy delivery (see **Fig. 1**). With optimal coaxial position of the Volt catheter and optimal electrode tissue proximity,

the baseline therapy can be sufficient for treatment of the vein. However, in instances where suboptimal positioning was observed, such as indicated by tissue proximity, additional applications were delivered (**Fig. 2**). At this investigational site, additional applications were also delivered at physician's discretion to ensure durable PV isolation and not transient tissue stunning was achieved.

When moving to subsequent veins, the Volt catheter was deflated and retracted into the Agilis, making sure it was back far enough to not interfere with the curve deflection of the Agilis. A combination of the deflection of the Agilis and advancing of the guidewire was used to gain access to the other veins. Once guidewire access was achieved, the Volt catheter was advanced and inflated. For the right PVs, every new position required pacing around each bipole pair of the Volt catheter to assess for phrenic nerve capture per clinical protocol. If phrenic nerve capture was observed and repositioning was not able to avoid capture, the therapy was switched to the low-voltage setting, which requires a baseline treatment of 3 applications with rotation to offset spline location after each treatment. Ablation was performed to target electrical isolation of the PVs. After all PVs had been treated with the Volt catheter, the catheter was exchanged for the HD Grid catheter. A postablation voltage map was created, and electrical isolation was confirmed using the HD Grid catheter

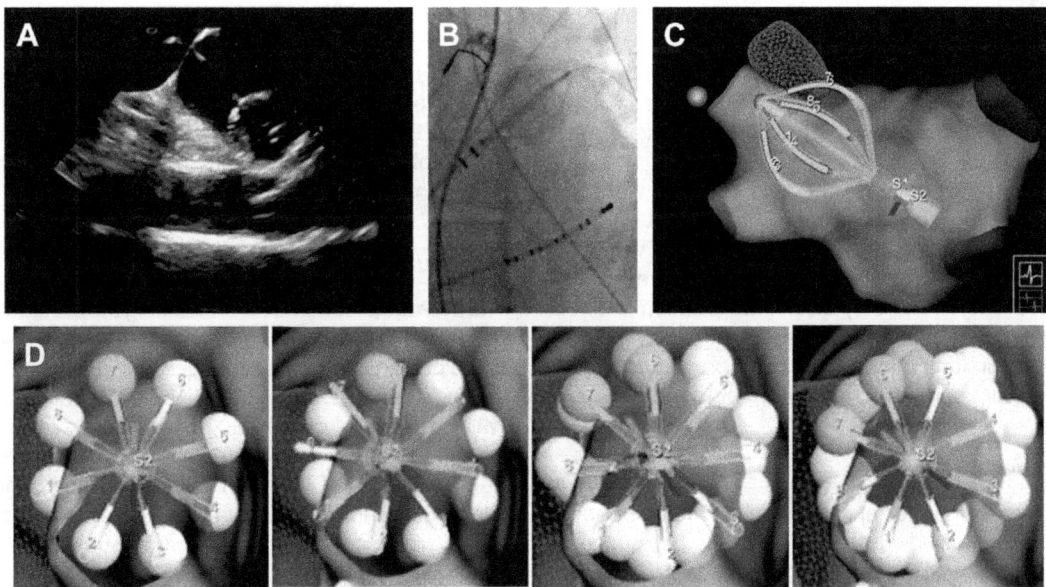

Fig. 1. Volt PFA catheter visualization on (*A*) intracardiac echocardiography, (*B*) fluoroscopy, and (*C*) 3D rendering via electroanatomical mapping system integration. (*D*) Mapping system integration allows visualization of electrode placement prior to ablation and therapy delivery via AutoMarks after therapy delivery. AutoMarks, colored to correspond with LivePoint assessed tissue proximity, allow visualization of catheter rotation for placement of subsequent therapy to achieve circumferential lesions.

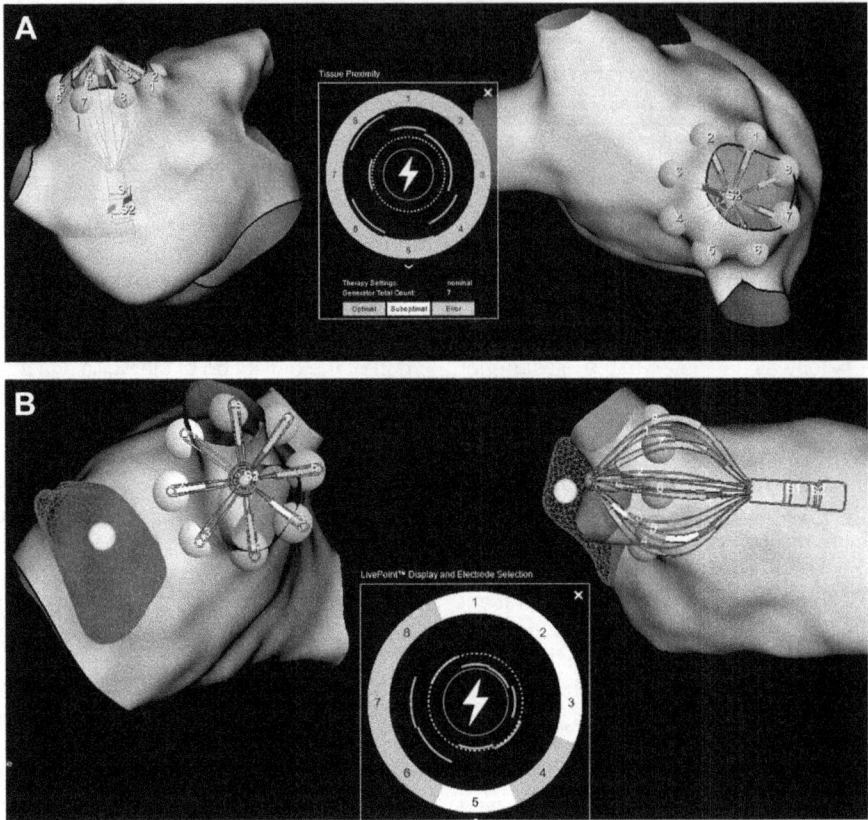

Fig. 2. Examples of (*A*) optimal coaxial alignment and (*B*) suboptimal catheter placement guided by electroanatomical mapping visualization and tissue proximity. The yellow dot marks the distal end of the guidewire used to assist in positioning of the catheter.

after a 20 minute wait period. In the event that isolation was not confirmed after the 20 minute wait, the Volt catheter was reinserted, and additional applications were delivered to achieve electrical isolation.

Additional ablations beyond the PVs were not allowed using the investigational system, and additional ablations with other devices were not allowed in the LA without constituting an effectiveness failure. The only additional ablation allowed was the treatment of cavo-tricuspid isthmus-dependent right atrial flutter that presented during the procedure using a market-approved device.

Subject Population

A single operator at the Arkansas Heart Hospital enrolled 47 subjects in the VOLT-AF IDE study between April 2024 and September 2024. This subset of subjects consisted of symptomatic, drug refractory paroxysmal atrial fibrillation (PAF; 55.3%, n = 26) and persistent atrial fibrillation (PersAF; 44.7%, n = 21) subjects indicated for de novo pulmonary vein isolation (PVI) ablation.

The subset population was 68.1% male (n = 32) with an average age of 62.6 ± 11.3 years. Baseline demographics and medical history are summarized in **Table 1**. All subjects have completed their index ablation procedure with the Volt PFA system and 12 month follow-up is ongoing.

Procedure Characteristics

The average procedure time, including the protocol-mandated pre-ablation and post-ablation phrenic nerve pacing and voltage mapping and a 20 minute waiting period, was 106.4 ± 21.1 minutes, with an average of 51.0 ± 23.1 minutes ablation catheter left atrial dwell time, 41.5 ± 14.8 minutes between first and last PFA therapy delivery, and 11.3 ± 5.1 minutes of fluoroscopy. The total number of PFA applications delivered per subject was 18.2 ± 3.1 applications. The breakdown of the total PFA applications per vein was 4.2 ± 1.2 in the left superior pulmonary vein (LSPV), 4.0 ± 0.9 in the left inferior pulmonary vein, 4.9 ± 1.2 in the right superior pulmonary vein, and 5.0 ± 1.0 in the right inferior pulmonary vein (RIPV). There were no

Table 1
Baseline demographics and medical history

Patient Characteristic	(N = 47)
Age (years)	62.6 ± 11.3
Sex (male)	68.1% (32)
Body mass index (kg/m²)	30.2 ± 5.0
Race	
White	97.9% (46)
Asian	2.1% (1)
CHA$_2$DS$_2$Vasc score	2.4 ± 1.4
LVEF (%)	55.9 ± 5.3
LA diameter (mm)	37.1 ± 6.9
Cardiovascular History	
Heart failure NYHA class I	4.3% (2)
Heart failure NYHA class II	8.5% (4)
Coronary artery disease	14.9% (7)
Diabetes	29.8% (14)
Heart failure	8.5% (47)
Hypertension	80.9% (47)
Myocardial infarction	4.3% (47)
Obstructive sleep apnea	4.3% (47)
Pulmonary disease	2.1% (47)
Stroke	2.1% (47)
Transient ischemic attack	2.1% (47)
Structural heart disease	8.5% (47)

Values are reported as mean ± SD or % (n).
Abbreviation: NYHA, New Your Heart Association.

ablations completed beyond the PVs for the subjects treated at this site. Phrenic nerve function via pacing and the absence of pericardial effusion via ICE was confirmed in all subjects at the end of the procedure.

Safety and Effectiveness

Safety and acute effectiveness have been assessed for all subjects. Comparison of preablation and postablation voltage maps demonstrates the isolation of PVs achieved at the end of the procedure (**Fig. 3**). Acute isolation, defined as the ability to isolate the targeted PVs using only the Volt PFA catheter for ablation as assessed by confirmation of electrical isolation via entrance block at a minimum after a minimum waiting period of 20 minutes, was achieved in 99.5% of treated veins (191 out of 192) in 97.9% of subjects (46 out of 47), where one LSPV in one subject was unable to be isolated after delivery of the maximum allowed 8 applications per vein specified in the clinical protocol. Mapping demonstrated that the PV connection was likely epicardial in origin. There

have been no repeat procedures in any subjects at this time, and long-term follow-up is ongoing.

The rate of subjects experiencing a primary safety endpoint event, defined as the rate of subjects experiencing a device and/or procedure-related serious adverse event with onset within 7 days of any ablation procedure (index or repeat procedure) that uses the Volt PFA system, was 2.1% (1 out of 47). One subject experienced pericarditis 3 days following the ablation procedure. One other serious adverse event was observed in this group of subjects, a new supraventricular tachycardia in a subject treated for PersAF. There were no deaths, stroke, coronary artery spasm, hemolysis, phrenic nerve damage, or other serious adverse events reported in these subjects.

Key Takeaways

When using this new PFA system, preprocedural CTs were found to be very helpful in reviewing the patient's anatomy prior to the procedure to help assess and plan for treatment of each vein, providing insight into the size of the veins, determining early branching, and planning the approach and placement of the Volt PFA catheter based on that branching.

There are many different techniques to maneuver the Volt system within the LA. At Arkansas Heart Hospital, the steerable sheath was primarily used for maneuvering with the wire accessing the veins, followed by delivery of the Volt catheter over the wire. Other investigators with early Volt PFA system experience have noted maneuvering the Volt PFA catheter using its bidirectional functionality while retracting the sheath back into the RA as a successful workflow to access the PVs. The system allows for the user to maneuver the Volt PFA system safely and effectively with their own preferred technique.

Use of a guidewire can be beneficial for maneuvering into the PVs. Two different 0.35 j-tip guidewires were used for these procedures (Merit (Merit Medical, USA) and Abbott Guide Right (Abbott, USA). The guidewire was connected to the EnSite X mapping system for visualization and used as a guide for maneuvering the catheter. Visualization of the guidewire by connecting to the mapping system helped to reduce fluoroscopy, to identify which PV and its branch the guidewire was accessing, and to confirm the stability and location of the Volt catheter.

During the first cases using the ablation catheter, additional focus was placed on ensuring the transeptal access puncture was low and anterior on the fossa ovalis to help access the RIPV. After the initial learning curve associated with becoming

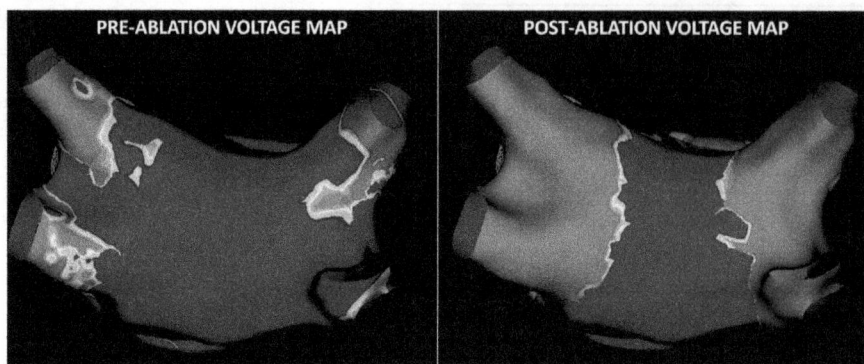

Fig. 3. Example of pre-ablation and post-ablation voltage maps demonstrating pulmonary vein isolation achieved after ablation with the Volt PFA system.

familiar with a new ablation technology and understanding how the sheath and ablation catheter interact, the transseptal access location was not as critical to help deliver the Volt catheter into the RIPV.

Lesion durability is a key factor in PFA therapy. The LivePoint tissue proximity display was critical to help understand the electrode interface with the tissue and was used in determining applications needed per vein. With coaxial placement of the Volt catheter in the vein and optimal circumferential contact (see **Fig. 2**), fewer applications were needed, resulting in a lesion application range closer to the baseline of 2 applications (typically 3–4). In the event of less-than-ideal contact and/or non-coaxial catheter placement, more treatments were delivered (typically 5–6) to ensure PV isolation.

Learning Curve From Radiofrequency to Single-Shot User

The single operator that performed these procedures at Arkansas Heart Hospital has over a decade of point-by-point RF ablation experience, currently using TactiFlex SE (Abbott, USA) as the preferred catheter for atrial fibrillation ablations. Switching from a point-by-point RF ablation to a single-shot PFA strategy was not difficult. The initial learning curve to overcome workflow changes, familiarize oneself with the Volt PFA catheter, and feel confident in the EnSite X mapping integration and location of the catheter was about 5 cases. Comfort managing the large-bore sheath was readily obtained given the similarity in managing large-bore sheaths with left atrial appendage closure and leadless pacemaker devices.

As a high-volume ablationist, effectiveness and efficiency of atrial fibrillation ablation using RF have already been achieved. In fact, the fluoroscopy time was increased with this initial PFA

experience. However, with PFA, concerns with esophageal temperature monitoring, PV stenosis, and phrenic nerve injury were eliminated. Often, the rate-limiting step for a safe, successful RF ablation is the wait time for the esophageal temperature to normalize before coming on ablation again. PFA offers a good solution to this issue.

Additionally, when good balloon-to-tissue proximity and contact (blue indication on LivePoint) is achieved, multiple applications or "insurance" lesions do not necessarily need to be applied to achieve durable isolation. PV potentials and electrograms disappear instantaneously. To ensure durability, up to 8 applications could be applied per vein. Initially, the strategy was to apply "insurance" lesions to make sure PV isolation was achieved at postablation mapping. However, through more experience with the catheter, as long as there was good coaxial alignment and tissue proximity, fewer applications actually led to shorter LA dwell time and potentially less pericardial irritation. Fluoroscopy time could also be further reduced or eliminated with improved confidence in the projection of the catheter onto the EnSite X geometry.

SUMMARY

The PFA technology is quickly being adopted into the field of electrophysiology due to the potential safety and efficiency benefits beyond traditional and well-established thermal ablation modalities. The case series presented here demonstrates a single operators' first experience with a novel PFA system. The clinical workflow and clinical study were designed to integrate lessons learned during preclinical development, such as the importance of the balloon to insulate electrodes and the blood pool while driving energy into the tissue, the importance of tissue proximity during energy delivery, and the role of coaxial positioning in achieving durable isolation. The learning curve for this new PFA technology was short due to similarities in the catheter ablation workflow, system features such as catheter form-factor, steering and guide-wire maneuverability, mapping integration, and tissue proximity. As demonstrated in this case series, the efficient adoption of this technology is safe and effective for the treatment of symptomatic drug refractory PAF and PersAF with minimal adverse events and high acute success.

CLINICS CARE POINTS

- Knowledge of tissue proximity was important in coaxial positioning of the PFA catheter and determination of therapy applications needed.
- The balloon-based PFA catheter can be maneuvered safely and effectively with an operator's preferred technique, which can include the use of preprocedural CTs, location of transeptal puncture, use of the steerable sheath, catheter steering, and guidewire placement.
- The use of this PFA system can be readily adopted into clinical practice with a short learning curve due to similarities in cardiac ablation workflow and compatibility with the use of electroanatomical mapping, fluoroscopy, and ICE.

DISCLOSURE

Dr M. Lo has served as a consultant, on advisory boards, and as a speaker for Abbott. A. Miller and K. Leverence are employed by Abbott. The VOLT-AF IDE Study is sponsored by Abbott.

REFERENCES

1. Tzeis S, Gerstenfeld EP, Kalman J, et al. European heart rhythm association/heart rhythm society/asia pacific heart rhythm society/Latin American heart rhythm society expert consensus statement on catheter and surgical ablation of atrial fibrillation. Heart Rhythm 2024;21(9):e31–149.
2. Anic A, Phlips T, Brešković T, et al. Pulsed field ablation using focal contact force-sensing catheters for treatment of atrial fibrillation: acute and 90-day invasive remapping results. Europace 2023;25(6).
3. De Potter T, Reddy V, Neuzil P, et al. Acute safety and performance outcomes from the inspIRE trial using a novel pulsed field ablation system for the treatment of paroxysmal atrial fibrillation. Eur Heart J 2021;42(Suppl_1). ehab724.0380.
4. Duytschaever M, De Potter T, Grimaldi M, et al. Paroxysmal atrial fibrillation ablation using a novel variable-loop biphasic pulsed field ablation catheter integrated with a 3-dimensional mapping system: 1-year outcomes of the multicenter inspIRE Study. Circ Arrhythm Electrophysiol 2023;16(3):e011780.
5. Reddy VY, Anic A, Koruth J, et al. Pulsed field ablation in patients with persistent atrial fibrillation. J Am Coll Cardiol 2020;76(9):1068–80.
6. Reddy VY, Anter E, Rackauskas G, et al. Lattice-tip focal ablation catheter that toggles between radiofrequency and pulsed field energy to treat atrial fibrillation. Circulation 2020;13(6).
7. Reddy VY, Dukkipati SR, Neuzil P, et al. Pulsed field ablation of paroxysmal atrial fibrillation: 1-year outcomes of IMPULSE, PEFCAT, and PEFCAT II. JACC Clin Electrophysiol 2021;7(5):614–27.
8. Reddy VY, Peichl P, Anter E, et al. A focal ablation catheter toggling between radiofrequency and pulsed field energy to treat atrial fibrillation. JACC Clin Electrophysiol 2023;9(8 Pt 3):1786–801.
9. Verma A, Boersma L, Haines DE, et al. First-in-human experience and acute procedural outcomes using a novel pulsed field ablation system: the PULSED AF Pilot Trial. Circ Arrhythm Electrophysiol 2022;15(1):e010168.
10. Verma A, Haines DE, Boersma LV, et al. Pulsed field ablation for the treatment of atrial fibrillation: PULSED AF pivotal trial. Circulation 2023;147(19):1422–32.
11. Turagam MK, Neuzil P, Petru J, et al. PV isolation using a spherical array PFA catheter: application repetition and lesion durability (PULSE-EU Study). JACC Clin Electrophysiol 2023;9(5):638–48.
12. Sanders P, Healy S, Emami M, et al. Initial clinical experience with the balloon-in-basket pulsed field ablation system: acute results of the VOLT CE mark feasibility study. Europace 2024;26(5).
13. Belalcazar A. Safety and efficacy aspects of pulsed field ablation catheters as a function of electrode proximity to blood and energy delivery method. Heart Rhythm O2 2021;2(6Part A):560–9.
14. Mittal L, Miller M, Fish J. PO-04-119 Impact of tissue contact impedance monitoring on pulsed field ablation lesion profile. Heart Rhythm 2024;21(5):S429–30.
15. Sundaram S, Nguyen JT, Friedman DJ, et al. PO-06-130 Chronic safety and efficacy of a novel balloon basket PFA catheter in a canine model with multi-level dosing. Heart Rhythm 2024;21(5):S633.

The VARIPULSE Pulsed Field Ablation Platform

Reshma Amin, MD, Mattias Duytschaever, MD, PhD*

KEYWORDS

- Pulsed field ablation • Variable loop circular catheter • Irreversible electroporation
- Pulmonary vein isolation • Atrial fibrillation

KEY POINTS

- The VARIPULSE pulsed field ablation (PFA) platform, by combining the benefits of mapping and pulsed field energy, is an emerging platform for AF ablation.
- Low rates of atrial arrhythmia recurrence have been demonstrated using the VARIPULSE PFA system for pulmonary vein isolation in patients with paroxysmal atrial fibrillation ablation.
- Safety profile is positive with no evidence of phrenic nerve, esophageal, or pulmonary vein injury found with use of the VARIPULSE system in either preclinical or clinical trials.

INTRODUCTION

Pulsed field ablation (PFA) is an emerging, nonthermal approach for AF ablation and more specifically pulmonary vein isolation (PVI). A novel PFA system, including a variable loop circular catheter (VLCC) integrated with a 3D mapping system, was developed to combine the benefits of PFA energy together with the advantage of electro-anatomical mapping.

THE VARIPULSE PULSED FIELD ABLATION SYSTEM

The VARIPULSE platform (Biosense Webster) includes the VARIPULSE Catheter, the TRUPULSE Generator, and the CARTO 3 Mapping System VARIPULSE Service Pack Software. The VARIPULSE Catheter (Fig. 1), is an 8.5 Fr bidirectional catheter with a variable (25 mm–35 mm) circular array of 10 3 mm-electrodes and 3 magnetic, single axis sensors.[1] The generator allows the delivery of biphasic PFA pulses (1800 V) in a bipolar configuration between skipped electrodes and between each of the adjacent electrodes between them. Nominal dosing is 1 ablation comprised of applications (250 ms, 10 s-time delay between applications) at each position (4 positions per vein). Integrated mapping allows real-time, nonfluoroscopic visualization and 3D lesion creation.

PRECLINICAL DATA

Multiple preclinical studies in porcine models have shown that the chosen waveform and catheter design, together with mapping leads, precisely deliver effective and durable atrial lesions without collateral injury.

Yavin and colleagues[2] assessed the performance of the VARIPULSE system in a right atrial line model, targeting linear block between the superior vena cava (SVC) and the inferior vena cava (IVC) (Fig. 2). In all but 1 animal where contact during ablation was challenging, PFA led to acute and chronic block (at 28 ± 3 days). In 6 animals, PFA was delivered close to the esophagus and phrenic nerve without evidence of collateral injury.

Hsu and colleagues assessed the performance of the VARIPULSE system in a left atrial pulmonary vein (PV) model, targeting PVI.[3] Multiple ablations (at supratherapeutic doses) were performed, including sites at nontherapeutic sites such as the right inferior PV lumen, right superior PV ostium, and adjacent to the esophagus and

Department of Electrophysiology, AZ Sint-Jan Hospital, Ruddershove 10, 8000 Brugge, Belgium
* Corresponding author.
E-mail address: Mattias.Duytschaever@azsintjan.be

Card Electrophysiol Clin 17 (2025) 259–265
https://doi.org/10.1016/j.ccep.2025.02.013
1877-9182/25/© 2025 Elsevier Inc. All rights are reserved, including those for text and data mining, AI training, and similar technologies.

Abbreviations	
AF	atrial fibrillation
CE	Conformite Europeenne
IVC	inferior vena cava
LA	left atrium
PAF	paroxysmal AF
PFA	Pulsed field ablation
PU	Polyurethane
PV	pulmonary vein
PVI	pulmonary vein isolation
RA	right atrium
RF	radiofrequency
SVC	superior vena cava
VLCC	variable loop circular catheter

phrenic nerve. PV narrowing was not observed acutely nor at follow-up. No injury was seen grossly or histologically in adjacent structures. All PVs were durably isolated, confirmed by bidirectional block at a remap procedure 30 days later.

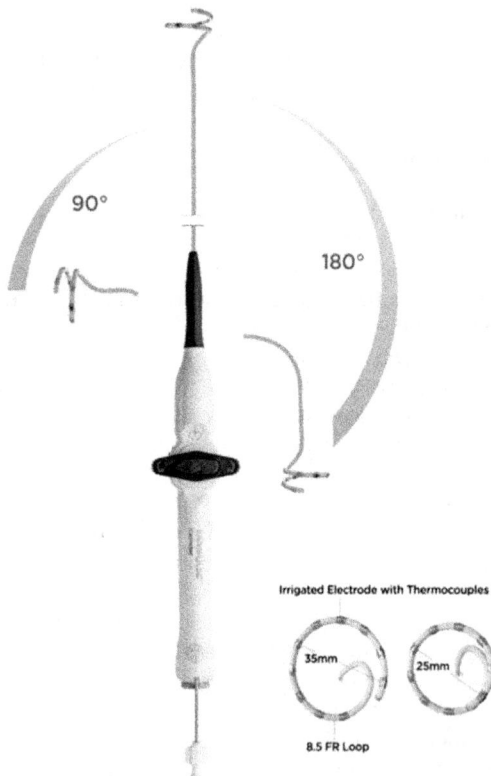

Fig. 1. The VARIPULSE variable loop catheter. The variable loop has a contraction range of 25 mm–35 mm, though it may deflect even further in the blood pool. The shaft has a bidirectional D-curve deflection. (*Reproduced from* Nair DG, Gomez T, De Potter T. VARIPULSE: A step-by-step guide to pulmonary vein isolation. J Cardiovasc Electrophysiol 2024;35(9):1817–27. https://doi.org/10.1111/jce.16366 under the CC BY license: https://creativecommons.org/licenses/by/4.0/.)

Histological examination showed complete, transmural necrosis around the circumference of the ablated PVs.[3] Similar results were observed by Grimaldi and colleagues[4] who performed PVI and SVC isolation with additional stacked applications in the left atrium (LA) roof and right atrium (RA) posterior wall, with successful acute ablation at all target sites in all animals and 100% lesion durability both at 7 and 30 days.

A further preclinical study in the left atrial model aimed to establish a dose response relationship to guide clinical study designs.[5] The animals were divided into 4 study groups; PFA at low dose (per vein 4 locations, per location 1 application, ie, 4 applications per PV); PFA at nominal dose (per vein 4 locations, per location 3 applications, ie, 12 applications per PV); PFA at high dose (per vein 4 locations, per location 6 applications, ie, 24 applications per PV). The fourth group underwent radiofrequency (RF) ablation (35 W or 50 W, $\leq$60 s). At 1-month, durable PVI was observed in 83.3% of RF animals whereas all animals that underwent PFA demonstrated chronic PVI. In the low dose PFA group, however, transmural lesions in regions outside the PV were observed less frequently (66% in the LA roof and posterior wall, LA appendage, and mitral annulus).

THE VARIPULSE-PULSED FIELD ABLATION SYSTEM FOR PULMONARY VEIN ISOLATION IN PAROXYSMAL ATRIAL FIBRILLATION: THE inspIRE STUDY

The InspIRE trial was a prospective, multicenter single-arm study aiming to evaluate the safety and efficacy of the VARIPULSE platform.[6,7] The study enrolled 226 patients with symptomatic, drug-resistant paroxysmal AF (PAF) in 13 centers across Europe and Canada. PFA applications were applied in a standardized manner with at least 12 applications per PV. The study was organized in 2 main phases. Wave I focused on assessing the system's initial safety and efficacy through extensive imaging (n= 40). Wave II, the pivotal phase, aimed to evaluate safety and efficacy over 1 year based on predetermined performance criteria (n=186). Results were described by Duytschaever[6] and De Potter[7] and colleagues. The PFA system resulted in isolation in 97.1% of veins. There were no primary adverse events in either phase (**Fig. 3**).[6] Additionally, there were no cases of esophageal injury, PV stenosis, or permanent phrenic nerve damage. Early detection of silent cerebral lesions in some patients during Wave I led to workflow modifications, such as a 10 second pause between PFA applications and minimizing catheter exchanges.

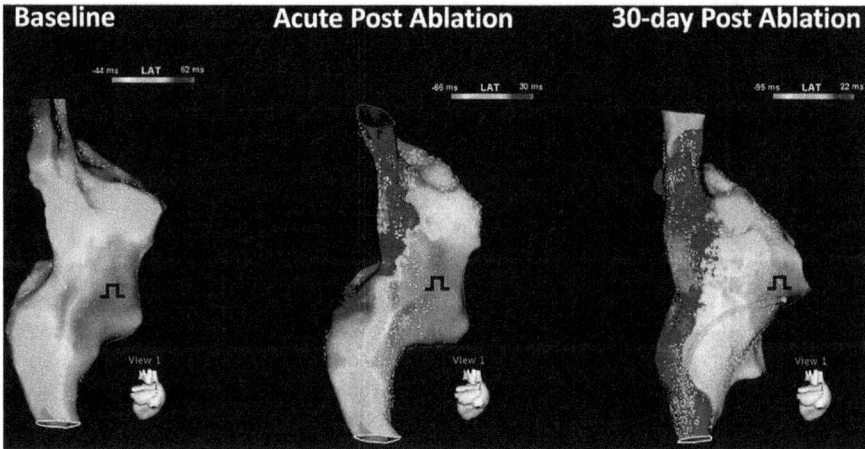

Fig. 2. The VARIPULSE platform in a preclinical right atrial line model. Feasibility and Durability of Right Atrial ablation line. The experimental model included a baseline activation map of the right atrium during pacing from the tricuspid annulus (*left*). PFA was then performed along the posterior wall from the SVC to the IVC. The presence or absence of activation line of block was examined by repeat mapping of the chamber during pacing from a similar location, immediately (*middle*) and 30-days (*right*) after ablation with the presence of a durable block noted. (*Reproduced from* Yavin H, Brem E, Zilberman I, et al. Circular Multielectrode Pulsed Field Ablation Catheter Lasso Pulsed Field Ablation. Circ Arrhythm Electrophysiol 2021;14(2). https://doi.org/10.1161/CIRCEP.120.009229.)

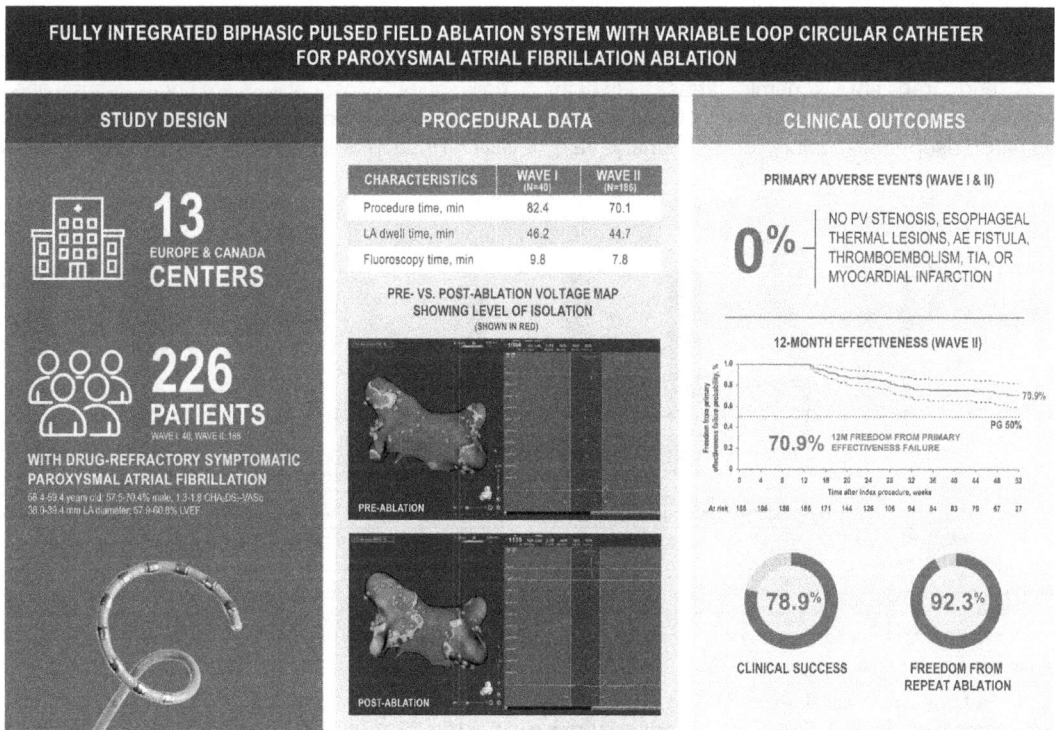

Fig. 3. The inspIRE study in PAF. No adverse events in the InspIRE study. (*Reproduced from* Duytschaever, De Potter, Grimaldi et al. Paroxysmal AF Ablation Using a Novel Variable-Loop Biphasic Ablation Catheter Integrated with a 3D Mapping system: 1-Year Outcomes of the Multicenter inspIRE study. Circ Arrhythm Electrophysiol. 2023; 16(3). https://doi.org/10.1161/CIRCEP.122.011780 under the CC BY license: https://creativecommons.org/licenses/by/4.0/.)

Freedom from any atrial arrhythmia recurrence at the 12-month mark was 75.6%.[7] Freedom from any recurrence as if would be obtained by standard clinical monitoring (without the trial's extensive protocol-driven rhythm monitoring) was estimated to be 85.8%. Efficacy was found comparable to recently published multicenter studies for PFA (**Fig. 4**).[7] Patients who received at least 12 PFA applications (4 ablations) per PV had a success rate of 79.2% at 12 months, compared to 57.1% in those who received fewer applications.

A total of 14 patients underwent repeat ablation. PV reconnections were noted in 37 of 51 veins (72.5%). Procedural efficiency was another notable result, with the average procedure time being 70.1 minutes, left atrial dwell time of 44.7 minutes, and minimal fluoroscopy time of 7.8 minutes.

THE VARIPULSE-PULSED FIELD ABLATION SYSTEM FOR PULMONARY VEIN ISOLATION IN PAROXYSMAL ATRIAL FIBRILLATION: THE admIRE STUDY

The admIRE trial was another prospective, multicenter single-arm study aiming to evaluate the safety and efficacy of the VARIPULSE-PFA system.[8] The study enrolled 277 patients with drug refractory PAF across 30 centers in the United States. Primary adverse event rate was 2.9%, primarily due to events such as pericardial tamponade and transient ischemic attacks (which resolved without lasting effects). Notably, no cases of esophageal injury or pulmonary vein

stenosis were observed, reinforcing the safety benefits of nonthermal ablation.

PVI was achieved in 100% of patients, with a first-pass isolation rate of 97.5% in targeted veins. At 12 months, with extensive protocol-driven rhythm monitoring, 75.4% of patients were free from any recurrence. Additionally, 91% of patients were free from repeat ablation during the follow-up period. Procedurally, the median PVI time was approximately 81 minutes, with zero or minimal fluoroscopy exposure in nearly a quarter of cases, highlighting the system's efficiency and low radiation requirements.

Quality-of-life assessments indicated significant improvement by 3 months, with scores sustained over 12 months. Cardiovascular-related hospitalizations and antiarrhythmic drug use both dropped sharply over the follow-up period, reflecting the clinical and lifestyle benefits of PFA in managing PAF.

Both the inspIRE and admIRE studies suggest that VLCC-PFA is a safe, effective, and patient-centered approach to treating PAF. Both studies were limited by the lack of a control group and protocol-mandated repeat evaluation at 3 months.

PROPOSED WORKFLOW FOR THE VARIPULSE PULSED FIELD ABLATION SYSTEM

The workflow was previously described by Nair and colleagues.[1] Most patients are under general anesthesia with a deep sedation protocol as an alternative.[9] Heparin is administered with anticoagulation

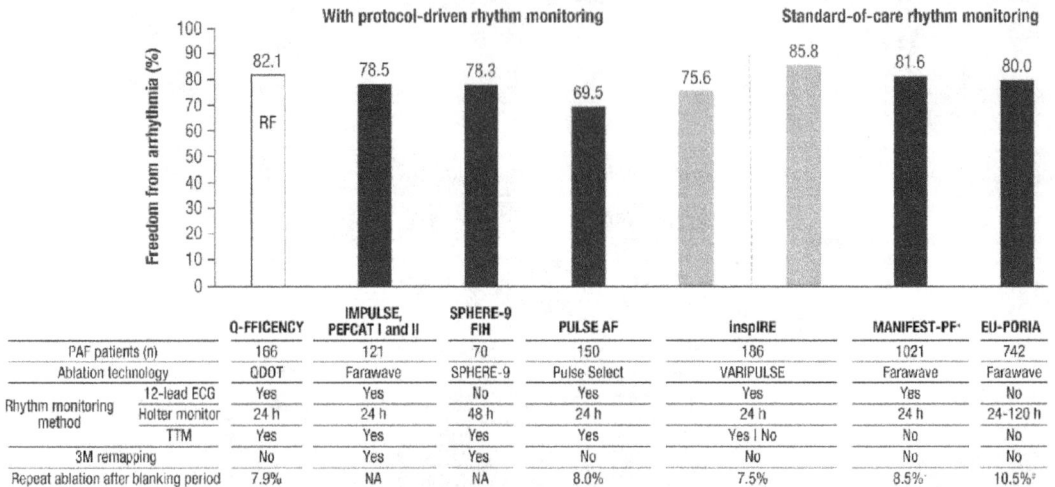

	Q-FFICENCY	IMPULSE, PEFCAT I and II	SPHERE-9 FIH	PULSE AF	inspIRE	MANIFEST-PF⁺	EU-PORIA
PAF patients (n)	166	121	70	150	186	1021	742
Ablation technology	QDOT	Farawave	SPHERE-9	Pulse Select	VARIPULSE	Farawave	Farawave
Rhythm monitoring method — 12-lead ECG	Yes	Yes	No	Yes	Yes	Yes	No
Rhythm monitoring method — Holter monitor	24 h	24 h	48 h	24 h	24 h	24 h	24-120 h
Rhythm monitoring method — TTM	Yes	Yes	Yes	Yes	Yes I No	No	No
3M remapping	No	Yes	Yes	No	No	No	No
Repeat ablation after blanking period	7.9%	NA	NA	8.0%	7.5%	8.5%	10.5%‡

Fig. 4. Freedom from atrial arrhythmia at 1 year in paroxysmal AF patients reported among recently published multicenter study for PFA. Freedom from any recurrence in the InspIRE study is comparable to recently published multicenter PFA studies. ‡ EU-PORIA repeat procedure rate calculated based on a study manuscript reporting 87 repeat ablations among 742 patients with PAF. (*Reproduced from* De Potter T, Grimaldi M, Duytschaever M, et al. Predictors of Success for Pulmonary Vein Isolation With Pulsed-field Ablation Using a Variable-loop Catheter With 3D Mapping Integration: Complete 12-month Outcomes From inspIRE. Circ Arrhythm Electrophysiol. 2024;17(5). https://doi.org/10.1161/CIRCEP.123.012667 under the CC BY license: https://creativecommons.org/licenses/by/4.0/.)

maintained at high levels (activated clotting time >350 s). After transseptal access, roving the VLCC creates a 3D electro-anatomical map of the LA and PVs. Due to the combination of mapping and size variability, the system can adapt to unique anatomical challenges, such as common ostia, middle veins, narrow posterior walls, and wide carinas.

Once positioned at the LA-PV junction with stable tissue contact (based upon the CARTO 3 Tissue Proximity Indication feature), ablation is performed with both closed and open loop configuration (**Fig. 5**).[1] Per standard, 12 PFA applications (4 ablations) per vein are given: 3 applications at each of 4 positions (ostial 1, ostial 2, antral 1, antral 2). Following ablation, entrance and exit block testing confirm PV isolation, and any remaining gaps are identified and treated through CARTO 3 mapping.

Initial experience with the mapping system (especially if combined with intracardiac echocardiography) indicates minimized fluoroscopy use.

Future optimizations may include indicators to streamline contact and ablation site selection, further refining its usability.

APPROVALS

In January 2024, the VARIPULSE platform received its first regulatory approval from the Japan Ministry of Health, Labor and Welfare for the treatment of symptomatic drug refractory recurrent PAF using PFA. In the US, the VARIPULSE Catheter and TRUPULSE Generator are currently investigational and are not approved by regulatory authorities. In Europe, the TRUPULSE generator received Conformite Europeenne (CE) mark in late 2023. The VARIPULSE Catheter received CE mark on FEBRUARY 28, 2024.

There was a voluntary recall of specific lots of the VLCC. The company found that a polymer used to bind the catheter electrodes to the catheter (Polyurethane, PU) had overrun the electrodes which

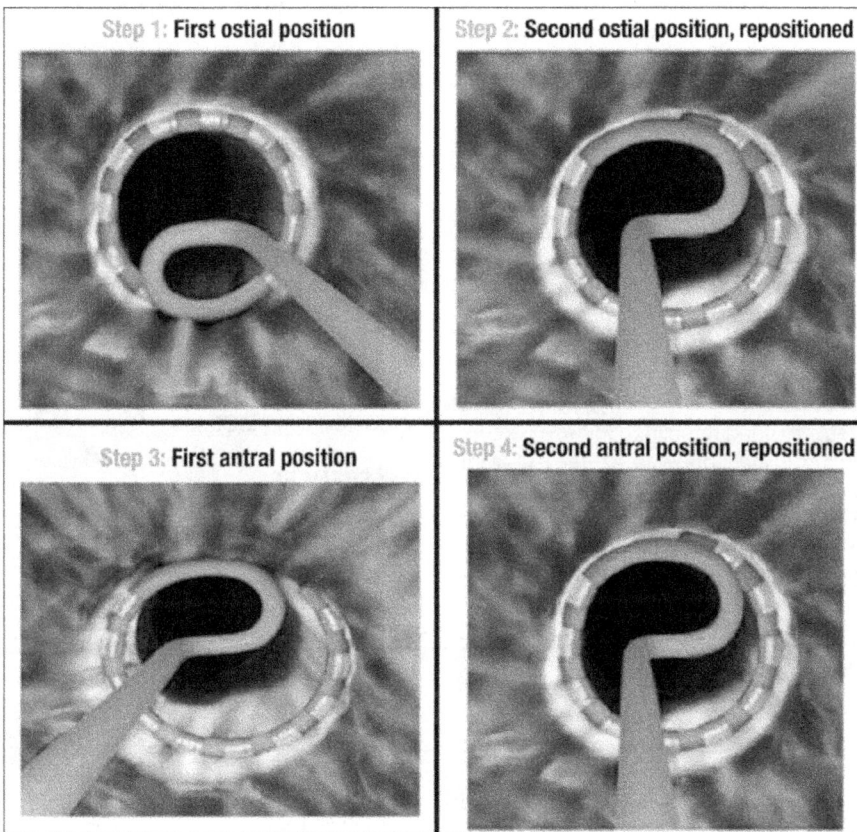

Fig. 5. Proposed workflow for PVI. The PVI workflow is performed in 4 steps. (1) Perform an ostial (closed loop) ablation. (2) Reposition the catheter to make a second ostial (closed loop) ablation. (3) Pull the catheter back, open the contraction, and reposition at an antral (open loop) position for a third ablation. Lastly, (4) make a final antral (open loop) ablation. (*Reproduced from* Nair DG, Gomez T, De Potter T. VARIPULSE: A step-by-step guide to pulmonary vein isolation. J Cardiovasc Electrophysiol 2024;35(9):1817–27. https://doi.org/10.1111/jce.16366 under the CC BY license: https://creativecommons.org/licenses/by/4.0/.)

has the potential to result in blocked irrigation holes, reduction in electrode surface area or PU extension beyond the electrode outside diameter, all leading to an increased risk of microbubbles and embolic events. VLCC sales resumed shortly after the recall upon resolution of the manufacturing issue.

THE VARIPULSE-PULSED FIELD ABLATION SYSTEM BEYOND PULMONARY VEIN ISOLATION AND PAROXYSMAL ATRIAL FIBRILLATION: ONGOING STUDIES

Because of the integrated mapping and the versatility of the catheter, the system might be appropriate for delivery of pulsed field energy outside the PVs, like the posterior wall, mitral isthmus or any other patient-specific target. The VIRTUE (Investigational Device Exemption [IDE]) study by Vivek Reddy and colleagues is a nonrandomized single center study which aims to assess safety and efficacy of the system to perform patient-specific AF/AT ablation in 150 patients with PAF, persistent AF, and atrial tachycardia. The POLARIS (IDE) trial is a prospective, nonrandomized study across 4 centers, led by Moussa Mansour and colleagues which aims to assess the safety and efficacy of the system to perform PVI and posterior wall isolation in 360 patients with paroxysmal and persistent AF. The SAFFICIENT trial, spearheaded by the Texas Cardiac Arrhythmia Research Foundation, is a multicenter, nonrandomized prospective study. It aims to recruit 2276 patients with both paroxysmal and persistent AF and is designed to compare the incidence of safety and efficacy of the system to perform PVI and posterior wall isolation in low volume (<100/y) compared to high volume (≥100/y) centers. The aFIRE trial is a multicenter registry conducted in 6 Chinese centers and will recruit 120 patients with AF for PVI, roof line, and posterior wall isolation. VARIPURE was recently initiated as a substudy of the SECURE Registry, a multicenter postmarket follow-up study. Over 15 European sites from more than 10 active countries initiated enrolling patients treated with the VARIPULSE platform as part of standard-of-care practice.

REAL WORLD DATA

To date, over 1700 cases using the VARIPULSE platform have been performed worldwide. No cases of esophageal injury, pulmonary vein stenosis, or phrenic nerve injury have been reported.

SUMMARY

As an emerging PFA system, the VARIPULSE platform shows considerable potential to become a standard approach in PVI for AF management. Its selective, low-risk ablation provides a compelling alternative to RF and cryoablation. Future studies are expected to further confirm its role in real-world settings, while upcoming modifications could enhance lesion durability and minimize recurrence, advancing the standard of care in AF ablation.

CLINICS CARE POINTS

- Use of the VARIPULSE platform has been found to be safe and feasible in the RA and LA in animal models.
- Preclinical data demonstrates that the VARIPULSE platform creates durable atrial lesions for PVI and other sites within the LA and RA.
- The VARIPULSE platform has been found to be safe and effective for PVI in patients with PAF.
- In patients who have undergone PVI for PAF with the VARIPULSE platform, there are low rates of atrial arrhythmia recurrence.
- There have been no cases of esophageal injury, phrenic nerve injury, or pulmonary vein stenosis with use of the VARIPULSE platform in clinical trials to date.

DISCLOSURES

R. Amin does not have any financial disclosures. M. Duytschaever has served on the speaker's bureau, is a consultant for Biosense Webster, Inc, and has received research support from Biosense Webster, United States.

REFERENCES

1. Nair DG, Gomez T, De Potter T. VARIPULSE: a step-by-step guide to pulmonary vein isolation. J Cardiovasc Electrophysiol 2024;35(9):1817–27.
2. Yavin H, Brem E, Zilberman I, et al. Circular multielectrode pulsed field ablation catheter lasso pulsed field ablation. Circ Arrhythm Electrophysiol 2021;14(2). https://doi.org/10.1161/CIRCEP.120.009229.
3. Hsu JC, Gibson D, Banker R, et al. In vivo porcine characterization of atrial lesion safety and efficacy utilizing a circular pulsed-field ablation catheter including assessment of collateral damage to adjacent tissue in supratherapeutic ablation applications. J Cardiovasc Electrophysiol 2022;33(7):1480–8.
4. Grimaldi M, Di Monaco A, Gomez T, et al. Time course of irreversible electroporation lesion development through short- and long-term follow-up in pulsed-field ablation–treated hearts. Circ Arrhythm

Electrophysiol 2022;15(7). https://doi.org/10.1161/CIRCEP.121.010661.

5. Hsu JC, Banker RS, Gibson DN, et al. Comprehensive dose–response study of pulsed field ablation using a circular catheter compared with radiofrequency ablation for pulmonary vein isolation: a preclinical study. Heart Rhythm O2 2023;4(10):662–7.

6. Duytschaever M, De Potter T, Grimaldi M, et al. Paroxysmal atrial fibrillation ablation using a novel variable-loop biphasic pulsed field ablation catheter integrated with a 3-dimensional mapping system: 1-year outcomes of the multicenter inspIRE Study. Circ Arrhythm Electrophysiol 2023;16(3). https://doi.org/10.1161/CIRCEP.122.011780.

7. De Potter T, Grimaldi M, Duytschaever M, et al. Predictors of success for pulmonary vein isolation with pulsed-field ablation using a variable-loop catheter with 3D mapping integration: complete 12-month outcomes from inspIRE. Circ Arrhythm Electrophysiol 2024;17(5). https://doi.org/10.1161/CIRCEP.123.012667.

8. Reddy VY, Calkins H, Mansour M, et al. Pulsed field ablation to treat paroxysmal atrial fibrillation: safety and effectiveness in the AdmIRE pivotal trial. Circulation 2024;150(15):1174–86.

9. Grimaldi M, Quadrini F, Caporusso N, et al. Deep sedation protocol during atrial fibrillation ablation using a novel variable-loop biphasic pulsed field ablation catheter. Europace 2023;25(9). https://doi.org/10.1093/europace/euad222.

Catheters and Tools with Pulsed Field Ablation
Pentaspline Farawave

Connor P. Oates, MD, Mohit K. Turagam, MD, FHRS*

KEYWORDS

• Pulsed field ablation • Farawave • Pentaspline catheter • Atrial fibrillation • Atrial flutter

KEY POINTS

- The Farawave pentaspline pulsed field ablation (PFA) catheter utilizes pulsed electrical fields to treat atrial fibrillation (AF), offering a reduced risk of complications such as esophageal injury, phrenic nerve paralysis, and pulmonary vein stenosis compared to thermal ablation.
- In treating paroxysmal AF, the Farawave pentaspline PFA catheter is noninferior to thermal ablation in the risk of 12-month recurrence of atrial arrhythmias when treating paroxysmal atrial fibrillation.
- Ongoing research is exploring the Farawave pentaspline PFA catheter for treating both atrial and ventricular arrhythmias.

INTRODUCTION

Over the past 2 decades, catheter ablation has become a standard therapy for atrial and ventricular arrhythmias. However, the safety and efficacy of these procedures have been limited by the energy sources used. Radiofrequency ablation and cryoablation, two well-established thermal energy techniques, not only target atrial or ventricular myocardium but also affect surrounding tissues, such as the esophagus, coronary arteries, and phrenic nerves. Additionally, the effectiveness of thermal energy ablation depends on prolonged catheter stability to create adequate lesions. Pulsed field ablation (PFA) technology is disrupting the treatment paradigms of catheter ablation.

One of the first commercially available PFA catheters is the Farawave pentaspline PFA catheter (Boston Scientific, Marlborough, MA). This device is a 12 F, over the wire, ablation catheter with 5 splines, each containing 4 electrodes per spline. These electrodes allow for pacing, recording of electrograms, and PFA. The pulse field itself is a bipolar, biphasic electrical pulse with programmable field strength from 1.8 kV to 2.0 kV applied over 2.5 seconds. The pentaspline catheter's unique design enables operators to deliver energy in different patterns (**Fig. 1**). These shapes include a "flower" (with splines spread at 90-degree angle from the catheter), the "basket" (forming a flattened, ovoid shape), and the "olive" (a rounded ball). The device is available in 31 mm and 35 mm sizes, referring to the diameter of the pentaspline catheter in the "flower" configuration, and is used exclusively with a steerable sheath.

The pentaspline catheter is designed for circumferential contact within the antrum of the pulmonary veins (PV). To perform pulmonary vein isolation (PVI), the catheter is first placed at the ostium of each PV in a basket configuration, and 2 sets of PFA treatments are administered. The catheter is then rotated to deliver 2 additional treatments in the same conformation to ensure full coverage. The catheter is then switched to a flower configuration, and 2 additional treatments are applied, followed by rotation and treatment with at least 2 additional pulses of PFA. Additional

Department of Cardiology, Helmsley Electrophysiology Center, Icahn School of Medicine at Mount Sinai, 1190 5th Avenue 1 South, New York, NY 10129, USA
* Corresponding author.
E-mail address: mohit.turagam@mountsinai.org

Card Electrophysiol Clin 17 (2025) 267–272
https://doi.org/10.1016/j.ccep.2025.02.014

Abbreviations	
AF	atrial fibrillation
HF	heart failure
$HF_{MR/rEF}$	heart failure with reduced or moderately reduced ejection fraction
HFpEF	heart failure with preserved ejection fraction
PFA	pulsed field ablation
PV	pulmonary veins
PVI	pulmonary vein isolation

treatments in various configurations can be performed at the operator's discretion and the PV anatomy.

PRECLINICAL ASSESSMENT OF THE FARAWAVE CATHETER

Preclinical studies have examined the cellular effects of PFA using the Farawave pentaspline catheter. When applied to the myocardium, this catheter creates discrete histologic lesions with sparing of extracardiac and connective tissues.[1] Unlike the thermal ablation lesions, PFA lesions do not continue to propagate over time. The duration needed for lesion creation depends solely on the time required to generate and deliver the pulsed electric field. While contact force is important for optimizing tissue penetration by the electrical field, it is not required for prolonged lesion formation.[2,3]

Notably, several preclinical studies have demonstrated that specific pulse characteristics

of PFA selectively targets myocardial tissue while minimizing risk of pulmonary vein stenosis, esophageal injury, and phrenic nerve paralysis. Preclinical models demonstrated that the use of the contemporary Farawave catheter in the PVs results in no significant PV stenosis.[4,5] Additionally, direct application of pulsed fields to the myocardium adjacent to the esophagus, as well as to the esophagus itself, has also demonstrated sparing of esophageal tissue.[6] These findings are starkly different from injuries that can occur during indiscriminate ablation with thermal energy.

SAFETY OF PULSED FIELD ABLATION WITH FARAWAVE IN THE ATRIA

In-vivo data from the Farawave catheter supports the preclinical findings that PFA has minimal effects on the esophagus and phrenic nerve compared to thermal ablation. In the ADVENT trial, which compared thermal ablation to PFA, PFA was associated with significantly less narrowing (−0.9% vs −12%, posterior probability >0.999) of the PVs.[7] A study by Cochet and colleagues used MRI before and after ablation to assess esophageal and phrenic nerve injury in patients treated with either PFA using the Farawave catheter or thermal ablation.[8] No esophageal injury or phrenic nerve injury were observed in the PFA group. Additionally, in the "real world" postapproval MANIFEST-PF (n=1758) and MANIFEST-17K (n=17,642) studies, no cases of esophageal injury, symptomatic PV stenosis or persistent phrenic nerve injury were reported.[9,10]

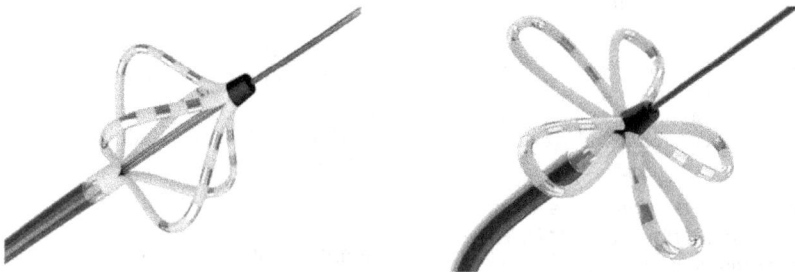

Study	Year of Publication	# Patients PFA	Type of Atrial Fibrillation	Follow-Up	12-Month Recurrence
Reddy et al: IMPULSE, PEFCAT, PEFCAT II Trials	2021	121	Paroxysmal	12 months	21.5%
Reddy et al: ADVENT Trial	2023	305	Paroxysmal	12 months	17.2%
Turagam et al: MANIFEST-PF Registry	2023	1,568	Paroxysmal (65%)/ persistent (35%)	12 months	21.9%
Kueffer et al; EU-PORIA Registry	2024	1,184	Paroxysmal (62%)/ persistent (38%)	12 months	26.0%

Fig. 1. Pulse field ablation using Farapulse catheter.

Other procedural complications, both major and minor, were comparable to those reported for contemporary thermal ablation: cardiac tamponade occurred in 1.0% of cases after PFA versus 0.8% after thermal ablation, stroke or TIA in 0.5% versus 0.4%, and vascular complications in 3.3% versus 1.4%.[9,11]

The effects of PFA on the coronary arteries are another key consideration. In a preclinical swine model, direct application of PFA to the coronary arteries using the Farawave catheter resulted in acute narrowing that resolved within 30 minutes, consistent with coronary vasospasm.[12] Over 80% of all treated arteries showed mild stenosis with neointimal hyperplasia and tunica media fibrosis after 4-weeks of survival. Histopathological analysis revealed that the lesions surround the coronary arteries and extend a few millimeters into the myocardium. These findings are similar to those seen in a swine model treated with radiofrequency ablation.[13]

During the initial clinical experience with PFA of the cavotricuspid isthmus using the Farawave catheter, subclinical coronary artery vasospasm was observed with ablation adjacent to coronary arteries.[14] The same authors identified that vasospasm was ameliorated with nitroglycerin. Ablation of the cavotricuspid isthmus using PFA has been noted to provoke moderate to severe angiographic vasospasm of the right coronary artery in up to 80% of patients.[15] Malyshev and colleagues found that episodes of vasospasm during ablation of the cavotricuspid isthmus were best minimized with multiple nitroglycerin (3 mg–2 mg every 2 minutes) boluses followed by an infusion strategy (1 mg/min).[15] Similar coronary artery vasospasm has also been identified angiographically during PFA of the postero-lateral mitral isthmus (7 of 17 patients, 41.2%), especially when mitral isthmus is situated superiorly (7 of 9 patients, 77.8%), a complication not typically observed with radiofrequency.[16] However, a small study showed that PFA-induced vasospasm does not result in new coronary stenosis, based on coronary angiogram performed at least 6 months after PFA.[15]

Overall, the incidence of coronary artery spasm is low, occurring at 0.14% (24 of 17,642 patients) as demonstrated in the MANIFEST-17K registry. The majority of these cases were proximity-related spasms, with 84% (21 of 24 cases) requiring intracoronary nitroglycerine for resolution.[9]

There is also growing evidence that PFA using the Farawave catheter affects the autonomic nervous system differently than thermal ablation. Parasympathetic innervation, which plays a key role in atrial fibrillation (AF) initiation and maintenance, can be affected during ablation.[17] Changes in baseline heart rates following ablation have been attributed to be evidence that ablation has had an effect on the autonomic nervous system that innervates the atria through the ganglionated plexi. Early feasibility studies comparing PFA using the Farawave catheter, radiofrequency ablation, and cryoablation showed that PFA had minimal effects on baseline heart rates, while thermal ablation was linked to increased heart rates due to reduced parasympathetic innervation of the ganglionated plexi.[18,19] In the ADVENT trial, patients treated with thermal ablation had significantly greater increases in mean heart rate compared to those treated with PFA.[20]

Lastly, hemolysis has been identified as a rare but notable complication of PFA with using the Farawave catheter. Ekanem and colleagues reported 5 cases (0.03%) of hemolysis-induced renal failure in an observational registry of 17,000 patients undergoing PFA.[9] Niles and colleagues identified a linear correlation between the number of PFA treatments and the occurrence of hemolysis, which is more likely when the PFA catheter is floating in the blood pool rather than being in direct contact with the myocardium.[21] Importantly, hemolysis has also been found to be more frequent in patients treated with PFA (with >70 PFA lesion) compared to those undergoing radiofrequency ablation.[22]

EFFICACY OF PULSED FIELD ABLATION WITH FARAWAVE FOR ATRIAL FIBRILLATION

IMPULSE, PEFCAT, and PEFCAT II demonstrated that PFA using the Farawave catheter is a safe and effective method for isolating the PV in patients with paroxysmal AF.[23,24] When using the Farawave catheter to perform PVI with an optimized waveform, durable PVI was achieved in 100% of patients at the 3-month follow-up using invasive remapping.[23,24] Long-term follow-up showed that atrial arrhythmias recurred in only 21.5% of patients after PFA with the Farawave catheter. The ADVENT trial, a randomized controlled study, confirmed that PFA with the Farawave catheter was noninferior to thermal ablation for atrial arrhythmia recurrence in patients with paroxysmal AF (17.2% vs 16.4%).[25] These findings were echoed in the post-approval MANIFEST-PF registry, which included 1568 patients from 24 European centers, showing a 78.1% success rate in maintaining arrhythmia freedom after 1 year, with a low 1.9% major adverse event rate.[10] Additionally, a sex-based analysis showed similar safety (1.5% vs 2.5%, $P = .19$) and effectiveness (79% vs 76.3%, $P = .28$) between men and women.[26]

Unlike the initial premarket studies, post-market data from the *EU-PORIA* registry showed PV durability rates of around 71%, with higher durability in procedures performed by operators with prior cryoballoon ablation experience compared to those with only point-by-point radiofrequency experience (76% vs 60%, *P*<.001).[27]

One of the most notable advantages of PFA with the Farawave catheter over thermal ablation is the increased procedural efficiency. In the *ADVENT* trial, PFA was significantly faster, with a procedure time of 105.8 ± 29.4 minutes compared to 123.1 ± 42.1 minutes for thermal ablation.[25] Registry data further supports this finding, suggesting that the procedural efficiency (median procedure time 61 minutes) using the Farawave catheter can be replicated in clinical practice beyond randomized clinical trial.[10]

There is promising data on the safety and feasibility of PFA using the Farawave catheter to perform left atrial posterior wall ablation. In the *PersAFOne* study, a two-center single-arm prospective trial using the Farawave catheter in patients with PersAF, safe and durable PVI and left atrial posterior wall alation were achieved in 96% of PVs and 100% of posterior walls upon invasive remapping at 3 months.[28] However, a subanalysis from the *MANIFEST-PF* registry showed no significant difference in freedom from atrial arrhythmia between patients who received PVI with posterior wall ablation and those who received PVI alone (66.4% vs 73.1%, *P*=.68) in a cohort of 547 patients with persistent AF with a comparable safety profile between both groups.[10]

Another important distinction between PFA and thermal ablation is the reduced burden of AF in patients treated with the Farawave catheter. In a pre-specified subgroup analysis of the *ADVENT* trial, patients with an AF burden greater than greater than 0.1% were associated with reduced quality of life and more interventions.[29] This threshold was previously proposed by Wechselberger and colleagues, based on the findings from the LINQ AF study, and it was linked to clinically significant outcomes in the CIRCA-DOSE trial.[30,31] PFA resulted in significantly more patients with a burden of atrial arrhythmias of less than 0.1% compared to thermal ablation (81.9% vs 74.8%, *P*=.035).[29]

Finally, limited data exists on the safety and effectiveness of PFA in patients with heart failure (HF). A *MANIFEST-PF* substudy using the Farawave catheter demonstrated that a 1-year freedom from atrial arrhythmia was significantly higher in patients without HF compared to those with heart failure with preserved ejection fraction (HFpEF) or heart failure with reduced or moderately reduced ejection fraction (HF$_{MR/R}$EF) (79.9%, 71.3%, and 67.5%; *P*<.001) but similar between patients with HF$_{MR/R}$EF and HFpEF (*P*=.26). Major adverse event rates were comparable across groups (1.9% for no-HF, 0% for HFpEF, and 2.5% for HF$_{MR/R}$EF).[32]

USE OF FARAWAVE IN THE VENTRICLES

Preclinical studies suggest that PFA can be effectively applied in the ventricle.[33,34] Data from animal models with ventricular scar indicate that PFA using the Farawave catheter can be performed over areas of preexisting ventricular scar.[35] PFA appears to effectively penetrate heterogenous ischemic scar tissue and successfully homogenize it with minimal gaps, as confirmed by histopathology.

Early clinical data suggests that PFA for PVC and VT ablations is safe and feasible. Several case reports have documented initial clinical experience using the Farawave catheter to perform PFA in the ventricles to treat scar based ventricular tachycardia.[36,37] Lozano and colleagues also recently demonstrated the feasibility of using the Farawave catheter to treat PVCs.[38] As with any new technology, unexpected clinical outcomes may arise, and further research is needed to establish safety and efficacy of PFA in ventricular applications.

FUTURE STUDIES USING FARAWAVE PULSED FIELD ABLATION CATHETER

There are several ongoing trials to evaluate the safety and effectiveness of Farawave PFA catheter in treating persistent AF. (i) *AVANT-GUARD* (NCT06096337) is a prospective, randomized trial comparing PFA versus antiarrhythmic drug therapy as first line treatment for persistent AF. Enrolling over 500 patients globally, the trial will assess the long-term safety and effectiveness of PFA, focusing on reducing AF burden and slowing disease progression. (ii) *ADVANTAGE AF* is a prospective, nonrandomized study (NCT05443594) including approximately 417 participants. This trial investigates PVI combined with empirical posterior wall ablation in drug-resistant persistent AF. The first phase of enrollment is complete, and the trial will assess safety and efficacy. An extension arm of this study also examines the use of the FARA-POINT PFA catheter for cavotricuspid isthmus ablation in patients with atrial flutter. These trials aim to expand the role of PFA in treating persistent AF by establishing its safety and long-term outcomes.

SUMMARY

Pulse field ablation using the Farawave pentasplie catheter is a promising technological advancement that has the potential to shift paradigms for the treatment of multiple atrial and ventricular arrhythmias. PFA allows for faster, safer treatment of paroxysmal and persistent AF with efficacy similar to that of thermal ablation. There is a tremendous amount of excitement in the field of electrophysiology surrounding PFA, and we look forward to the future investigations that will determine how to best use the Farawave pentasplie catheter to improve patient care.

CLINICS CARE POINTS

- Pulsed field ablation is an emerging technology in cardiac electrophysiology that uses pulsed electrical fields to precisely target myocardial tissue.

- Pulsed field ablation of the pulmonary veins using the Farawave pentaspline catheter to perform pulmonary vein isolation has been associated with a reduced risk of complications such as esophageal injury, phrenic nerve paralysis, and pulmonary vein stenosis compared to thermal ablation.

- The use of the Farawave pentaspline PFA catheter to treat paroxysmal atrial fibrillation is noninferior to thermal ablation in the risk of 12-month recurrence of atrial arrhythmias when treating paroxysmal atrial fibrillation.

- Future studies are needed to determine the safety and efficacy of pulse field ablation using the Farawave pentaspline PFA catheter to treat other atrial and ventricular arrhythmias.

DISCLOSURES

M.K. Turagam is a consultant for Boston Scientific, Medtronic, Abbott, Biosense Webster, and Sanofi.

REFERENCES

1. Koruth JS, Kuroki K, Kawamura I, et al. Focal pulsed field ablation for pulmonary vein isolation and linear atrial lesions: a preclinical assessment of safety and durability. Circ Arrhythm Electrophysiol 2020;13(6): e008716.
2. Nakagawa H, Farshchi-Heydari S, Maffre J, et al. Evaluation of ablation parameters to predict irreversible lesion size during pulsed field ablation. Circ Arrhythm Electrophysiol 2024;17(8):e012814.
3. Nakagawa H, Castellvi Q, Neal R, et al. Effects of contact force on lesion size during pulsed field catheter ablation: histochemical characterization of ventricular lesion boundaries. Circ Arrhythm Electrophysiol 2024; 17(1):e012026.
4. Koruth J, Verma A, Kawamura I, et al. PV isolation using a spherical array PFA catheter: preclinical assessment and comparison to radiofrequency ablation. JACC Clin Electrophysiol 2023;9(5):652–66.
5. Koruth J, Kuroki K, Iwasawa J, et al. Preclinical evaluation of pulsed field ablation: electrophysiological and histological assessment of thoracic vein isolation. Circ Arrhythm Electrophysiol 2019;12(12): e007781.
6. Koruth JS, Kuroki K, Kawamura I, et al. Pulsed field ablation versus radiofrequency ablation: esophageal injury in a novel porcine model. Circ Arrhythm Electrophysiol 2020;13(3):e008303.
7. Mansour M, Gerstenfeld EP, Patel C, et al. Pulmonary vein narrowing after pulsed field versus thermal ablation. Europace 2024;26(2):euae038.
8. Cochet H, Nakatani Y, Sridi-Cheniti S, et al. Pulsed field ablation selectively spares the oesophagus during pulmonary vein isolation for atrial fibrillation. Europace 2021;23(9):1391–9.
9. Ekanem E, Reddy VY, Schmidt B, et al. MANIFEST-PF Cooperative. Multi-national survey on the methods, efficacy, and safety on the post-approval clinical use of pulsed field ablation (MANIFEST-PF). Europace 2022;24(8):1256–66.
10. Turagam MK, Neuzil P, Schmidt B, et al. Safety and effectiveness of pulsed field ablation to treat atrial fibrillation: one-year outcomes from the MANIFEST-PF Registry. Circulation 2023;148(1):35–46.
11. Oates CP, Basyal B, Whang W, et al. Trends in safety of catheter-based electrophysiology procedures in the last 2 decades: a meta-analysis. Heart Rhythm 2024;21(9):1718–26.
12. Higuchi S, Im SI, Stillson C, et al. Effect of epicardial pulsed field ablation directly on coronary arteries. JACC Clin Electrophysiol 2022;8(12):1486–96.
13. Viles-Gonzalez JF, de Castro Miranda R, Scanavacca M, et al. Acute and chronic effects of epicardial radiofrequency applications delivered on epicardial coronary arteries. Circ Arrhythm Electrophysiol 2011;4(4):526–31.
14. Reddy VY, Petru J, Funasako M, et al. Coronary arterial spasm during pulsed field ablation to treat atrial fibrillation. Circulation 2022;146(24):1808–19.
15. Malyshev Y, Neuzil P, Petru J, et al. Nitroglycerin to ameliorate coronary artery spasm during focal pulsed-field ablation for atrial fibrillation. JACC Clin Electrophysiol 2024;10(5):885–96.
16. Zhang C, Neuzil P, Petru J, et al. Coronary artery spasm during pulsed field vs radiofrequency catheter ablation of the mitral isthmus. JAMA Cardiol 2024;9(1):72–7.
17. Sharifov OF, Fedorov VV, Beloshapko GG, et al. Roles of adrenergic and cholinergic stimulation in

spontaneous atrial fibrillation in dogs. J Am Coll Cardiol 2004;43(3):483–90.

18. Musikantow DR, Neuzil P, Petru J, et al. Pulsed field ablation to treat atrial fibrillation: autonomic nervous system effects. JACC Clin Electrophysiol 2023;9(4):481–93.

19. Lemoine MD, Mencke C, Nies M, et al. Pulmonary vein isolation by pulsed-field ablation induces less neurocardiac damage than cryoballoon ablation. Circ Arrhythm Electrophysiol 2023;16(4):e011598.

20. Gerstenfeld EP, Mansour M, Whang W, et al. Autonomic effects of pulsed field vs thermal ablation for treating atrial fibrillation: subanalysis of ADVENT. JACC Clin Electrophysiol 2024;10(7 Pt 2):1634–44.

21. Nies M, Koruth JS, Mlček M, et al. Hemolysis after pulsed field ablation: impact of lesion number and catheter-tissue contact. Circ Arrhythm Electrophysiol 2024;17(6):e012765.

22. Osmancik P, Bacova B, Herman D, et al. Periprocedural intravascular hemolysis during atrial fibrillation ablation: a comparison of pulsed field with radiofrequency ablation. JACC Clin Electrophysiol 2024;10(7 Pt 2):1660–71.

23. Reddy VY, Dukkipati SR, Neuzil P, et al. Pulsed field ablation of paroxysmal atrial fibrillation: 1-year outcomes of iMPULSE, PEFCAT, and PEFCAT II. JACC Clin Electrophysiol 2021;7(5):614–27.

24. Reddy VY, Neuzil P, Koruth JS, et al. Pulsed field ablation for pulmonary vein isolation in atrial fibrillation. J Am Coll Cardiol 2019;74(3):315–26.

25. Reddy VY, Gerstenfeld EP, Natale A, et al. Pulsed field or conventional thermal ablation for paroxysmal atrial fibrillation. N Engl J Med 2023;389:1660–71.

26. Turagam MK, Neuzil P, Schmidt B, et al. Clinical outcomes by sex after pulsed field ablation of atrial fibrillation. JAMA Cardiol 2023;8(12):1142–51.

27. Kueffer T, Bordignon S, Neven K, et al. Durability of pulmonary vein isolation using pulsed-field ablation: results from the multicenter EU-PORIA Registry. JACC Clin Electrophysiol 2024;10(4):698–708.

28. Reddy VY, Anic A, Koruth J, et al. Pulsed field ablation in patients with persistent atrial fibrillation. J Am Coll Cardiol 2020;76(9):1068–80.

29. Reddy VY, Mansour M, Calkins H, et al. Pulsed field vs conventional thermal ablation for paroxysmal atrial fibrillation: recurrent atrial arrhythmia burden. J Am Coll Cardiol 2024;84(1):61–74.

30. Andrade JG, Deyell MW, Macle L, et al. Healthcare utilization and quality of life for atrial fibrillation burden: the CIRCA-DOSE study. Eur Heart J 2023;44(9):765–76.

31. Wechselberger S, Kronborg M, Huo Y, et al. Continuous monitoring after atrial fibrillation ablation: the LINQ AF study. Europace 2018;20(FI_3):f312–20.

32. Turagam MK, Neuzil P, Schmidt B, et al, MANIFEST-PF Cooperative. Safety and effectiveness of pulsed field ablation for atrial fibrillation in patients with heart failure: a MANIFEST-PF Sub-analysis. JACC Clin Electrophysiol 2024. S2405-500X(24)00351-7.

33. Koruth JS, Kuroki K, Iwasawa J, et al. Endocardial ventricular pulsed field ablation: a proof-of-concept preclinical evaluation. Europace 2020;22:434–9.

34. Kawamura I, Reddy VY, Santos-Gallego CG, et al. Electrophysiology, pathology, and imaging of pulsed field ablation of scarred and healthy ventricles in Swine. Circ Arrhythm Electrophysiol 2023;16(1):e011369.

35. Im SI, Higuchi S, Lee A, et al. Pulsed field ablation of left ventricular myocardium in a swine infarct model. JACC Clin Electrophysiol 2022;8(6):722–31.

36. Peichl P, Bulava A, Wichterle D, et al. Efficacy and safety of focal pulsed-field ablation for ventricular arrhythmias: two-centre experience. Europace 2024;26(7):euae192.

37. Zhang Z, Xiao Y, Wang C, et al. Pulsed field ablation: a promising approach for ventricular tachycardia ablation. Int J Cardiol 2024;407:131985.

38. Lozano-Granero C, Hirokami J, Franco E, et al. Case series of ventricular tachycardia ablation with pulsed-field ablation: pushing technology further (Into the Ventricle). JACC Clin Electrophysiol 2023;9(9):1990–4.

Catheters and Tools with Pulsed Field Ablation— Pulmonary Vein Isolation and Nanosecond Pulse Field Ablation

Jan Petru, MD*, Moritoshi Funasako, MD, PhD, Petr Neuzil, MD, PhD

KEYWORDS

- Nanosecond • Pulsed field ablation • nsPFA • Atrial fibrillation ablation • Electroporation
- Pulmonary vein isolation

KEY POINTS

- Nanosecond PFA (nsPFA) has potential advantages over microsecond pulses such as deeper penetration of the electric field into tissue, creating larger lesions while depositing less overall energy, faster treatment, and less muscle and nerve stimulation.
- Rather than generating permanent pores in cell membrane leading to necrosis, nsPFA (which can permeabilize even very small organelles inside the cells, including the mitochondria) generates smaller (~1 nm wide), transient pores which initiate regulated cell death.
- Excellent safety, lesion consistency, and durability of ablation lesion sets created with nsPFA have been demonstrated in preclinical studies and early phases of clinical testing.

INTRODUCTION

As the need for more effective and safer options for cardiac ablation to treat atrial fibrillation has grown, energy modalities with "nonthermal" mechanisms of cell death have emerged as promising alternatives. Pulse field ablation (PFA) has gained attention in this field as one of these energy modalities and the initial PFA systems have demonstrated excellent safety and efficacy profiles.[1,2]

PFA uses pulsed electric fields to ablate tissue utilizing irreversible cell electroporation as the mechanism of cell death. The first commercial system was introduced in 2004 for the ablation of soft tissue (NanoKnife System, AngioDynamics, NY). The NanoKnife System utilized pulse durations of 100 microseconds and voltage amplitudes of up to 3000 V utilizing 2 or more needle electrodes deployed in a parallel configuration.[3] The cell death mechanism of PFA is the electroporation of the cell membrane, or creation of pores with enough pulses that the pores do not reseal, causing irreversible damage or cell death.[4] The pores are large enough to allow ATP and many other important cellular molecules to leak out of the cell, which leads very quickly to cellular necrosis. This nonthermal cell death mechanism has the advantage of preserving acellular structures within the tissue being ablated, which can lead to improved healing.[5,6]

One of the disadvantages of PFA can be strong muscle contraction and nerve capture during treatment due to the relatively long pulse durations and high voltages utilized, leading to the need for

Department of Cardiology, Charles University, Na Homolce Hospital, Roentgenova 2, 150 30, Prague 5, Prague, Czech Republic
* Corresponding author.
E-mail address: jan.petru@homolka.cz

Card Electrophysiol Clin 17 (2025) 273–285
https://doi.org/10.1016/j.ccep.2025.02.015
1877-9182/25/© 2025 Elsevier Inc. All rights are reserved, including those for text and data mining, AI training, and similar technologies.

Abbreviations

CT	computed tomography
EAM	electroanatomical mapping
EFT	electric field threshold
FEA	finite element analysis
ICE	intracardiac echocardiography
IVC	inferior vena cava
nsPFA	nanosecond PFA
PFA	pulse field ablation
PV	pulmonary vein
RCD	regulated cell death
RSPV	right superior pulmonary vein
SVC	superior vena cava
TTE	transthoracic echocardiography

muscle paralytic drugs. PFA systems have more recently utilized different pulsing strategies in an attempt to minimize muscle contraction and nerve capture but this continues to be an issue with systems today, and some of these newer strategies are limited by thermal effects when used with ablation catheters.

NANOSECOND PULSED FIELD ABLATION

Nanosecond PFA (nsPFA) utilizes pulsed electric fields with ultrashort pulses that are less than a microsecond in duration, typically tens to hundreds of nanoseconds in duration, or several orders of magnitude shorter in duration than initial PFA systems. The initial use of nanosecond pulsed electric fields in biology was published by Shoenbach and colleagues in 2001.[7] They showed that nsPFA pulses could permeabilize very small organelles inside of the cells, including the mitochondria. Rather than generating permanent pores leading to necrosis, nsPFA generates smaller (~ 1 nm wide), transient pores which initiate regulated cell death (RCD). RCD is the pathway cells utilize to self-destruct when they reach the end of their useful life and encounter a lethal gene mutation or an injury that they are unable to repair.[8] Regulated cell death (RCD) is characterized by rapid nuclear pyknosis,[9] intracellular Ca^{2+} increases,[10] DNA fragmentation,[11] reactive oxygen species (ROS) formation,[12] caspase-3 activation[13] to hydrolyze proteins, and mitochondrial swelling.[14]

The novel mechanism of nsPFA has shown to have several advantages over microsecond PFA. The ultrashort pulse duration enables the use of higher amplitude pulses that can lead to deeper penetration of the electric field into tissue, creating larger and deeper ablation zones while depositing less overall energy into the tissue. The lower energy exploited by nsPFA during an ablation leads

to less heat deposited than microsecond PFA, and also enables larger footprint electrode designs that can lead to more reliable and faster overall treatments. These potential treatment benefits of nsPFA are achieved while also minimizing muscle stimulation or nerve capture due to the ultrashort duration pulses. The recognition of these advantages led to the development of an nsPFA system called the CellFX System (Pulse Biosciences, Inc) and a number of clinical applications, including cardiac catheter ablation for the treatment of atrial fibrillation (AF), have been developed and used clinically.

CellFX TECHNOLOGY INTRODUCTION AND CLINICAL APPLICATIONS

The CellFX system is a software tunable nsPFA platform that enables the delivery of nsPFA treatments with user selectable pulse duration, pulse amplitude, number of pulses, and pulse frequency

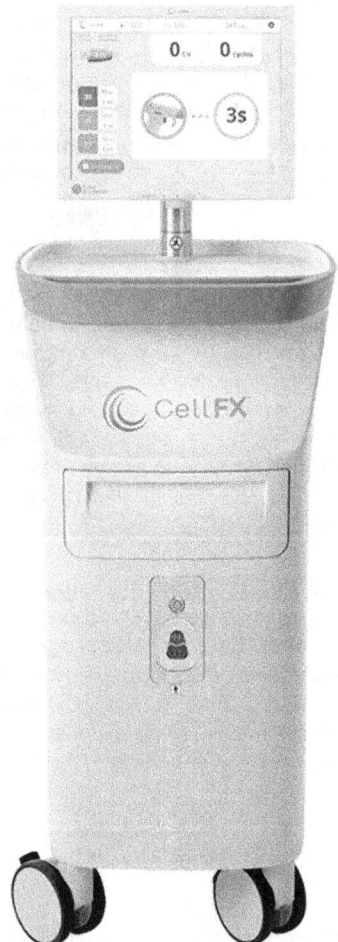

Fig. 1. CellFX system. (*With permission from* Pulse Biosciences, Inc.)

(Fig. 1). The treatments are selected through the graphical user interface on the console. The CellFX Console has an electrode interface connector on the front where application-specific devices are plugged in and utilized in the clinical setting.

In 2021, the CellFX System received an Food and Drug Administration (FDA) clearance and Conformité Européene (CE) mark for the treatment of benign skin lesions in dermatology. Over 7000 patients have been treated to date with no serious adverse events.[15–19] In the dermatology setting, patients receive only a small injection of local anesthesia at the treatment site and treatments last 5 to 15 seconds per lesion. Example dermatologic applications include the removal of sebaceous hyperplasia and seborrheic keratosis and the treatment of basal cell carcinoma[17] (Fig. 2), to name a few.

In 2024, the CellFX System received an FDA clearance for an nsPFA percutaneous electrode for soft tissue ablation in a surgical setting (Fig. 3). The electrode can be used under computed tomography (CT) or ultrasound guidance to deliver a volumetric ablation in solid organs. The initial application is in the treatment of benign thyroid nodules. Clinical use of nsPFA with the percutaneous electrode has occurred in an office or outpatient setting with fully conscious patients that require only a local injection of anesthesia.

CellFX TECHNOLOGY FOR ATRIAL FIBRILLATION TREATMENT

More recently, CellFX devices for the treatment of atrial fibrillation have been developed including a bipolar surgical clamp with parallel jaws to enable the Cox-Maze procedure for the treatment of atrial fibrillation in cardiac open-heart surgery (Fig. 4). Each jaw of the clamp integrates one of the electrode bipoles. With the clamp, nsPFA treatments are delivered across thick myocardial tissue in a few seconds without any clinically relevant thermal rise. The cardiac surgery bipolar clamp has demonstrated very good transmural contiguous ablations in a preclinical porcine model[20,21] and is currently being used in a feasibility first-in-human study in concomitant cardiac surgery.

CellFX 360° CATHETER FOR ENDOCARDIAL ABLATION

The application of nsPFA for endocardial cardiac ablation for the treatment of atrial fibrillation holds significant promise for the delivery of a safe, effective, and efficient procedure. The 360° catheter (Figs. 5 and 6) is designed to deliver nsPFA energy to endocardial locations in the atria, mainly in the pulmonary veins to create electrical isolation as a cornerstone to treat atrial fibrillation. The nonirrigated catheter consists of a 125 cm long, 11.5-F shaft that can be connected to a compatible, commercially-available electroanatomical mapping (EAM) system with both magnetic-based and electrical impedance-based localization capabilities. The catheter is a bidirectionally steerable dual-purpose ablation and mapping catheter with 2 flexible, concentric Nitinol wire ablation electrodes on its distal active portion. An outer 30 mm diameter ring and an inner 22 mm diameter ring act as a bipole electrode pair. An electrical field is generated across the 2 wire electrodes, leading to the creation of a radially uniform toroidal ablation field. A standard dose of energy is

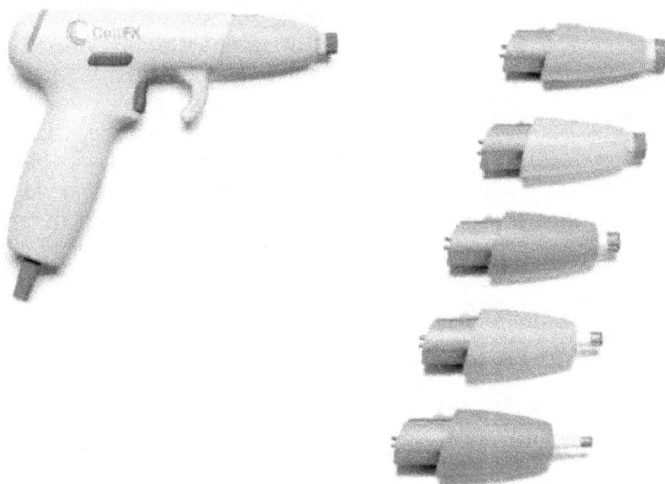

Fig. 2. CellFX dermatology handpiece. (*With permission from* Pulse Biosciences, Inc.)

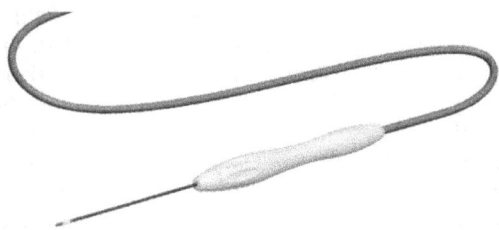

Fig. 3. CellFX percutaneous electrode. (*With permission from* Pulse Biosciences, Inc.)

delivered over a 5-s application and is designed to generate a transmural and circumferential lesion at the target site. A faster ~2-s dose is being investigated clinically as well. The catheter has 12 sensing electrodes for electroanatomic mapping and tissue contact sensing.

The distal end of the catheter with ablative electrodes can be placed in the antrum or ostium of a target pulmonary vein in an "umbrella" configuration (**Fig. 7**) to facilitate the generation of a complete circumferential lesion that is capable of isolating a vein in a single application. Similarly, ablative rings may also be placed flat against endocardial tissue (**Fig. 8**) such as the left atrial posterior wall to generate lesions for electrical isolation of larger areas of the myocardium. Pairs of sensing electrodes located on each strut of the electrode assembly as well as the shaft of the catheter can be used to monitor tissue contact and ablation efficacy by assessment of local electrograms and can also be used with EAM systems as mentioned earlier for localization and mapping. Due to the "nonthermal" nature of nsPFA, which results in much less thermal effects than microsecond PFA, no irrigation is required for this catheter design.

PRECLINICAL ASSESSMENT OF CellFX 360° CATHETER

To demonstrate the efficacy of the CellFX 360° Catheter system, ablations were carried out in a porcine endocardial model.[19] The catheter was advanced into the heart through a 12-F sheath

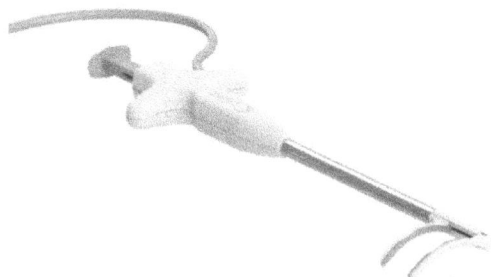

Fig. 4. CellFX cardiac surgical clamp. (*With permission from* Pulse Biosciences, Inc.)

and energy was delivered to a variety of intracardiac targets including the superior vena cava (SVC), mitral isthmus, pulmonary veins, left and right ventricle, and atrial wall tissue to investigate the tissue response following nsPFA delivery at these locations. Fluoroscopy, intracardiac echocardiography (ICE), and 3-D mapping were used to confirm the location of the catheter for each ablation site (**Fig. 9**).

Gross assessment of ablated endocardial tissue at 1-month post procedure in a porcine model clearly demonstrates that the CellFX system generates persistent, uniform circumferential lesions with sharp boundaries at the intended target sites, including the SVC, the right superior pulmonary vein (RSPV), and the mitral isthmus (**Fig. 10**). The lesion appearance is not consistent with a thermal injury, instead presenting as a pale band with well-demarcated borders. Slight central hemorrhage is observed acutely and resolves by 30 days post ablation. The lack of a thermal component to the ablation was further confirmed by MRI and histopathological assessments of the target sites.

Intracardiac electrograms were consistently significantly diminished or absent after nsPFA with the CellFX 360° Catheter demonstrating an immediate effect on electrical activity at the ablation site. These findings, including level of isolation, were demonstrated by 3D EAM acutely and as well rechecked at the termination of the experiment at 2 or ~30 days post procedure.

Electroanatomical mapping of the left atrium of the animals which underwent pulmonary vein isolation using the CellFX 360 Catheter demonstrated complete electrical isolation of the treated pulmonary veins immediately post ablation and remained isolated at 1-month post procedure (**Figs. 11** and **12**). This demonstrates the functional durability of the lesions observed by gross assessment during necropsy.

Histopathological assessment of ablated veins (SVC, pulmonary veins) demonstrated complete circumferential and transmural ablation of the vessel lumen in all instances. Lesions appeared to remain circumferential and transmural both acutely and at up to 30 days post ablation, suggesting that reconnection did not occur during the subsequent healing process after ablation. Lesion depth was bounded by the wall thickness of the target vein and was reported as 5.5 ± 0.5 mm for pulmonary veins and 3.6 ± 0.6 mm for SVC. Lesion widths were 17.9 ± 1.4 mm and 15.7 ± 1.4 mm for the pulmonary veins and SVC, respectively.

Histopathological assessment of ablations performed in the mitral isthmus were uniformly transmural, with an average lesion depth of $6.4 \pm$

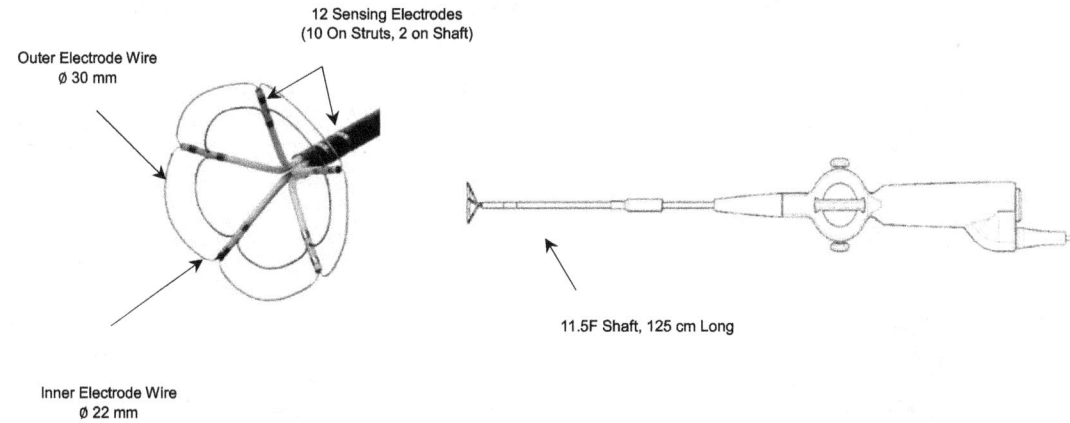

Fig. 5. CellFX 360° catheter.

0.4 mm and an average lesion width of 18.6 ± 1.1 mm. Coronary vessels within the ablated region of the mitral isthmus including the coronary sinus and left circumflex artery were well preserved, and there was no sign of stenosis or thrombosis. The valve remained fully intact within the ablated zone, with no significant histologic changes after direct ablation of the valvular tissue.

Histopathological assessment of ablations applied to the ventricles was also performed to confirm the maximum ablation depth which could be achieved using the CellFX 360° Catheter. Ventricular lesion depth was 7.1 ± 1.3 mm and lesion width was 14.7± 4.5 mm. Depth is bounded by transmurality in 27% of ventricular lesions assessed, suggesting that this average depth is an underestimate of the maximum lesion depth

that is reproducibly achievable by the CellFX 360° Catheter.

Phrenic nerve palsy was probed acutely post procedure and at termination for all animals by pacing. No phrenic nerve palsy was observed after intracardiac ablation acutely or at the scheduled termination time point, establishing that even when performing ablations in the SVC, the phrenic nerve is not affected.

Moderate coronary spasm was noted by angiography in one animal which was ablated immediately adjacent to the right coronary artery; however, this observation resolved with the application of nitroglycerine and was without any sequela. There is no evidence of coronary stenosis in any animal at the time of termination by angiography or histopathological assessment of vessels near the ablation zone.

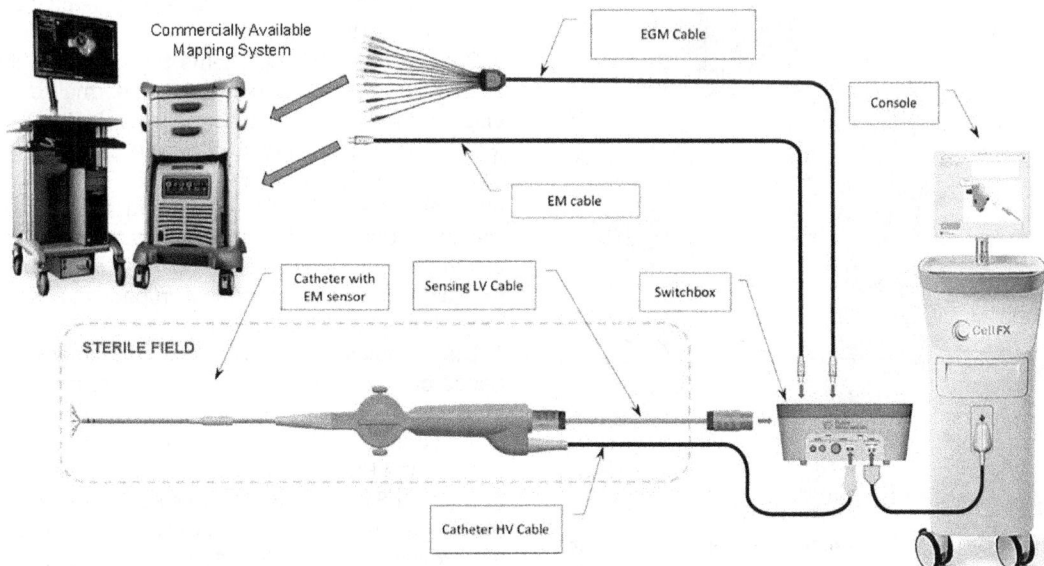

Fig. 6. CellFX 360° catheter system. (*With permission from* Pulse Biosciences, Inc.)

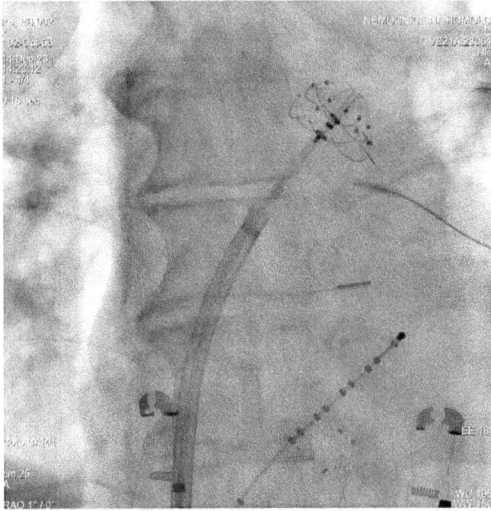

Fig. 7. CellFX 360° catheter positioned in left superior pulmonary vein with ablative electrodes inverted into an "umbrella" configuration.

Esophageal safety was also evaluated by performing ablations in the inferior vena cava (IVC) while the esophagus was mechanically deviated to contact the vessel to simulate a "worst-case" scenario in the preclinical model. At 2-days post procedure, shallow crescent-shaped lesions were present histologically in the esophagus of animals where the tissue was brought into direct contact with the IVC during ablation. These lesions did not impact the mucosa, and at 30-days post procedure, there were no significant histologic observations in the esophagi, demonstrating the esophageal safety of nsPFA even when administered extremely close to the esophagus.

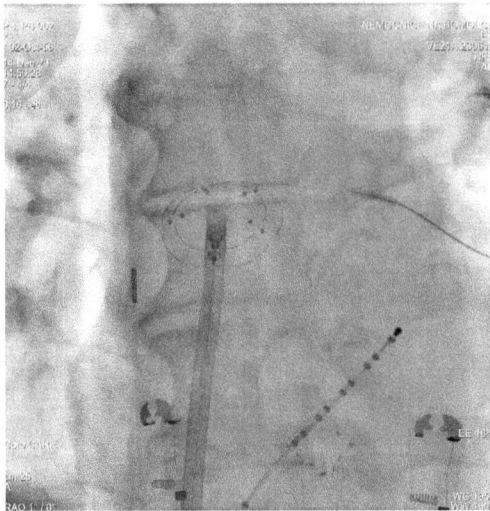

Fig. 8. CellFX 360° catheter positioned against left atrium posterior wall with Ablative Electrodes in a Flat Configuration.

FINITE ELEMENT MODELING OF CellFX 360° CATHETER

The size of the static electric field generated by the CellFX 360° Catheter was calculated using COMSOL Multiphysics (version 6.0) finite element analysis (FEA) software. Three-dimensional (3D) models were created to represent the electrodes of the CellFX 360° Catheter engaged with the ostium of a 6-mm thick pulmonary vein (PV) that was modeled as cardiac tissue. Blood occupied the volume within the PV, and either fat or connective tissue (or pulmonary artery) occupied the volume outside of the PV.

The 3D model is shown later (**Fig. 13**) where the catheter's electrodes are in intimate contact with PV and the radial support struts are modeled in an inverted "mushroom" configuration that is observed when the electrodes are pushed into the ostium of the PV.

A cross-section plane was taken along the axis of the PV to view the finite element analysis (FEA) results within the wall of the pulmonary vein. In the **Fig. 14** depicted later, the cross-sectioned PV is shown in blue along with other details of the FEA model, note that the cross-sectioned electrodes are shown to scale.

The FEA results were calibrated utilizing histopathological data from preclinical experiments using a porcine model [ref to Mt. Sinai data from 2023 HRS poster]. The maximum depth of the ablation zones in the preclinical experiments was compared to the FEA analysis to determine the effective electric field threshold (EFT). Electric fields greater than or equal to the EFT will induce cell death. Conversely, electric fields less than the EFT are assumed to not cause cell death (cells will remain viable).

Because the EFT represents the border of the ablation zone, the EFT was used to normalize the electric field results. The normalized electric field (E*) is defined as $E^* = E/EFT$, where E is the electric field (calculated by FEA), and EFT is the effective field threshold. By calibrating to a mean treatment depth and normalizing to the EFT, any electrical transmission line losses or voltage reflection inefficiencies do not impact the accuracy of the presented results.

The predicted nsPFA ablation dimensions based on the COMSOL FEA results are provided in **Table 1** presented later for 2 conditions: (1) with connective tissue or pulmonary artery backing the PV, and (2) with fat backing the PV.

The 2D FEA estimates of the electric field within the PV during nsPFA with the CellFX 360° catheter are provided later in **Figs. 15** and **16** for 2 conditions: (1) with connective tissue or pulmonary

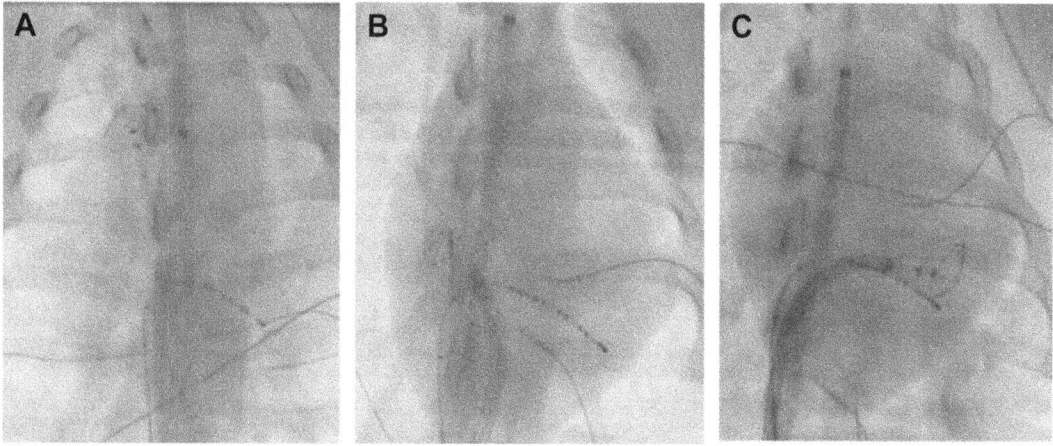

Fig. 9. Representative catheter placement and conformation assessed by fluoroscopy during ablation in (*A*) the superior vena cava (SVC) (*B*) the right superior pulmonary vein (RSPV), and (*C*) at the mitral isthmus.

artery backing the PV, and (2) with fat backing the PV.

Finally, a single 3D FEA estimate of the electric field within the PV during nsPFA with the CellFX 360° catheter is provided later in **Fig. 17** to show that the static electric field is uniform and fully circumferential around the PV during nsPFA with the CellFX 360° Catheter.

INITIAL CLINICAL EXPERIENCE

Based on the FEA analysis and demonstrated safety and effectiveness of the CellFX 360 catheter system in preclinical studies, a first-in-human feasibility study was initiated at Na Homolce Hospital, Prague, Czech Republic in December 2023. The study design is a prospective, nonrandomized, open labeled, single-arm feasibility study to evaluate the initial clinical safety and device performance of the endocardial ablation catheter system for global mapping and ablation of left atrium for the treatment of paroxysmal atrial fibrillation.

Up to 60 subjects will be included in the study. Detailed inclusion and exclusion criteria are in **Box 1**. All subjects should undergo an electroanatomical remapping procedure at 3 months post index procedure to assess the durability of PV isolation and other lesion sets. The follow-up will last 12 months with visits at 7 days, 1 month, 3 months, 6 months, and 12 months with a blanking period for recurrent atrial fibrillation or atrial tachycardia of 3 months following endocardial catheter ablation procedure. Rhythm monitoring consist of weekly (or during symptoms) transmitted reports from transtelephonic monitor (TTM) event recorders and two 24-hour Holter ECG monitors at 6 and 12 months.

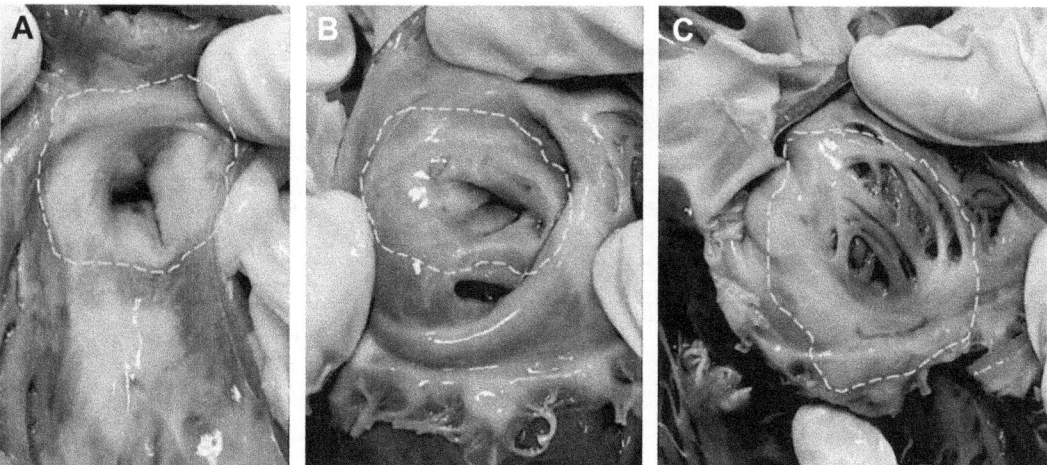

Fig. 10. Gross pathology at 1-month post ablation shows circumferential lesions in the (*A*) SVC, (*B*) RSPV, and (*C*) mitral isthmus. Lesions present as a circumferential ring of pale tissue surrounding the lumen of the vessel.

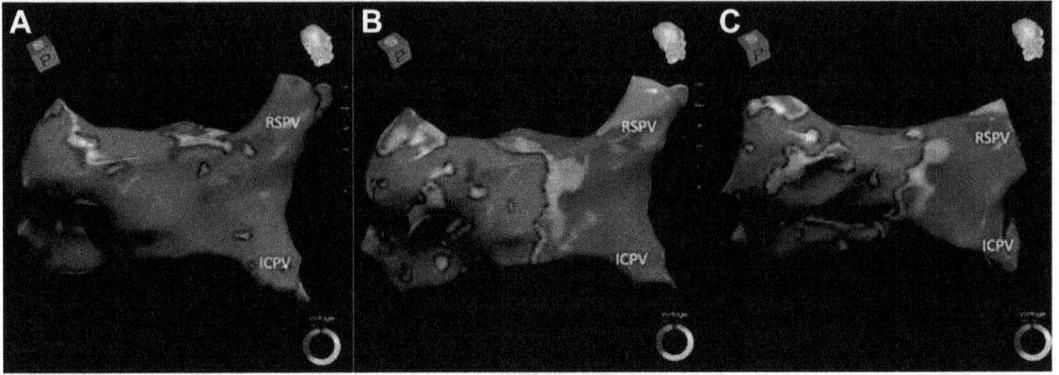

Fig. 11. Animal model—EA maps (iMAP 3-D mapping system) of the left atrium: (*A*) Preablation; (*B*) immediately post ablation; (*C*) 1-month post ablation. Red regions indicate electrical isolation (IEGMs below threshold 0.1 mv). EA, electroanatomical; iMAP, the name of the mapping system; IEGMs, intracardiac electrograms.

ENDOCARDIAL ABLATION PROCEDURE

Procedures are typically performed under general anesthesia or deep sedation with uninterrupted anticoagulation. After the administration of heparin and under fluoroscopy and ICE guidance, transseptal puncture is done, ideally in the anteroinferior part of the septum which allows easier manipulation with this relatively large ablation device in the left atrium (LA). An EA map of the LA is then created using a standard EAM System. CardioNXT iMap, CARTO 3 System and the EnSite X have all been used in this study. The CellFX 360 ablation catheter is then introduced into the LA through a deflectable 13-F sheath. activated clotting time (ACT) should be above 350s before PFA delivery. The catheter is positioned into the ostium and antrum of each vein. Only one application is made in each position. Depending on the anatomy and size of the pulmonary veins, the catheter is used as a single shot device or as a catheter for segmental ablation to cover the entire antrum of the pulmonary veins (eg, left common trunk or large RSPV).

In the study, the application of a default dose (5 sec) and a low dose (2.5 sec) have been tested. Examples of the catheter viewed using fluoroscopy and ICE are shown in **Fig. 18**. The representation of the catheter in EA maps serves only for rough orientation of the catheter in the atrium. Depending on the clinical situation (extensive substrate of the left atrium, AF organization into atrial tachycardia, etc.) and after individual assessment by the operator, it is possible to ablate additional locations in the LA (and/or right atrium [RA]) outside of the pulmonary veins, for example, posterior wall, mitral isthmus, or cavo-tricuspid isthmus. After ablation, the extent of ablation is evaluated by remapping.

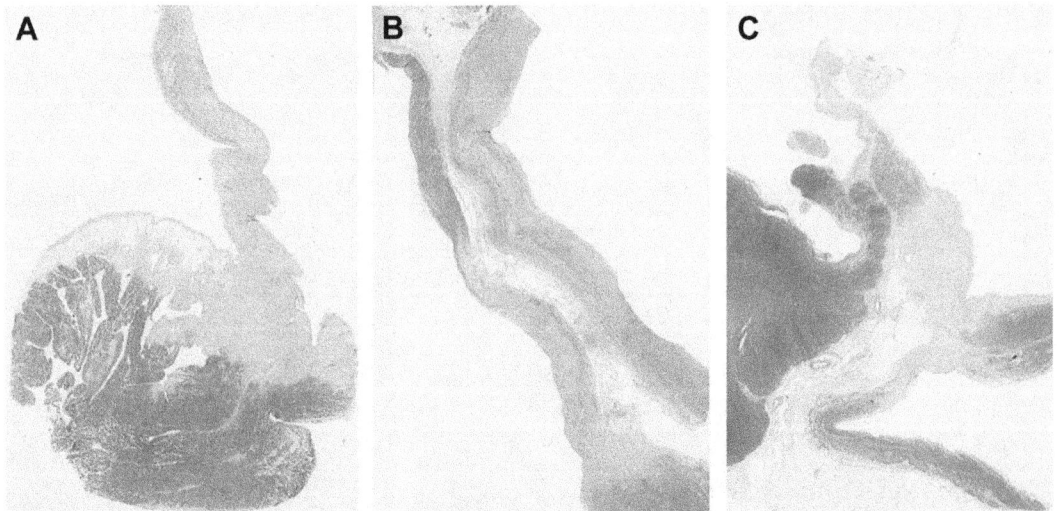

Fig. 12. Typical histologic sections of intracardiac tissue stained with Gömöri's Trichrome (*A*) SVC, (*B*) RSPV, (*C*) mitral isthmus. Blue regions indicate tissue which has undergone a loss of viable myocardium due to ablation.

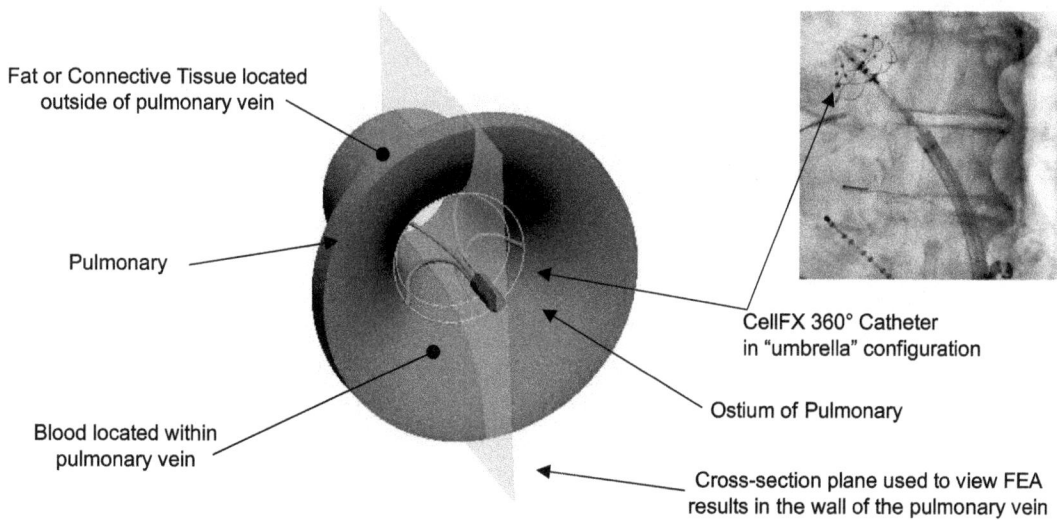

Fat or Connective Tissue located
outside of pulmonary vein

Pulmonary

Blood located within
pulmonary vein

CellFX 360° Catheter
in "umbrella" configuration

Ostium of Pulmonary

Cross-section plane used to view FEA
results in the wall of the pulmonary vein

Fig. 13. 3D COMSOL model for the CellFX 360° Catheter in the ostium of a pulmonary vein.

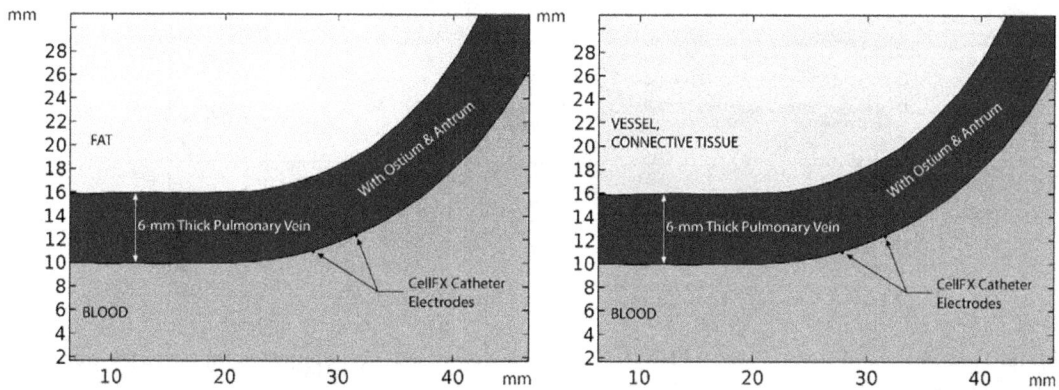

Fig. 14. Cross section of COMSOL model showing pulmonary vein in blue. Note the small size of the Nitinol (NiTi) wire electrodes, which are shown to scale.

Table 1
Predicted nanosecond pulse field ablation zone dimensions for the CellFX 360° catheter

Condition Simulated	Ablation Depth (mm)	Ablation Width at Endocardial Surface (mm)	Ablation Width at Epicardial Surface (mm)	Notes
Connective tissue or pulmonary artery backing PV	6.0	14.2	4.5	Transmural, so depth limited by 6-mm PV wall thickness
Fat backing PV	6.0	12.3	7.0	Transmural, so depth limited by 6-mm PV wall thickness

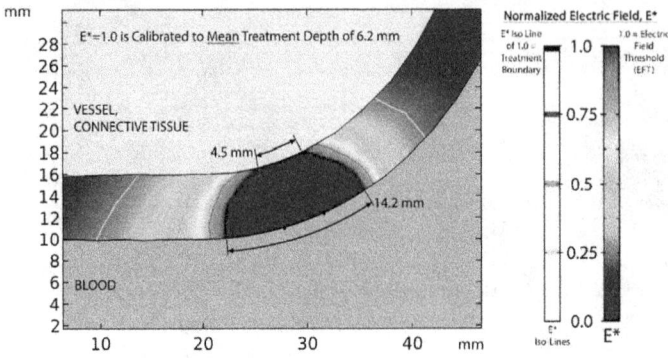

Fig. 15. Predicted nanosecond pulse field ablation (nsPFA) electric field within the PV for the CellFX 360° Catheter when connective tissue backs the pulmonary vein.

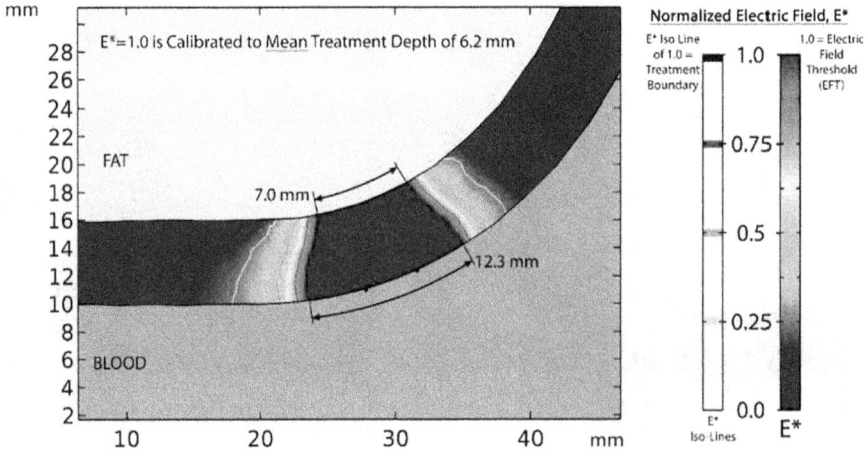

Fig. 16. Predicted nsPFA electric field within the PV for the CellFX 360° Catheter when fat backs the pulmonary vein.

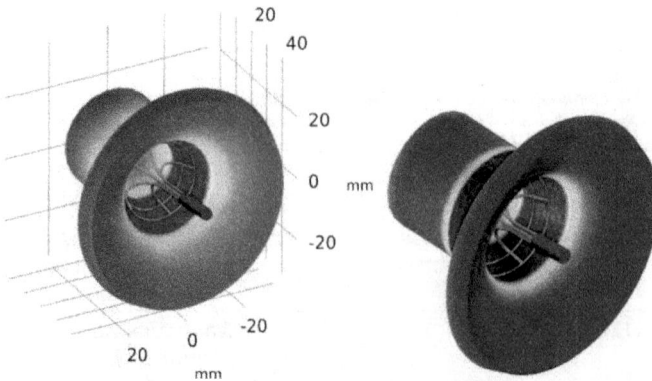

Fig. 17. Predicted nsPFA electric field within the PV for the CellFX 360° Catheter when fat backs the pulmonary vein.

Candidates must meet *ALL* the following criteria:

1. Subject must be $\geq$ 18 and $\leq$ 75 years of age on the day of enrollment.

2. Subject is willing and capable of providing informed consent to undergo study procedures and participate in all examinations and follow-up visits and tests associated with this clinical study.

3. Subjects with paroxysmal atrial fibrillation who have had at least one AF episode documented within 1 year prior to enrollment. Documentation may include ECG, transtelephonic monitor (TTM), Holter monitor (HM), or telemetry strip.

4. Subjects who have failed at least 1 antiarrhythmic drug (AAD; class I or III, or AV nodal blocking agents such as beta blockers and calcium channel blockers) as shown by recurrent symptomatic AF, or intolerance to the AAD or atrio-ventricular (AV) nodal blocking agents.

5. Antero-posterior left atrial diameter $\leq$ 5.5 cm as documented by transthoracic echocardiography (TTE) or CT within 3 months prior to the procedure.

6. Left ventricular ejection fraction $\geq$ 40% as documented by TTE within 12 months prior to the procedure.

An example EA acute and remap of one of the study subjects is shown in **Fig. 19**.

PREPROCEDURAL AND POSTPROCEDURAL ASSESSMENT

There are also other substudies within the clinical trial. For example, in a selected number of patients, endoscopy of the upper part of the digestive system is performed to evaluate the effect of nanopulses on the esophageal mucosa. Great emphasis is also placed on the evaluation of possible silent strokes and other findings (brain MRI before and after ablation) or PV stenosis using CT.

PRELIMINARY DATA AND EXPERIENCE

At the time of this writing, 54 patients with paroxysmal atrial fibrillation have been enrolled in the feasibility study and all index procedures have been completed successfully by 4 experienced operators in one center in Na Homolce Hospital Prague. The vast majority of procedures were performed under general anesthesia combined with paralysis. However, in patients treated under sedation, it appears that the muscle stimulation during the nsPFA delivery is not as pronounced as when using commercially available microsecond PFA systems, and similarly, the provocation of cough is not as excessive or limiting. All pulmonary veins were

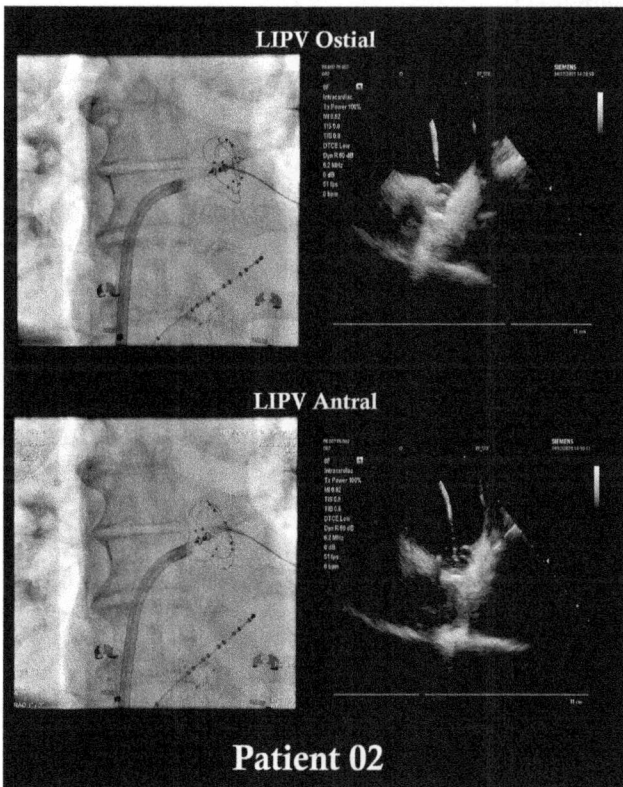

Fig. 18. Fluoroscopy and intracardiac echo images: The CellFX 360 catheter is placed in the left inferior pulmonary vein (LIPV) Ostia and on the LIPV Antrum. The ring electrodes and sensing electrodes are clearly visible in fluoroscopy and on ICE the cross section of the catheter in the vein is also clear.

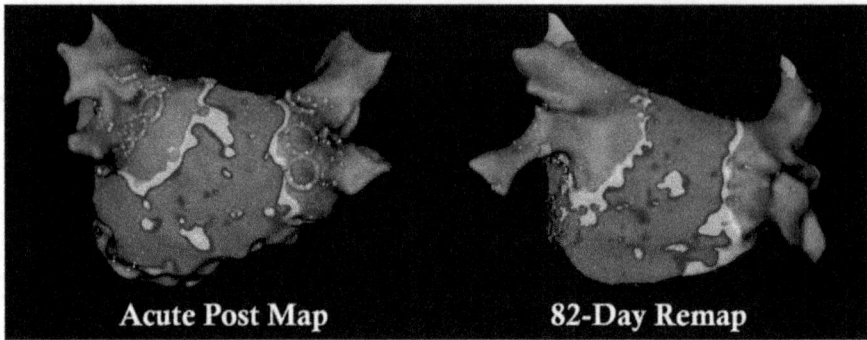

Fig. 19. An example of a pre and post procedure electroanatomical mapping that shows pulmonary vein isolation acutely and at an 82-day remap.

successfully electrically isolated during the index procedure using the tested catheter and 2 to 3 applications per vein. No acute complications have been reported. One patient developed a pericardial effusion 4 days after the procedure, which was treated by pericardicentesis due to inflammation. In the examined patients, no mucosal damage to the esophagus was detected endoscopically, and there was no evidence of pulmonary vein narrowing after ablation. Brain MRI findings before and after ablation are currently being evaluated. Patient recruitment is expected to be completed soon and the remapping part of the clinical trial continues smoothly.

SUMMARY

Although the use of PFA has been shown to increase the speed, efficiency, and safety of catheter ablation compared to conventional thermal (radiofrequency, cryo) energies, there remain unmet needs to be addressed for the procedure improvement and better outcomes of AF ablation. The CellFX Catheter System with nsPFA is another emerging technology which could play an important role in this field. Excellent lesion consistency and durability of ablation lesion sets created by nsPFA have been proven in preclinical studies and the early results of this study suggest the results will translate well to human use. Moreover, less muscle stimulation and cough provocation can contribute to procedural simplification and ease of use. Our preliminary experience with catheter performance is encouraging. For an overall evaluation, it is necessary to wait for the results of the ongoing feasibility study.

CLINICS CARE POINTS

- During the short period of use, the safety, speed, and effectiveness of PFA in catheter treatment of atrial fibrillation have been demonstrated with plenty of advantages over thermal conventional energies.

- Pulmonary vein isolation is achievable with only 2 or 3 applications per vein, so the technology can truly be called as a single shot ablation.
- There is no need to apply nsPFA to the same location multiple times to create durable and effective lesion as with other technologies.

DISCLOSURE

J. Petru: research grant—Pulse Biosciences, Inc, United States. M. Funasako: The author has nothing to disclose. P. Neuzil: research grant—Pulse Biosciences, Inc.

REFERENCES

1. Reddy & Ekanem, et al. Multi-National Survey on the Safety of the Post-Approval Clinical Use of Pulsed Field Ablation in 17,000+ Patients (MANIFEST-17K). AHA 2023.
2. Emmanuel E, et al. "Multi-national survey on the methods, efficacy, and safety on the post-approval clinical use of pulsed field ablation (MANIFEST-PF)." Europace 24.8 (2022): 1256-1266.
3. Davalos RV, Mir IL, Rubinsky B. Tissue ablation with irreversible electroporation. Ann Biomed Eng 2005; 33:223–31.
4. Onik G, Mikus P, Rubinsky B. Irreversible electroporation: implications for prostate ablation. Technol Cancer Res Treat 2007;6:295–300.
5. Phillips MA, Narayan R, Padath T, et al. Irreversible electroporation on the small intestine. Br J Cancer 2012;106:490–5.
6. Arena CB, Sano MB, Rossmeisl JH, et al. High-frequency irreversible electroporation (H-FIRE) for non-thermal ablation without muscle contraction. Biomed Eng Online 2011;10:102.
7. Schoenbach KH, Beebe SJ, Buescher ES. Intracellular effect of ultrashort electrical pulses. Bioelectromagnetics 2001;22:440–8.

8. Tang D, Kang R, Berghe TV, et al. The molecular machinery of regulated cell death. Cell Res 2019;29:347–64.

9. Nuccitelli R, Pliquett U, Chen X, et al. Nanosecond pulsed electric fields cause melanomas to self-destruct. Biochem Biophys Res Commun 2006;343:351–60.

10. Vernier PT, Sun Y, Marcu L, et al. Calcium bursts induced by nanosecond electric pulses. Biochem Biophys Res Commun 2003;310:286–95.

11. Nuccitelli R, Chen X, Pakhomov AG, et al. A new pulsed electric field therapy for melanoma disrupts the tumor's blood supply and causes complete remission without recurrence. Int J Cancer 2009;125:438–45.

12. Nuccitelli R, Lui K, Kreis M, et al. Nanosecond pulsed electric field stimulation of reactive oxygen species in human pancreatic cancer cells is Ca^{2+}-dependent. Biochem Biophys Res Commun 2013;435:580–5.

13. Ren W, Sain NM, Beebe SJ. Nanosecond pulsed electric fields (nsPEFs) activate intrinsic caspase-dependent and caspase-independent cell death in Jurkat cells. Biochem Biophys Res Commun 2012;421:808–12.

14. Nuccitelli R, McDaniel A, Connolly R, et al. Nanopulse stimulation induces changes in the intracellular organelles in rat liver tumors treated in situ. Laser Surg Med 2020;52:882–9.

15. Nuccitelli R, Wood R, Kreis M, et al. First-in-human trial of nanoelectroablation therapy for basal cell carcinoma: proof of method. Exp Dermatol 2014;23:135–7.

16. Hruza GJ, Zelickson BD, Selim MM, et al. Safety and efficacy of nanosecond pulsed electric field treatment of seborrheic keratoses. Dermatol Surg 2020;46:1183–9.

17. Munavalli GS, Zelickson BD, Selim MM, et al. Safety and efficacy of nanosecond pulsed electric field treatment of sebaceous gland hyperplasia. Dermatol Surg 2020;46:803–9.

18. Ross AS, Schlesinger T, Harmon CB, et al. Multicenter, prospective feasibility study of Nano-Pulse Stimulation™ technology for the treatment of both nodular and superficial low-risk basal cell carcinoma. Front Oncol 2022;12:1044694.

19. Katz BE, Nestor MS, Nuccitelli R, et al. Safety and effectiveness of nano-pulse stimulation™ technology to treat acne vulgaris of the back. J Cosmet Dermatol 2023;22:1545–53.

20. Yu Jakraphan, Yi J, Nikolaisen G, et al. Efficacy of a surgical cardiac ablation clamp using nanosecond pulsed electric fields: an acute porcine model. J Thorac Cardiovasc Surg 2024;24.

21. Nies M, Watanabe K, Kawamura I, et al. Ablating myocardium using nanosecond pulsed electric fields: preclinical assessment of feasibility, safety, and durability. Circulation 2024;17(7).

Moving?

Make sure your subscription moves with you!

To notify us of your new address, find your **Clinics Account Number** (located on your mailing label above your name), and contact customer service at:

Email: journalscustomerservice-usa@elsevier.com

800-654-2452 (subscribers in the U.S. & Canada)
314-447-8871 (subscribers outside of the U.S. & Canada)

Fax number: 314-447-8029

Elsevier Health Sciences Division
Subscription Customer Service
3251 Riverport Lane
Maryland Heights, MO 63043

*To ensure uninterrupted delivery of your subscription, please notify us at least 4 weeks in advance of move.

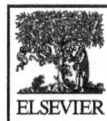

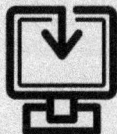

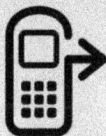

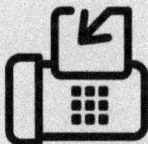

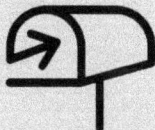

ELSEVIER